A History of Modern Immunology

A History of Modern Immunology

The Path Toward Understanding

Zoltan A. Nagy

AMSTERDAM • BOSTON • HEIDELBERG • LONDON
NEW YORK • OXFORD • PARIS • SAN DIEGO
SAN FRANCISCO • SINGAPORE • SYDNEY • TOKYO

Academic Press is an Imprint of Elsevier

Academic Press is an imprint of Elsevier
32 Jamestown Road, London NW1 7BY, UK
225 Wyman Street, Waltham, MA 02451, USA
525 B Street, Suite 1800, San Diego, CA 92101-4495, USA

Notice
No responsibility is assumed by the publisher for any injury and/or damage to persons
or property as a matter of products liability, negligence or otherwise, or from any use or
operation of any methods, products, instructions or ideas contained in the material herein.
Because of rapid advances in the medical sciences, in particular, independent verification
of diagnoses and drug dosages should be made

British Library Cataloguing-in-Publication Data
A catalogue record for this book is available from the British Library

Library of Congress Cataloging-in-Publication Data
A catalog record for this book is available from the Library of Congress

ISBN: 978-0-12-416974-6

For information on all Academic Press publications
visit our website at www.store.elsevier.com

Typeset by TNQ Books and Journals

Printed and bound in United States of America

14 15 16 17 18   10 9 8 7 6 5 4 3 2 1

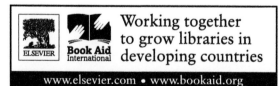

In memory of my friends
Rodney Langman and
György Fehèr

Contents

Introductory Words About Science, Scientists, and Immunology

Before we set out to follow through the events of a very exciting era in the history of immunology, I feel I owe the reader at least an attempt to define what science, and more specifically, immunology is all about.

There are several different ways to define science, but if we want to grasp its essence, the following simple statement is adequate: Science is an intellectually driven, often experimental activity, whose goal is to gain insight into the works of the universe.

Hence ideally a scientist is a person, who is blessed (or damned) with a restless mind, and an overdose of curiosity, which properties literally force him/her to keep asking all those What?, Why?, and How? questions that down-to-earth people only ask in their childhood. Not that scientists would be more infantile than others, but their extremely critical mind makes them reject all answers that they have been given by others. It is thus not surprising that the greatest reward for scientists is the moment, when their hard work and good fortune permit them a glimpse into a new facet of reality, be it even a tiny little one that has not been seen by anyone else before. Such rare moments set them into a state of euphoria that cannot be achieved by any other way, for example, by a tenure position at a famous university or even by a Nobel Prize (although these may also be good to have).

Unfortunately, this little sketch I have just drawn of science and its players deviates grossly from the picture that the mass media prefer to convey to the public. According to media representation, science is a very logical and very dry (i.e., boring) undertaking with the final goal of donating a significant benefit to mankind. The problem with this perception is that it confounds science with its potential utility. Undoubtedly, usefulness is an important aspect, and nobody is more aware of it than scientists themselves, particularly when they try to apply for a research grant. Nevertheless, the driver and the final goal of science is understanding and not utility.

For example, physicists, when they started to study nuclear fission hoped for a new insight into the structure of matter, and certainly did not intend to build nuclear power stations, let alone atomic bombs. The sad fact, however, that finally they were the ones to point out that nuclear fission can be used for a bomb, and indeed they participated in the construction of the bomb cast a dark and long-lasting shadow over the public image of science. This example also reveals that, although utility is a side-effect rather than the goal of science, it can sometimes change the life of mankind significantly, and in an often unforeseeable direction. This is why science is usually considered to be dangerous by the public. However, the statement that science itself is a purely mental pursuit remains valid, danger arising only from its uncontrolled applications. The important thing to keep in mind is that all qualities human beings can enjoy nowadays, beyond the ones given by nature, have resulted from either science or arts (and not from money, as most would think at the dawn of the third millennium).

Of course, the media, in order to avoid inconsistency with the picture they painted of science, also try their best in creating a false image of scientists. Accordingly, scientists who are selected to appear in public must look very stern and serious (although they can still be somewhat handsome), they must emanate unusual mental power, and their behavior must resemble that of a high priest in ancient Egypt. Admittedly, some colleagues like to use this image as a respectable disguise, but most scientists are not like this. Indeed, they are just like other people: they can be aggressive or timid, egomaniac or humble, dictatoristic or self-enslaving, careeristic or modest, political or naïve, business-like or puristic, conformistic or anarchistic, opportunistic or revolutionary, but they all have one thing in common: their inability to stop asking questions and seeking answers.

Let us turn now to immunology that, based on the foregoing discussion, is easily defined as the particular branch of life sciences, whose aim is to understand how the immune system functions. This definition has always been valid, even at times when the immune system existed solely as an assumption, and immunology appeared to be equal to vaccination, or antibodies, or serological reactions, and it will remain valid until the last piece of stone is placed into the wall of the knowledge tower of the immune system.

As the title of this book indicates, I shall attempt to summarize here the major events in the construction of the immunology tower during a period roughly corresponding to the last third of the twentieth century. There were several reasons for choosing this period. First, this era followed immediately the so-called 'immunological revolution', and was thus the time when most questions about the biology of the immune system were raised and also found their answers. Second, because I had the privilege to be an immunologist in this period, I shared all the excitement associated with it, and can thus convey its events to the reader on the basis of personal experience. Finally, the time that has elapsed since then provides one with the wisdom of hindsight, as well as sufficient distance to cool down and look back with sharper, more critical eyes.

Although the book was originally planned to summarize the history of immunology from about 1970 onward, I realized that the story would remain 'hanging mid-air' without at least a short résumé of the preceding 10–15 years, when most knowledge was generated on which modern immunology has been based. Furthermore, the language spoken by immunologists also originated from this time. Therefore, the highlights of this fruitful era are included, for the sake of non-immunologists, as a 'pre-history'. The science then generated can now be found in every immunology textbook, and the detailed history of this era is well covered in Arthur Silverstein's book.[1]

To return to the metaphor used above, I should point out that the immunology tower has not been built of uniform bricks, but rather of individually carved stones of different shapes and sizes, similarly to the Inca buildings in Matshupitshu and Sachsahuayman. But unlike the Inca buildings, the construction of the immunology tower has not been led by a chief architect, and thus every single stone reflects the idea of its mason about the best fit. Consequently, many (or perhaps most) of the stones would not fit. Nevertheless, ideas and data that have, in retrospect, turned out to be misfits will also be included here, because nothing illustrates better the development of a cognitive process than the errors made on the way. Not to mention that the omission of errors and inclusion of only the highlights would have reduced the book to an 'executive summary'. Nonetheless, this book is not meant to be a complete historical account of all immunological research conducted during the last third of the twentieth century. To keep a better focus, I will only cover topics that appeared most central for our understanding, corresponding largely to what was considered 'mainstream' immunology at that time.

Another, perhaps unusual feature of this book is that it will not only deal with science, but also with the personalities of scientists. I have always found it a great injustice to remember only the names of scientists in conjunction with their contributions, and not their personality, although the latter was often more interesting than the former. This applies all the more to immunology that has abounded in interesting, colorful personalities. In an attempt to correct this injustice at least to some extent, I included short comments or anecdotes about many of the participants of the immunology game. More often than not, these comments just represent snapshots that have, for inexplicable reasons, remained stuck in my memory. At this place, I apologize to those colleagues, who may not agree with their snapshots. My only excuse is my good intention to preserve at least a fragmentary image of their personalities, without becoming either insulting or flattering.

Also, to render the text more 'palatable', whenever it comes to personal experience or views, I will pass on the narrative to an imaginary 'Doctor G' (who is the author in singular first person, in analogy to 'K' in Franz Kafka's 'Castle'). This arrangement permits a clear distinction between objective and subjective/interpretative passages, and also a more direct colloquial style for the latter.

The language of the book is kept intentionally simple, to facilitate understanding of the complicated scientific content. In the referencing, I did not strive for completeness, but selected primary publications that first described a key discovery important for understanding of the topic discussed.

Despite all efforts for clarity and simplification, an appropriate background will be mandatory for full comprehension of the text, and thus the readership for whom I would recommend this book is, on the first place, research and clinical immunologists, as well as students and teachers of immunology. Novices in any of the covered subdisciplines may make particularly good use of the book, as they could get the complete background information of the respective area, with all key discoveries, references and interpretations by a short reading. For the same reason, the book may be useful for research managers in the pharma and biotech industry, who are running or planning to run immunology projects. Of course, immunology aficionados with a biomedical background are also welcome, in general all those, whose interest – beyond merely gathering chronologically ordered information – is in the process of how our understanding of the immune system has evolved.

At this place I would like to express my deep thanks to many colleagues, who helped me along the way. I am most indebted to Melvin Cohn for his following the development of the manuscript with interest and providing invaluable comments, references and encouragement. I thank Arthur Silverstein for reviewing the manuscript and commenting on it from the perspective of the historian. I owe a debt to Hugh McDevitt for reviewing part of the manuscript and giving valuable advice. Finally I thank Christophe Benoist, Zlatko Dembic, Donald Forsdyke, Robert Huber, Robert Kerbel, Paul Lehmann, Sebastian Meier-Ewert, Hans-Georg Rammensee, Thomas Revesz, Edward Rosloniec, and Ronald Schwartz for their help in refreshing my memories and providing references.

REFERENCE

1. Silverstein AM. *A History of Immunology*. San Diego: Acad. Press; 1989.

Pre-history with Far-reaching Consequences

Chapter 1

The Immunological Revolution

Those who received their biomedical education around 1960 could not even have suspected that one of the most significant revolutions in life-sciences was taking place at that time: the transformation of serology-centered immunology into immunobiology. Students could not have possibly been informed about this, as the university textbooks at that time were only allowed to contain solid, well-established facts of science, notably those that had survived at least a decade without being refuted. Thus little wonder that the students missed out the birth of immunobiology. As a matter of fact, immunology at that time was not considered as a science in its own right, it usually occupied a single chapter in the students' microbiology textbook, describing at most vaccination, antibodies, serological reactions, and the use of antibodies for typing of bacteria. The most sophisticated piece of science included was the description of how to render antisera 'monospecific' by sequential absorption. Concerning the possible nature and origin of antibodies, a single laconic statement was made, namely that they were localized in the gamma-globulin fraction of serum, implying cautiously that not all gamma-globulins were necessarily antibodies. Indeed, the bulk of gamma-globulins was thought to represent 'normal' serum proteins that were probably produced in the liver (by the motto that substances of unknown nature and origin are best to be blamed on the liver; nota bene, even old, conservative textbooks could contain not all that solid facts!). Naturally, nothing about the cellular basis of immunity passed the inclusion criteria, since the first discoveries in this direction were at most a couple of years old. It is not surprising that the biologically interested student, after reading through the chapter, might have concluded: 'All this may well be very useful, but rather boring.'

Consequently, chances were meagre that creative students would have decided to join immunology research, the few exceptions were those who attained the new knowledge by self-education.

At this point, the reader may wonder why self-evident questions, such as the cellular origin of immunity, were not addressed long before 1960. The explanation lies in what one could rightly call a historical artefact. Namely, immunology in the preceding 50 years had dealt only with antibodies, and immunologists had been convinced that clarifying the nature of antibodies and of their interaction with antigen would answer all outstanding scientific questions. In accordance with this notion, the approach to immunology was predominantly chemical,

A History of Modern Immunology. http://dx.doi.org/10.1016/B978-0-12-416974-6.00001-6

biological concepts hardly having a chance to penetrate the field. Therefore, the designation of this era by historians as the 'dark ages of immunology'[1] is not quite unfounded, although important contributions were also made at this time, in particular to serology. The prevailing paradigm blindfolded immunologists so strongly that new facts, not accounted for by the effect of antibodies, were needed to change their mind.

The earliest 'heretical' phenomenon was delayed-type (or tuberculin-type) hypersensitivity (DTH; its history is amply described[1]). It had been known for some 50 years that *Mycobacterum tuberculosis*, when administered intradermally in small amounts, caused a local inflammatory reaction, which was also widely used as a reliable diagnostic marker for previous infection. Although it was noted that the reaction developed in the absence of circulating antibodies against the bacteria, it was easier to 'sweep it under the carpet' by postulating that it represented a local, non-immunological reaction against toxic bacterial products. But this proposition became untenable some 20–30 years later, when it was demonstrated that DTH could also be induced with a variety of simple proteins. Soon became the immunological nature of the reaction also evident, and the finding that it could be passively transferred with blood cells of sensitized donors to naïve recipients[2] marked the birth of cellular immunology.

Studies on the mechanism of skin-graft rejection were even more revealing. Thanks mostly to Peter Medawar and his group, the immunological nature of graft rejection was proven quickly and beyond any doubt,[3,4] and it was also observed that the majority of cells infiltrating the graft were lymphocytes, providing the first hint to an immunological role for this abundant but thus far functionless blood cell population. Further, it was shown that graft rejection was not accompanied by antibody formation against donor erythrocytes, and that the immunizing antigens were on donor leukocytes.[5] Finally, the demonstration by Mitchison[6] and Billingham et al.[7] that transplantation immunity could be adoptively transferred with cells but not with the serum of sensitized donors placed graft rejection into the category of cellular immunity together with DTH. Thus, here were two, well-established immunological phenomena that had nothing to do with antibodies.

A major eye-opener was also the discovery of immunological tolerance[8,9] that could not be explained by the then-fashionable instructive models of antibody production (the latter proposed that antigen would instruct, or even serve as a template for antibody synthesis). Finally, the accumulation of new evidence alerted immunologists to wake up from their 'sleeping beauty slumber', and start asking all those questions that would have been due long ago. These were the most important preparatory steps to what is usually referred to as 'the immunological revolution'.

1.1 THE CLONAL SELECTION THEORY

If immunologists were asked to name one single event that marks the beginning of the immunological revolution, most of us would vote for the appearance of 'The Clonal Selection Theory of Acquired Immunity'[10] by Macfarlane Burnet in 1959. This theory provided, for the first time, a biology-based conceptual framework for the development of immune responses, and its main theses have remained valid to date, so it has rightly become the alphabet of immunological thinking, and it is now 'in the blood' of every immunologist.

Of course, the clonal selection theory did not come 'out of the blue', it was indeed preceded by two major selectional hypotheses, namely the side-chain theory[11,12] of Paul Ehrlich in 1897, and the natural selection theory[13] by Niels Jerne in 1955 (the gap in between was filled with instructional theories of the 'dark ages'). Common to all three concepts is the basic postulate that antibodies are natural components of the body, produced at a slow, constant rate, independent of antigen challenge (a sharp demarcation from the instructionists' view). The role of antigen is then to select and bind to the appropriate specific antibody (out of a mixture of many), and this triggers the production of large amounts of the same antibody. The distinctive features of the three theories lie in the assumed place of selection and the subsequent events.

Ehrlich placed the antibodies as 'side-chains' onto the surface of cells. In his view, a single cell possesses many different side-chains, but only those binding antigen will be overproduced and shed into the blood. In contrast, Jerne's natural antibodies were assumed to circulate in the blood, and the ones binding antigen would then be transported to specialized cells capable of producing the very same antibody. How this transport and the subsequent triggering of specific antibody production would occur have remained unexplained.

Burnet's concept that also incorporated new knowledge about protein synthesis was the one to hit the nail on the head. Burnet realized that neither antigen nor antibody could carry specific information to a cell to induce antibody formation, what they could do at most is to signal a pre-programmed machinery for protein synthesis. Thus he placed the natural antibody of Jerne back onto the cell surface as a receptor, similarly to Ehrlich. And here came the stroke of genius: he postulated that each specific antibody receptor was only expressed on a single cell and its descendants, i.e., a cell clone. This statement implied that cells of each clone had been programmed to produce one single antibody specificity. Specific binding of antigen would trigger only the cells of the relevant clone to expand (proliferate) and differentiate into antibody-secreting cells (Fig. 1.1).

Besides being essentially correct, Burnet's theory offers several advantages. First, it allows the body to run several different immune responses simultaneously, a definitive advantage in a pathogen-ridden world. Furthermore, the postulated clonal expansion accounts nicely for the observed continued antibody production after elimination of the antigen, as well as for the enhanced antibody response upon repeated immunization ('booster effect'). To explain the improved quality of antibodies after booster ('affinity maturation'), Burnet invoked minor somatic mutations in the antibody-encoding gene, an aspect that was further elaborated by Lederberg.[14] The newly discovered phenomenon of self-tolerance could also be explained by the deletion of self-reactive clones early in ontogeny.

Resting lymphocytes | Proliferation | Differentiation | Antibody secretion

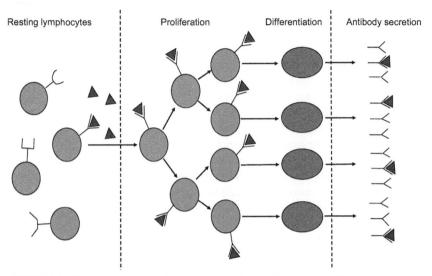

FIGURE 1.1   Schematic representation of Burnet's clonal selection theory. Resting lymphocyte clones (circles) express different receptors. Antigen (triangles) finds a clone with the appropriate receptor. The selected clone proliferates, differentiates into plasma cells (ellipses) and the latter secrete antibody of the same specificity. Based on Reference 1.

From the experimentalists' point of view, the most attractive aspect of the theory was that many of its postulates were testable. For example, with the development of the new immunofluorescence technique, it became easy to demonstrate that the precursors of antibody-forming cells (now B cells) indeed carried immunoglobulin receptors on their surface. Indirect evidence also accumulated to support the one-cell-one-antibody thesis. First, each B cell was shown to express antibodies of a single molecular species, i.e., the same heavy and light chain class of immunoglobulin, and in animals heterozygous for immunoglobulin allotypes (allelic variants of immunoglobulin) either one or the other allotype but not both.[15] The latter finding has indicated that mechanisms must exist in the lymphocyte that inactivate the immunoglobulin gene in one of the two parental chromosomes ('allelic exclusion'), pointing again in the direction of lymphocyte monospecificity. Second, using radiolabeled antigens, specific antigen binding was demonstrated to only very small fractions of lymphocytes,[16] suggesting clonality of their antigen receptors. Third, the use of heavily radioactive antigens permitted selective killing of antigen-binding cells by local radiation, and the remaining cell population was shown to be incapable of responding to the same antigen, whereas it responded to other antigens normally.[17] The latter, so called 'antigen-suicide' experiments provided the strongest indirect evidence for the clonality of immune response. But the final evidence came from the discovery of monoclonal antibodies,[18] whose very existence would be impossible, if lymphocytes were not monospecific. The proposal that clonal deletion should be a mechanism of immunological tolerance was also proven experimentally, some 30 years later.[19–21]

Besides his theoretical contributions, Burnet had another important achievement, namely, that he managed by his knowledge and personal charisma to turn the Walter and Eliza Hall Institute in Melbourne into one of the most prominent immunological sites of the world, a Mecca of immunologists, for many years to come. It was thus more than deserved that Macfarlane Burnet was awarded with the Nobel Prize (together with Peter Medawar), even though he received the prize for the discovery of immunological tolerance that he did not really discover himself.

No concept has ever existed in science without inciting opposing views, and thus clonal selection had its opponents too. Of the numerous arguments brought up against it, the funniest one is the so-called 'elephant–tadpole paradox'. It goes as follows: The clonal selection theory implies that a large animal with a vast number of lymphocytes must have many more clones than a small animal, and consequently, an elephant should be much better protected against infections than a tadpole, which is not only absurd but is also not observed in reality. Even funnier is that this argument could not be refuted, and thus the paradox had stayed with us until its explanation almost 30 years later.[22] Fortunately, tadpoles were meanwhile investigated, and found to have a sufficiently large antibody repertoire,[23] so we need not worry too much about them.

1.2 THE BIRTH OF B AND T LYMPHOCYTES

Perhaps the most obvious sign for the one-sided thinking in the 'dark ages' was that nobody asked the question: What cells are responsible for the immune response? It was taken for granted that upon immunization, highly sophisticated, specific antibodies arose in the body, whose chemical structure and specificity were worth the scientific pursuit, but the cellular origin of these highly rated substances did not raise curiosity in anybody.

The first important step toward clarification of the cellular basis for immunity was taken as late as in 1956, when Bruce Glick and his colleagues reported that the removal of bursa of Fabricius (a curious little gland-like organ on the dorsal site of the cloaca) from chicken embryos resulted later in a failure to produce antibodies.[24] Unfortunately, not a single immunologist took notice of his results for several years. The reason was that he published this epoch-making finding in *Poultry Science*, a journal highly unlikely to be found in the library of immunological institutions. The finding was then seized upon by several groups, and the chicken became the favorite animal model in immunology for a while. The details were soon worked out: bursectomy shortly before hatching has been shown to result in either a complete loss of antibodies or only IgM antibodies were made,[25] whereas cell-mediated immunity (e.g., delayed-type hypersensitivity, allograft rejection, graft versus host reaction) remained unaltered.[26] Bursectomy combined with irradiation caused, in addition, total agammaglobulinemia, but cell-mediated immunity was only minimally affected.[27] The time point of bursectomy appeared important: bursectomy performed on day-old chicks or later led only to partial unresponsiveness to antigens[25,28] and the serum gamma-globulin level also tended to normalize with age.[29] Thus it appeared that precursors of antibody-forming cells left the bursa already in the late embryonic life, at first the IgM-producing cells. The cellular basis for the functional deficiency was shown to be a complete absence of the antibody-forming cell lineage (surface immunoglobulin-positive cells,[30] plasmoblasts, preplasmocytes, plasma cells[31]), and a loss of germinal centers and periellipsoidal lymphoid tissue[31] in the peripheral lymphoid organs (i.e., spleen). The transfer of histocompatible bursa cells into bursectomized, irradiated chicken led to the restoration of all these deficiencies.[27,32] Taken together, these results have indicated that the bursa serves as a 'nursery school' for early precursors of a distinct lymphoid cell lineage that eventually develops into antibody-forming plasma cells. This lineage of lymphoid cells was then termed bursa-derived lymphocytes.

Of course, this discovery launched a chase for the mammalian equivalent of the bursa of Fabricius, which was more difficult to find, as a discrete organ for this purpose is not available in mammals. On the basis of experimental data, two organs could compete for the bursa-equivalent title, namely the bone marrow[33] and the fetal liver.[34] Finally, the bone marrow won the race, and because its initial is also 'B', the subset of lymphocytes responsible for antibody production could be termed B lymphocytes (or B cells), to the great relief of nomenclature committees.

A few years later, one of the giants of the 'Australian school', Jacques Miller started a quest for an immunological role of the thymus, another mysterious organ that had been held for an endocrine gland, but it seemed to be comprised of lymphoreticular tissue. At that time, the thymus was considered to be immunologically inert, because, first, no plasma cells and germinal centers were found there after antigenic stimulation, and second, adult thymectomy had no effect on antibody response. Miller might have thought, brilliant as he has been, that the thymus, similarly to the bursa of Fabricius, might be an originator of immunocompetent cells in embryonic life. And he was right, as he was also later in so many instances. To test this hypothesis he performed neonatal thymectomy in mice, and found a severe depletion of lymphocytes and a loss of cellular immunity in the mature animals. He published his observations as a one-and-a-half-page-long preliminary communication in Lancet,[35] and this modest paper marked the birth of a new cell lineage. Later similar deficiencies were reported in the chicken after neonatal thymectomy.[36] The new cell lineage responsible for cellular immunity was therefore termed thymus-dependent, or T lymphocytes (or T cells, for short).

The bursa/bone marrow and thymus were then coined the 'central lymphoid organs' to emphasize their decisive role in the ontogeny of lymphocytes, whereas the sites where the functionally mature lymphocytes migrate subsequently, e.g., the spleen and lymph nodes, were referred to as 'peripheral lymphoid organs' or simply 'the periphery'.

Later on it was demonstrated that the two lymphoid cell lineages not only differ in their development and function, but are also distinguishable by cell surface markers. The pioneering work on lymphocyte markers was done by Martin Raff, a Canadian neurobiologist (and former star quarterback football player for McGill University) upon his sabbatical leave at Mitchison's famous laboratory at the Department of Zoology, University College, London. He showed that B cells expressed readily detectable amounts of immunoglobulin (Ig) on their surface,[37] and thus, surface Ig could be considered as a B cell marker, although not a distinguishing one, because it was unclear at that time, whether T cells also expressed Ig in small amounts or failed to express it altogether. The first marker that enabled a clear distinction between T and B cells was the 'theta' alloantigen, a nerve cell antigen that Raff found to be expressed also on the cell membrane of T cells,[38] but not of B cells. The theta antigen exists in two allelic forms in mice, a rare allotype (later termed Thy-1.1) in strain AKR and a frequent one (Thy-1.2) in all other known mouse strains. Thus, immunization of AKR mice with thymocytes of other strains (e.g., CBA or C3H that are identical at major histocompatibility loci with AKR) resulted in a Thy-1.2-specific alloantibody (or anti-Thy1.1 in the opposite strain combination), which turned out to be an extremely useful tool in T-cell studies. Martin Raff's contributions also affected his own life, in that he has never returned to Canada, he remained in England permanently. What he did return to, however, was neurobiology, at least this can be assumed, because he disappeared after a while from the hectic show-stage of immunology.

The identification of B and T lymphocytes was perhaps the most important discovery in the history of immunobiology. Yet, the fathers of T and B cells have never been considered for a Nobel Prize. The ways of the Nobel Committee are sometimes inscrutable.

1.3 T-B CELL COLLABORATION

By the early 1960s, immunologists had a good reason to be satisfied with themselves: they seem to have finally found, in the dualistic build-up of the immune system, an appropriate model to answer many longstanding questions. In fact, all known immunological phenomena (except allergy) could now be ascribed to either T-cell-mediated cellular or B-cell-dependent humoral immunity. Since the T and B cell lineages not only performed different tasks, but also followed distinct developmental pathways, it was logical to view them as separate systems that functioned completely independent of one another. Therefore, the first demonstration of a cross-talk between them created more annoyance than happiness in the immunological community.

The trouble had started earlier, with a mysterious finding by Benacerraf and Gell.[39] These authors studied the minimal antigenic requirements of a

DTH response by adopting Landsteiner's classical experimental system, i.e., using a small chemical compound (hapten) coupled to an immunogenic protein (carrier). It had been well established that immunization with a hapten-carrier conjugate yielded antibodies exquisitely specific for the hapten, irrespective of what carrier it was coupled to. Benacerraf and Gell found, however, that this rule was not applicable to DTH: here, the response induced by, for example, hapten 'X' coupled to carrier 'A' could only be elicited with the same, 'X-A' conjugate, but not with the same hapten 'X' coupled to another carrier, e.g., protein 'B'. This finding, termed 'carrier effect' incited wild speculations, of which still the most logical was the one proposed by the same authors, namely, that the combining site involved in DTH was larger than that of an antibody to encompass, in addition to the hapten, also part of the carrier protein. But eventually all speculations succumbed to Mitchison's findings[40] demonstrating that indeed two different cell types participated in the responses to hapten–protein conjugates, namely, an effector cell recognizing the hapten and a 'helper' cell recognizing the carrier.

Subsequently, Claman and colleagues[41] observed a synergy between thymus and bone marrow cell populations in antibody production. But it was again Jacques Miller together with his student Graham Mitchell, who firmly established the helper role of T cells in the production of IgG antibodies by B cells, in two ground-breaking papers in the *Journal of Experimental Medicine*.[42,43]

Although at a scientific meeting in 1968, Miller was accused of overcomplicating immunology, later on, most immunologists had to admit that what they had viewed as a nuisance turned out to be the birth of a new, exciting concept: the regulation of immune responses by cell to cell interactions. This concept opened up a fury of research activity that almost overdominated immunology in the subsequent 25 years. As we will see later, this research produced many important pieces of data but also some problematic ones.

1.4 THE STRUCTURE OF IMMUNOGLOBULINS

It was an interesting coincidence that the 60-year-old quest for the structure of antibodies and the nature of their interaction with antigen was crowned with success exactly during the period of the immunological revolution. This enabled a happy union of old established immunochemistry with newborn immunobiology to finally become one single discipline.

As always in science, the spectacular advance in immunochemistry owed a lot to certain novel techniques that had become available to biochemical studies, e.g., ultracentrifugation, electrophoresis, and immunoelectrophoresis. These new tools permitted the separation of antibody molecules by size and charge. The early results did not make the lives of researchers any easier, as it turned out that antibodies were heterogeneous in size, the majority being smaller (7S by sedimentation in the ultracentrifuge), whereas some antibodies appeared much larger (19S). In addition, a substantial heterogeneity was seen also in terms of their migration in electric field. The only light in the darkness was the observation that certain biological characteristics (e.g., complement binding) appeared to correlate with one or another physical property. Most helpful was in the molecular characterization of antibodies (by then called immunoglobulins, and later simply Ig) the finding that their cleavage by certain enzymes[44] (i.e., papain and trypsin) or by reduction[45] resulted in stable fragments of different sizes. It was then shown by Edelman and Poulik[46] that Ig molecules were made up of two kinds of polypeptide chains, a larger one of ~50 000 molecular weight (heavy or H chain) and a smaller one of ~20 000 molecular weight (light or L chain). These results allowed Porter[47] to propose a basic structure for Ig-s, consisting of two disulfide-bonded H chains, and two L chains, each joined to one H chain with a disulfide bond. Porter could also hypothesize that the antigen-binding site might possibly be formed by parts of both H and L chains (Fig. 1.2).

Edelman[48] was then the one who came up with a more comprehensive structural interpretation, largely based on studies with myeloma proteins[49] that turned out to be practically 'monoclonal' immunoglobulins, and were thus

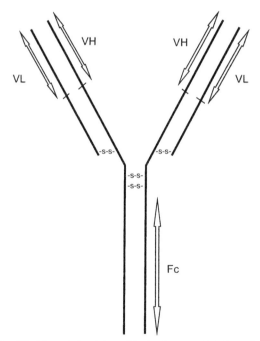

FIGURE 1.2   A simplified four-chain stick model of an immunoglobulin molecule. The molecule consists of two identical heavy and light chains, joined by disulfide bonds (-S-S-). The amino terminal portions of heavy and light chains are variable (VH, VL), whereas the remaining portions are constant. The two VH–VL pairs form two identical antigen-binding sites. The carboxy terminal ends of heavy chain constant regions form the Fc portion responsible for immunological effector functions. Based on References 47, 48.

suitable to protein sequencing. The final picture that emerged depicted Ig-s as being composed of two light chains (either κ or λ), and two heavy chains, γ for IgG, μ for IgM (a pentameric macroglobulin), δ for IgD (exists only in membrane bound form), α for IgA (mono- or dimeric), and ε for IgE (responsible for allergies). The amino-terminal V (variable) portions of H and L chains were proposed to form the antigen-combining site, thus, each monomeric Ig was bivalent (possessing two binding sites). The carboxy-terminal, constant (C) part of the H chains (called Fc portion) was found to be responsible for the biological effector functions of the molecule (e.g., binding to Fc receptors, and fixation of complement). For their ground-breaking discovery, Edelman and Porter were awarded the Nobel Prize almost instantaneously.

The assembly of more and more amino acid sequences of Ig-s permitted Wu and Kabat[50] to gain a more precise idea about the antigen-combining site. They plotted the number of amino acid variations at each position of the molecule (the ever-since famous 'Wu-Kabat plot'), and found that within the V region of H and L chains there are, beside relatively conserved sections, three hypervariable regions that they assumed to fold into a single binding site. Subsequent X-ray crystallography studies[51] confirmed this hypothesis.

Thus, the old dream of immunochemists finally came true. But what has the structure of immunoglobulins actually revealed? First of all, it has revealed itself, and second, it has substantiated our view of Ig-s as being 'intelligent' molecules with a specific portion to target a pathogen, and at the opposite end carrying the 'weapon', the immunological effector mechanism to rid the pathogen. Actually this had been assumed before. Evidently, the knowledge of Ig structure is absolutely essential for immunology, and it has also been instrumental for the development of future antibody technologies. But the expectation of the 'dark ages' that the structure of immunoglobulins would answer all questions of immunology was naturally not fulfilled.

1.5 ALLERGY: FROM DISEASE SYMPTOMS TO IGE

It has been known since the end of the eighteenth century that immune responses in certain instances are accompanied by adverse reactions ranging from local skin irritation to lethal anaphylactic shock. These conditions are lumped together under the umbrella of 'hypersensitivity', a term reflecting the earlier interpretation that they represent an overreaction to toxic components of the antigen. However, it had soon become clear that non-toxic substances, such as serum injected from one individual into another could also cause similar symptoms, hinting at an immunological rather than toxic mechanism. That certain human conditions, now known as allergies, including hay fever and asthma belong to the group of hypersensitivities was also proposed in the early twentieth century (for the early history of hypersensitivities see Silverstein[1]). The idea, however, that immune responses might cause disease appeared to be irreconcilable with the protective function of immunity, and as a consequence, hypersensitivity research was left to clinicians, and has remained outside of 'mainstream' immunology for a long time.

Allergies usually triggered by otherwise harmless 'environmental' antigens represent the most frequent type of hypersensitivity. Their pathomechanism was a matter of heated debates in the first decades of the twentieth century.[1] Interestingly, some of the early assumptions, e.g., that allergy is caused by a special class of antibodies (called reagins), and that such antibodies are cytotropic, have later been confirmed experimentally. Perhaps the most important early contribution to understanding allergy was the Prausnitz-Künstner experiment.[52] One of the authors, Künstner, was sensitive to cooked fish flesh, although his serum showed no reactivity in vitro with the allergen. But a small amount of his serum injected in Preusnitz's skin provoked a local reaction upon injection of fish extract to the same site 24 h later. This experiment was the first clear demonstration that allergy can be passively transferred with serum into an insensitive recipient.

A major problem in the early phase of allergy research was that 'reaginic' antibodies were present at so low concentrations in the blood that they usually remained undetectable by available methods. The first sensitive method for their detection, an often overlooked achievement, was 'passive cutaneous anaphylaxis' (PCA) developed by Zoltan Ovary. He studied, together with Guido Biozzi in Rome, the role of histamine in vascular permeability and allergic reactions.[53] The simple and efficient in vivo assay he developed for this purpose consisted of intradermal injection of a small serum sample into a test animal, e.g., a guinea pig, followed (after a sensitization period) by intravenous injection of the antigen together with a blue dye. Local histamine release due to the antigen–antibody interaction caused increased vascular permeability, and the dye leaking from the blood appeared as a blue-stained spot in the skin of the animal within a matter of minutes.[54] The novelty of this test was that it assayed 'reaginic' antibodies through a defined biological activity, and in addition, it was extremely sensitive, permitting the detection and quantitation of nanogram amounts of antibody. The PCA assay was then used in countless studies of allergy all over the world.

Dr. Ovary was one of the many exile Hungarians, who had to leave their home country because of the absurdities of twentieth century politics. His name – despite its orthographic identity with an English word – is Hungarian: its approximate translation is 'old castle'. Zoltan Ovary, in contrast to most exile Hungarians, made the best out of his status. He lived in Rome, Paris, and New York, he was a connoisseur in arts, music, architecture, practically in everything that culture could offer. And being a pleasant and cultured man, almost everybody who counted in twentieth century science and culture was his friend or personal acquaintance, from Jacques Monod to Baruj Benacerraf, and from Bela Bartok to Salvador Dali.[55] In the last ~45 years of his career, he was Professor at the New York University Medical School, where he was honored as a living classic, and remained active until the age of 98 years! Zoltan Ovary was one of the last renaissance personalities, after whose depart the Earth has become a bleaker place to live.

The decisive step in unravelling the secret of allergy was taken by the husband–wife team of Kimishige and Teruko Ishizaka, two outstanding experimenters, in 1966. They prepared a rabbit antiserum against the reagin-rich fraction of a serum from a ragweed-sensitive patient, and found that this antiserum neutralized the reaginic activity, and reacted with an immunoglobulin (Ig) that was different from all known Ig isotypes.[56,57] The new Ig class was designated γE, later IgE.

The discovery of IgE permitted for the first time to ask relevant questions about the mechanism of allergy, e.g., why the isotype switch of Ig is shifted toward IgE, and what kind of environmental and genetic factors predispose to elevated IgE levels. Furthermore, the very existence of IgE as a distinct class of Ig implied that IgE-triggered effector mechanisms must have been selected to fulfill a special protective function. Indeed, it is conceivable that repeated exposure of the airways to pollen, molds, insect products, etc., could have been sufficiently noxious to select a distinct effector mechanism for the elimination of these allergens. But the protective effect of IgE responses has been difficult to assess, because allergens are neither toxic nor are they part of the fast-growing pathogens, and thus the harm that would be caused by a deficient IgE response may not be immediately obvious. Therefore, studies of the protective role of IgE fell short in allergy research compared to IgE-induced immunopathology. Along this line of reasoning, the allergic reaction can be regarded as an exaggerated form of a useful effector response as foreseen by Clemens von Pirquet[58] as early as 1910.

REFERENCES

1. Silverstein AM. *A History of Immunology*. San Diego: Acad. Press; 1989.
2. Landsteiner K, Chase MW. *Proc. Soc. Exp. Biol. Med.* 1942;**49**:688.
3. Medawar PB. *J. Anat.* 1944;**78**:176.
4. Medawar PB. *J. Anat.* 1945;**79**:157.
5. Medawar PB. *Br. J. Exp. Pathol.* 1946;**27**:15.
6. Mitchison NA. *Proc. R. Soc. London Ser. B* 1954;**142**:72.
7. Billingham RE, Brent L, Medawar PB. *Proc. R. Soc. London Ser. B* 1954;**143**:58.
8. Owen RD. *Science* 1945;**102**:400.
9. Billingham RE, Brent L, Medawar PB. *Nature* 1953;**172**:603.
10. Burnet FM. *The Clonal Selection Theory of Acquired Immunity.*. London: Cambridge Univ. Press; 1959.
11. Ehrlich P. *Klin. Jahrb* 1897;**60**:199.
12. Ehrlich P. *Proc. R. Soc. London* 1900;**66**:424.
13. Jerne NK. *Proc. Natl. Acad. Sci. USA* 1955;**41**:849.
14. Lederberg J. *Science* 1959;**129**:1649.
15. Pernis B, Chiappino G, Kelus AS, PGH Gell. *J. Exp. Med.* 1965;**122**:853.
16. Sulitzeanu D, Naor D. *Int. Arch. Allergy Appl. Immunol.* 1969;**35**:564.
17. Ada GL, Byrt P. *Nature* 1969;**222**:1291.

18. Köhler GF, Milstein C. *Nature (London)* 1975;**256**:495.
19. Kappler JW, Roehm N, Marrack P. *Cell* 1987;**49**:273.
20. Kappler JW, Staerz U, White J, Marrack PC. *Nature* 1988;**332**:35.
21. MacDonald HR, Schneider R, Lees PK, Howe RC, Acha-Orbea H, Festenstein H, Zinkernagel RM, Hengartner H. *Nature* 1988;**332**:40.
22. Langman RE, Cohn M. *Mol. Immunol.* 1987;**24**:675.
23. du Pasquier L. *Curr. Top. Microbiol. Immunol.* 1973;**61**:37.
24. Glick B, Chang TS, Jaap RG. *Poultry Sci.* 1956;**35**:224.
25. Cain WA, Cooper MD, Good RA. *Nature* 1967;**217**:87.
26. Warner NL, Szenberg A, Burnet FM. *Aust. J. Exp. Biol. Med* 1962;**40**:373.
27. Cooper MD, Schwartz ML, Good RA. *Science* 1966;**151**:471.
28. Glick B. *Proc. Soc. Exp. Biol. Med.* 1968;**127**:1054.
29. Arnason BG, Jankovic BD. *J. Immunol.* 1967;**99**:917.
30. Alm GV, Peterson RDA. *J. Exp. Med.* 1969;**129**:1247.
31. Cooper MD, Peterson RDA, Good RA. *Nature* 1965;**205**:143.
32. Toivanen P, Toivanen A, Good RA. *J. Exp. Med.* 1972;**136**:816.
33. Cooper MD, Lawton AR. In: Hanna Jr MG, editor. *Contemporary Topics in Immunobiology.* New York, London: Plenum Press; 1972, . p. 49. 1.
34. Owen JJT, Cooper MD, Raff MC. *Nature* 1974;**249**:361.
35. Miller JFAP. *Lancet* 1961;**II**:748.
36. Aspinall RL, Meyer RK, Graetzer MA, Wolfe HR. *J. Immunol.* 1963;**90**:872.
37. Raff MC, Sternberg M, Taylor RB. *Nature* 1970;**225**:553.
38. Raff MC, Wortis HH. *Immunol.* 1970;**18**:931.
39. Benacerraf B, Gell PHG. *Immunol.* 1959;**2**:53.
40. Mitchison NA. In: Landy M, Braun W, editors. *Immunological Tolerance.* New York: Acad. Press; 1969. p. 149.
41. Claman HN, Chaperon EA, Triplett RF. *Proc. Soc. Exp. Biol. Med.* 1966;**122**:1167.
42. Miller JFAP, Mitchell GF. *J. Exp. Med.* 1968;**128**:801.
43. Mitchell GF, Miller JFAP. *J. Exp. Med.* 1968;**128**:821.
44. Porter RR. *Biochem. J.* 1950;**46**:473.
45. Edelman GM. *J. Am. Chem. Soc.* 1959;**81**:3155.
46. Edelman GM, Poulik MD. *J. Exp. Med.* 1961;**113**:861.
47. Porter RR. *Br. Med. Bull.* 1963;**19**:197.
48. Edelman GM. *Biochemistry* 1970;**9**:3197.
49. Kunkel HG. *Am. J. Med.* 1965;**39**:1.
50. Wu TT, Kabat EA. *J. Exp. Med.* 1970;**132**:211.
51. Poljak RJ, Amzel LM, Avey HP, Chen BL, Phizackerly RP, Saul F. *Proc. Natl. Acad. Sci. USA* 1973;**70**:3305.
52. Prausnitz C, Künstner H. *Zentralbl. Bakteriol.* 1921;**86**:160.
53. Biozzi G, Mene G, Ovary Z. *Boll. Soc. Ital. Biol. Sper.* 1950;**26**:327.
54. Ovary Z. *Boll. Soc. Ital. Biol. Sper.* 1951;**27**:308.
55. Ovary Z. *Souvenirs: around the world in ninety years.* New York: India Ink Press; 1999.
56. Ishizaka K, Ishizaka T. *Allergy* 1966;**37**:169.
57. Ishizaka K, Ishizaka T, Hornbrook MM. *J. Immunol.* 1966;**97**:75.
58. von Pirquet C. *Allergie.* Berlin: Springer-Verlag; 1910.

Part II

The History

By the end of the immunological revolution in the late 1960s, the major questions of immunology appeared to have been answered.[1] Indeed, more knowledge accumulated in this short period about the immune system than during the entire preceding history of immunology. What seemed to remain was just 'to sort out some mechanistic details'. But as is well known, the devil is always in the detail, and thus some of the remaining puzzles have proven extremely difficult to crack, and others have persisted to date. Furthermore, as usually happens in science, the new discoveries have not only provided answers, but also posed new questions (an aspect that renders scientific quest an endless enterprise). As a result, the forthcoming 20–30 years have turned out to be just as exciting as, but much more contradictory than, the immunological revolution itself. As a matter of fact, the revolution, in retrospect from the turn of the millennium, appears to have just been the 'picking of low-hanging fruits'.

In 1970, the major outstanding questions seemed to be the following:
1. The mechanism(s) of the generation of antibody diversity
2. The behavior of T lymphocytes
3. The role of the major histocompatibility complex in immune responses
4. The mechanism(s) of acquired immunological tolerance
5. The regulation of immune response.

On the way, these topics have revealed their internal complexities, ramifications, and even some unexpected, fanciful outgrowths, and all these expanded their history enormously.

As far as the experimental approaches are concerned, the 1970s were dominated by cell biology, which provided some important insights, but at the same time also created a huge amount of not always useful phenomenology. The 1980s then witnessed the massive entry of molecular biology into the field, and this has become a success story, so that molecular biology has remained ever since a permanent member in the immunological toolbox. Another victory of this era was that human immunology stepped out of the clinic, and claimed its place in basic science.

The experimental models have also undergone significant technical development. At the beginning were the genetically characterized inbred mouse and rat strains, followed by bone marrow chimeras, and toward the end came transgenic and gene knock-out animals.

At this point, the chronicler would like to introduce 'Doctor G', an active participant in the field, who is invited to provide interpretations and details that would have remained hidden for everyone else but the insider. His contribution is expected to facilitate understanding of this complex, fast-growing science.

REFERENCE

1. Jerne NK. Cold Spring Harbor Symp. *Quant. Biol.* 1967;**32**:601.

Chapter 2

A Very Special Location: The Basel Institute for Immunology

It was one of those wonderful summer mornings that can linger long in memory. The sun stood still low above the horizon, and radiated a warm light onto half of the garden, while the eastern half remained under the long shadows of cypresses in the neighboring lot. Doctor G woke up this morning earlier and less tired than usual.

'What a megalomaniac idea to plant sky-scraping trees on such a small lot!' was his first thought, and he felt a slight indignation at his late grandfather, who had sold that lot some 40 years ago. But after having his usual quadruple espresso, he became more positively tuned, and finally came the long-hatched decision in the bathroom during shaving: he will do research in immunology!

Until then, Dr. G's special field of research had been experimental pathology, although it was not necessarily his field of interest. He got involved in it by chance, after he had received his DVM degree with summa cum laude qualification, but he could not find a job. He kept returning to a research institute of the Academy of Sciences asking about a possible opening, when one day the director said to him: 'Our pathologist just walked out of my office, he will move to take a university position. So, if you are interested in pathology, you will have a job, if not, you won't.' 'Of course, I am interested' answered Dr. G immediately.

He was already used to take what he got, because it was made clear to him early enough that he was born into the wrong social class, and so he could, at best, expect to be tolerated, but not to be supported by the political system. His idea to go to research also had a political taint: namely, he had to choose an activity, for which the membership of the Socialist Worker Party (that he missed) was alone not sufficient. Furthermore, Dr. G learned everything with little effort, and also realized that occupations other than research would bore him to death.

'After all, it would not hurt to learn some pathology' he thought. But a few years and publications later, he could no longer envisage himself looking at histological sections eight hours a day for the rest of his life. His interest in immunology was awakened by his failure to distinguish between physiological and pathological conditions in sections of lymphoid organs. So he went to the

A History of Modern Immunology. http://dx.doi.org/10.1016/B978-0-12-416974-6.00002-8

library and soon became familiar with all major findings of the immunological revolution.

'A science where new cells are still being discovered is not only exciting, but also something to which I could contribute' he thought and so he did.

Researchers at the Academy had the privilege of applying once a year for a foreign fellowship in the West. What bothered Dr. G most was that his applications had been flatly turned down for eight years in a row, while his party-member colleagues returned already from their second Western stay with boosted egos, and some convertible money. Thus in the ninth year, he was the one to be surprised most that a 10-month Swiss fellowship was granted to him. 'The comrades at the Academy must have lost their vigilance' he said sarcastically.

In the application form he had to list two Swiss institutions, where he would like to spend his time of fellowship. At the first place, he named an institute, where immunohistology research was conducted, and to the second place he put, after some hesitation, the Basel Institute for Immunology. Although the latter filled him with panic-like fear, because he had seen many publications coming out of there, and hardly understood a word of them. And as it happened, his first choice did not materialize, however, he soon received a nice letter from Niels Jerne, the Director, to personally inform him that he had been elected to be a Member of the Basel Institute for Immunology for the duration of his fellowship. The decision was probably based on a paper that Dr. G had published in *Nature New Biology* (a short-lived *Nature* branch) on his chicken immunology studies. (The choice of chicken fitted well with the profile of his Institute, and as an added benefit, the experimental animals were edible.) Thus, Dr. G had to face the fact that, whether he wanted or not, he would fall into the deep water of 'big science' immunology, like Pilatus into the *Credo*, so to say.

At first sight of the Basel Institute, his uneasy feelings got worse, if that were possible. It was, for the early 1970s, an ultra-modern building, made of glass and aluminum, with a work of techno-art, a revolving spiral on a long bowed metal stalk by Jean Tinguely at the entrance. (Tinguely was a Swiss artist famous for his complicated mechanical constructions, every part of which was moving and busily doing some absurdly useless work.) Dr. G had a hard time to find the entrance itself, because none of the aluminum-framed glass units had a door-handle. The interior of the Institute was just as confusing: a maze of laboratories without doors, interconnected with stairs and gaps between movable walls. Later on he learned that this was meant to promote communication, and to prevent researchers from encapsulating themselves in private cells. This, of course, made good sense, nevertheless the place remained frightening, like a futuristic nightmare-vision. It was a relief for Dr. G that at least the restrooms had doors.

Upon his arrival, Dr. G was led to Niels Jerne's roof-top office by his secretary. Jerne's person acted on him almost as disquietingly as the building. First of all, he did not fit the internal image Dr. G had of great scientists. He was slender, very well dressed, and moved quickly and energetically, like a corporate top-manager. He had an impressive mane of well-combed grayish hair, almost too much for a man of his age. His voice was cold and commanding, and he spoke fast with an undertone of urgency that further strengthened his top-manager image. His face was a curious mixture of tough and almost childish soft features, and as the only scientist-like requisite, he wore fashionably designed but strong glasses.

'This man seems to have been assembled of many incompatible parts' was Dr. G's first impression.

His deputy, Ben Pernis, the discoverer of allelic exclusion, was also present. Ben made a somewhat more familiar impression on Dr. G. He was bald-headed and bulky, also very well dressed, and because he was an Italian, he could also smile. He spoke very fast, as many Italians do, but he did it in an impeccable English, a very non-Italian trait.

Jerne asked Dr. G a few quick questions, and received some embarrassed stuttering answers, until one topic developed into a firework-like scientific discussion between Jerne and Ben, which made them completely forget about Dr. G's presence. Finally they realized that they were not alone, told Dr. G that he would work in Ben's lab, and also recommended him to go and look at the town now, because later on he would hardly have time to do so. This is how Dr. G's first and last personal discussion with Jerne ended.

The Basel Institute for Immunology was founded and supported by Hoffmann–La Roche, one of the pharma giants in Basel. Because it was a family-owned firm, it could afford such extravagancies, and even more. For example, Mr. Sacher, a family member, formerly an artist himself, had strong Maecenas inclinations, and filled the company areal and buildings with pieces of modern art. The Institute also owed him the Tinguely work. Furthermore, he established the Scola Cantorum Basiliense, a meanwhile world-famous music school in Basel. Thus, Mr. Sacher was a good man, and as such lived a happy, and over 90 years long life.

The purpose of the Basel Institute was to provide talented scientists with a place, where they could work in complete academic freedom and with full financial support. A scientist's Fairyland, so to say. Little wonder that the Institute, almost instantaneously after its opening became the number-one immunology site in Europe, and one of the leaders in the world. All the mother company asked for in return was the right for potential practical applications, and this was not too much. Another expected benefit was that scientists trained at the Institute could then be employed at the company's own research department.

The Institute had no structural hierarchy: there was the Director and all others were Members. Another strict policy was that permanent memberships were non-existent, with a few exceptions. One was, for example, Dr. Trnka, a jolly, well-nourished, white-haired man, originally from Czechoslovakia. Trnka did some experimental work, but his major function was to run the administration of the Institute. So if it came to financials, it was advisable to be in good terms with Trnka, because he made all these decisions. But Trnka was such a friendly person that it would have been really difficult not to be in good terms with him. Another permanent member was Ivan Lefkovits, a nice, relaxed and good-mannered man with an ever-youthful face, also from Czechoslovakia. Ivan took the fancy of constructing complicated, automated devices for bio-assays, e.g., for limit-dilution analysis, used to study the size of immune cell repertoires (one of Jerne's prime interests), and later for the automated analysis of two-dimensional electrophoretic 'fingerprints'. Ivan spoke a series of languages (including Hungarian), and all with a unique accent that could not be accorded to his mother tongue, and so it must have been his own individualized one. Dr. G assumed that these two men might have belonged to the court of Jerne's previous kingdom, and they accompanied him to Basel.

There were also a few returning visitors, who spent part of every year at the Institute, and after a while assumed some special, 'institutionalized' role. One of them was Steve Fazekas de St. Groth, a very dignified and serious, pipe-smoking Australo-Hungarian virologist in his early fifties. He was the discoverer of a phenomenon that he termed 'original antigenic sin'. This was the observation that persons infected with flu virus 20 years back or longer, kept making antibodies against the first virus upon every re-infection, although the newly infecting virus meanwhile mutated far away from the original one. Dr. G has been unable to understand this phenomenon to date. Steve, by the way, turned out to have, behind the serious façade, an excellent humor and a ruthless sarcasm. He was famous for expressing himself in highly sophisticated English, but with a strong Hungarian accent. He usually refused to speak Hungarian for no good reason, because he could immediately be spotted by his ex-fellow countrymen on the basis of his accent. Steve's role at the Institute was unclear, but since he was extremely intelligent, he might have been one of Jerne's regular discussion partners. Dr. G could not find out whether Steve also conducted his own research there, as a matter of fact, he saw Steve only once sitting in front of a sterile hood, repairing his shoe inside.

Another returning figure was Ruggiero Ceppellini, an Italian transplantation geneticist. He was an aggressive man of power, the type of professor whom Italians call 'baroni'. Almost everybody in the Italian transplantation scene owed Ceppellini the beginning (or the end) of his or her carrier. He often gave seminars in Basel about the genetics of HLA, the human major histocompatibility complex (MHC), that most immunologists failed to understand, partly because they were not familiar with the topic, but mostly for acoustic reasons, due to Ceppellini's extremely strong Italian accent. Jerne kept him at the Institute, probably because his almost infallible intuition suggested to him that the mysterious role of MHC in immunity might turn out to be something interesting. Besides, Ceppellini provided the majority of personnel for the Institute's small transplantation immunology group.

But the most interesting 'commuter' was Melvin Cohn, a top theorist beside Jerne, who came from the Salk Institute for about 6 months every year. Mel was very sociable, Dr. G could always see him somewhere in discussion with somebody, with a wide, provocative smile on his face. Mel's role at the Institute was tutorial on the surface, as he gave regular seminars on immunological theory or new intriguing findings. But in reality, he was a mind-teaser. He always managed to raise tremendous opposition to what he said, and then skilfully channeled the aggression of his colleagues into scientifically meaningful directions. He was, in a way, similar to those life-size smiling puppets in entertainment parks, which everybody was allowed to hit as hard as he could, but they kept smiling, just a lamp lit up to show the strength of the blow. Dr. G admired Mel for his courage to take up this role that was certainly not imposed on him, he must have identified it for himself. Later on they came to know each other better, and have remained on friendly terms ever since.

There were many more interesting personalities around, who will be mentioned later on, in connection with their work. But most of the Members were very well-trained, aggressive and overexcited youngsters from Western Europe and the USA. Dr. G looked upon them as being the pampered products of the decadent West, but deep inside he envied them for their superior education, good English, and the freedom in behavior that they could afford. On top of these, they were all younger than himself, and so Dr. G felt sometimes to be literally nothing in comparison to them.

Most Members had 2-year contracts, just about enough time to complete a small piece of research work. But some contracts were extended to semi-permanency provided that the particular Member was working on a key project of Jerne's interest. With his 10-month stay, Dr. G felt severely handicapped, not to mention that, in addition to the work, he also had to catch up with the science and with new methods during this short time: 'Either I shall half-kill myself and make it, or just get peacefully forgotten' was Dr. G's attitude.

As a result of the fast-turnover policy, a whole generation of immunologists has grown up, almost every member of which spent some time at the Institute. They are often referred to as 'The Basel Family'.

All Members, permanent or temporary, young or old, female or male, were united in one respect: they all worshipped Jerne. This attitude was further supported by the fact that Jerne never appeared in the crowd, although he was always present, and anybody could go to his office and discuss things with him.

'This is a good method to maintain mysticism' thought Dr. G, but he was unfair, as the reason behind Jerne's isolation was his shyness. Nevertheless, he gave a seminar every now and then, where he revealed some interesting facets of his personality. For example, he turned out to be completely apolitical and sincere like a child. He made statements, such as: 'I published only 16 papers in my life, and most of them were wrong', for which the youth found him even more adorable. The Jerne cult finally culminated in a two-volume large 'Festschrift' for his seventieth birthday,[1] in which every Member submitted his contribution as an offering on the Jerne altar. At this point Jerne retired, moved to his villa in the Province, and broke contact with all immunologists except Ivan Lefkovits.

The most important event in the lives of Members was the appearance of the 'Annual Report of the Basel Institute for Immunology'. It was awaited with an impatient anticipation, as is Christmas by children. The report contained abstracts of the Members' results, and an impressive list of usually several hundred publications. But the most important part was Jerne's introduction, in which he described, in his crisp, clear and provocative way, his thoughts and reflections on the results of the year. Members whose contributions were dealt with in the introduction felt as happy as sportsmen upon winning an Olympic medal. But Jerne could sometimes also be skeptical making statements such as: 'Immunology resembles more and more the science of meteorology: we have an ever-increasing number of parameters, but cannot tell what the weather will be like tomorrow in Basel.'

After Jerne's retirement, Fritz Melchers, a leading B-cell immunologist and long-term Member took over the Director position. Fitz was rather arrogant on the surface, but otherwise a good person. He came from a strongly patriarchal family, and paternal rigor might have had molded him into what he became. His father was Emeritus Professor of Plant Genetics at the Max-Planck-Institute of Biology in Tübingen, a real old-fashioned German professor, six and a half feet tall, beyond 80 still erect and strong; a man made of steel and authority. Fritz had extremely high respect for his father. When he gave a lecture in Tübingen, his father was usually sitting in the first row, and Fritz addressed the audience thus: 'Ladies and Gentlemen, Dear Father'. Under Melchers's directorship the Institute had survived for almost another two decades. Around the turn of the millennium Hoffmann–La Roche lost interest in immunology, closed down the Institute, and sold the facilities for a nominal price of one Swiss Franc to an affiliated company.

But in the memory of all former Members the Institute lives on as a beautiful, exotic pearl among scientific institutions, and they cannot but regret that it is all over now.

REFERENCE

1. The Immune System. Festschrift in honor of Niels Kaj Jerne on the occasion of his 70th birthday. In: Steinberg CM, Lefkovits I, editors. Basel, New York: Karger; 1981.

Chapter 3

Immunological Specificity

Specificity is generally considered to be the all-pervasive principle that is effective when two entities interact, irrespective of whether the latter are atoms, macromolecules, cells, or human beings. Specificity has therefore been a preferred substrate for thinking in a number of disciplines including chemistry, biology, psychology, and, last but not least, philosophy.

In immunological thinking, specificity has occupied a prominent place ever since the discovery of antibodies and their capability to distinguish between pathogens more than 130 years ago. With some exaggeration, one could even regard the history of immunology as a continued quest for the meaning and the basis of immunological specificity. Of course, the concept of specificity has undergone many changes over the past 130 years, depending on the actual stand of experimental immunology. Based on the state of scientific-technological progress, the conceptual development of immunological specificity falls roughly into three periods.

1. The archaic period (~1880–1920), when hypotheses of specificity were created in the absence of structural information about either antigen or antibody.
2. The chemical period (~1920–1975), when experimental data accumulated on antigens and antibodies, culminating in the determination of immunoglobulin (Ig) structure, and the X-ray crystallography of antigen–antibody complexes.
3. The biological period (~1975–2000), starting with the discovery of how antibody diversity is generated and concluding with concepts that attempt to place the available information into a biological-evolutionary context.

Immunological specificity in the sense used here is confined to describe the interaction between antibody and antigen. The specificity of the T-cell antigen receptor (TCR), a molecule similarly variable to Ig, differs in important details from that of Ig, and thus merits separate discussion. Furthermore, the history of TCR started in 1984, and thus skipped most detours of the first and second period. The focus of this discussion will be on how the modern concept of antibody specificity has evolved. Earlier concepts will be described to the extent needed for understanding the contemporary view. Interested readers will find the detailed history of immunological specificity, in particular the history of the first and second period, in Arthur Silverstein's book.[1]

A History of Modern Immunology. http://dx.doi.org/10.1016/B978-0-12-416974-6.00003-X

The first coherent hypothesis of immunological specificity was set forth by Paul Ehrlich in his famous side-chain theory.[2,3] Ehrlich considered specificity to be the consequence of interaction between chemically defined complementary molecular structures, and consequently, the antigen–antibody interaction, a strong, irreversible chemical bonding. Although his view incited heated debates over the following decades, in particular, concerning the irreversible nature of antigen–antibody interactions, the concept had remained essentially unchallenged until Karl Landsteiner published his work on synthetic haptens. In these studies, Landsteiner and Lampl[4,5] investigated the specificity of antibodies raised against proteins substituted with two series of small chemical compounds (haptens). They found that a given antibody reacted most strongly with the immunizing hapten, but showed reactions of graded affinities also with chemically related haptens. While Ehrlich's concept envisaged a one-to-one relationship between antigen and antibody, and cross-reactivity was explained by sharing a determinant (epitope) by two different antigens, Landsteiner's data demonstrated that one antibody can react to a number of related epitopes with different affinities, which ruled out the requirement for a perfect fit.

Curiously, this was not the message that caught the fancy of most immunologists in connection with the Landsteiner study. Instead, they were amazed that antibodies could be produced against compounds that had never existed before in nature. Since the number of naturally occurring antigens alone was extremely large, with the added number of antigenic chemical compounds it was almost impossible to imagine that a vertebrate host could carry prior information for the production of all these antibodies. This view then led to 'instructionist' hypotheses, according to which antigens somehow mold the structure of antibodies to achieve a close fit. The idea of an almost infinite number of antibodies, often referred to as the 'Landsteiner legacy', was another unwanted outgrowth that lingered on in immunology for quite a while.

But the Landsteiner study also had long-lasting positive impacts. First, it has raised the possibility for the first time that antigenicity may not be determined by the chemical nature of the ligand. And second, haptens became important research tools of immunology to be used over the next 50–60 years. In contrast to the hapten study, Landsteiner's other important contributions (the ABO blood group system for which he received the Nobel Prize, the first autoantibody, serodiagnosis of syphilis and poliomyelitis, transfer of delayed-type hypersensitivity with leukocytes, and many more) were treated as dry historical facts, taken for granted. Thus it is not surprising that Landsteiner himself felt he would have deserved the Nobel Prize for the hapten work instead of the ABO system.[1]

Until the 1950s, the problem of specificity could only be approached reasonably from the ligand's side, because organic chemistry was sufficiently developed to be able to synthesize a variety of small antigenic compounds, whereas protein chemistry was still in its infancy so that the antibody molecule remained unknown besides that it was a globulin. Experiments with small organic molecules yielded important though indirect information about the size and possible shapes of the antigen-combining site, and suggested that most antibodies were bivalent. Furthermore, they revealed another complexity, namely that any given antiserum could contain a number of different antibodies reacting to the same antigen. The latter finding inspired David Talmage[6] to propose for the first time in history that the repertoire of antibodies may not be as vast as earlier assumed. According to his argument, if the epitopes were distributed on antigens combinatorially, then an antibody repertoire for a relatively small number of epitopes could react with a vast number of different antigens. At the same time, the idea of an enormous repertoire was criticized also from the cellular selectionist's point of view by Lederberg.[7] He pointed out that the antibody repertoire could not reasonably be larger than the number of B cells an animal can have. These ideas were important seeds for later concepts aiming at the definition of a biologically relevant size of antibody repertoire.

The period from about 1960 to the mid-1970s witnessed the breakthrough of determining the structure of Ig, and its interaction with antigen (see Section 1.4). These studies translated the mystic concept of immunological specificity into a close structural complementarity which permits the formation of a number of non-covalent interactions (hydrogen bonds, ionic interactions, van der Waals forces, hydrophobic interactions) between the epitope and the Ig combining site. It has also become clear that there is nothing special about epitopes: they can be any three-dimensional patch on the molecular surface of antigen. Thus epitopes do not determine antigenicity, it is the Ig combining site that selects the fitting epitope. The physical-chemical definition of antibody specificity was thus complete, what remained was to place this information back into biology.

By the mid-1970s, advances in molecular biology permitted investigation of the next important question: how is antibody diversity generated? As discussed later in detail (Section 5.2), this happens in two stages. First, during B cell ontogeny one of many variable (V) region genes is rearranged to other gene segments to form a complete gene encoding the Ig variable region, which is then joined to a constant (C) region gene.[8] Second, after contacting antigen the Ig molecule undergoes further somatic mutations.[9]

The discovery that Ig gene segments rearrange combinatorially tempted immunologists to assess the repertoire size by sequence diversity arising through rearrangements. However, the number obtained ($\sim 10^{19}$ excluding somatic mutations, see Section 5.2) was far too high to translate into biological relevance, if for no other reason than because of the Lederberg argument, i.e., that there is no animal on this planet that would have so many B lymphocytes (a mouse has $\sim 10^8$, man 10^{11}, and elephant 10^{14} B cells). Thus the numerology exercised with sequence diversity revived the old idea of an excessively large repertoire for another while.

The biological approach to estimating the size of repertoire was based on functional and evolutionary considerations. The starting point was a very simple thesis, which was so self-evident that most immunologists were embarrassed for not coming to it before. This was the following: 'antibodies function concentration dependent'. Considering that the lowest antibody concentration required for the elimination of antigen is ~10 ng/ml, in body fluids with 10 mg/ml of Ig there is room for at most 10^6 different functional antibodies, provided that each individual antibody is represented at threshold concentration.[10] Because the immune system is selected through the efficiency of its effector function (capability to eliminate pathogens), antibodies below the effective concentration would be unselectable. For the production of 10 ng/ml/day of antibody, ~500 Ig-secreting plasma cells/ml of body fluid are required. Assuming that B cells divide every 0.75 day, and that the time interval between the first encounter with a pathogen and the production of an effective antibody concentration should not exceed 5–6 days, at least 10 B cells/ml of body fluid specific for a given pathogen must be present prior to antigen encounter. The number of B cells calculated for volume of body fluid is in the order of 10^7/ml in all vertebrates, which permits the immune system to deal effectively with maximum 10^6 different antigens (or probably less) at a time. These calculations have led to the definition of 'protecton',[10,11] which corresponds to the smallest B cell number that provides the animal with ~90% protection. This is ~10^7 B cells in 1 ml of body fluid in the smallest vertebrate (hummingbird). Implicit is that larger animals must have repeated units of the same protecton (e.g., an elephant should have 10^7 protectons).

Of course, the very same idea can also be expressed differently, namely, that the size of individual B cell clones should be proportional to the size of animal (more exactly the volume of body fluid) in order to ensure a functional concentration of antibodies. This implies that big animals do not possess more clones than small ones, but more cells per clone.

One conclusion from the protecton concept that surprised many immunologists concerned the size of the functional, evolutionarily selectable antibody repertoire: this was postulated to be much smaller than anticipated on the basis of experimental results and sequence diversity. At first sight such a repertoire appeared too small to recognize the antigenic universe. However, this was likely to be an illusion, because antibodies recognize epitopes that should be distributed combinatorially on different antigens (the Talmage principle[6]). Thus a repertoire recognizing 10^5 epitopes, and at average ten epitopes per antigen would be able to distinguish $10^5 C_{10} = 10^{43}$ different antigens.[12]

'The protecton idea came up against massive resistance on the part of most immunologists' comments Dr. G. 'The basis for this was the collective experience that one could make antibody to just about anything. Surely this can be achieved, but only by using granuloma-provoking mycobacteria, slow release emulsions, repeated boosting, etc., which over time permit the expansion of rare clones, i.e., these specificities are selected artificially and not by evolution. Such experiments say something about the size of the *potential* repertoire, but are not relevant for the *available* repertoire that protects against infection. Nevertheless, immunologists have remained somewhat split-minded concerning the question of repertoire size up to these days.'

The next important question was how specific antibodies should be. The biological approach to this problem was based on the appreciation that antibodies activate biodestructive effector mechanisms (complement, phagocytosis, etc.) that are indiscriminatory on their own, and therefore, antibodies must 'tell' them what to destroy and what to spare. Consequently, antibodies must be sufficiently specific to direct the effector mechanisms to the intruder (pathogen, non-self) and away from the body (self). In other words, the evolutionary selective pressure on antibody specificity is the necessity to make self–non-self (S–NS) discrimination, and it is exercised through the destructive effector mechanisms.[12,13] The resulting specificity should be a compromise between two extremes: if antibodies bound to everything (specificity zero), the host would destroy the pathogens as well as itself, and if specificity were 'infinite', S–NS discrimination would be perfect, but the repertoire would be immense and thus the response to a pathogen would be too slow, and the host would die of infection. A compromise in between is reached, when the specificity is just appropriate to make S–NS discrimination with an acceptably low frequency of mistakes. In this case the repertoire would also be sufficiently small to be able to respond rapidly. It is perhaps useful to emphasize here that the distinction between different pathogens cannot drive specificity, because it does not make any difference for the outcome of a response whether the antibody recognized a 'private' epitope of a certain pathogen or a 'public' one shared by a number of different pathogens. Antibodies distinguish between pathogens to the extent that they discriminate S from NS.

According to this concept, specificity can be expressed as a constant, K, which is defined as the probability that a change in recognition would be anti-S. The question then arises: upon what properties is evolution selecting to arrive at a functional K value? Here we have to reiterate that the selection pressure is on the effector response: it must be sufficiently specific to eliminate the pathogen without debilitating the host (S–NS discrimination). The specificity of effector response depends on four factors:[12]

1. Specificity of the Ig combining site itself
2. The number of different binding sites per Ig
3. The number of different antigen receptors per cell
4. The range over which the activation signal operates in T–B cell collaboration.

In case of factor 1, evolution is likely to select for the size of the combining site.[14] Obviously, if the latter could only interact with a single amino acid, S–NS discrimination would be impossible. Conversely, if it were too large, there would be no cross-reactivity, but the repertoire would be non-functional and thus unselectable. The size of combining site that could make sufficient S–NS discrimination is estimated to encompass epitopes of ~5 amino acids, or a monosaccharide. Factors 2 and 3 are selected to have one specificity per Ig (allelic exclusion) and one receptor per cell (clonality). The selection pressure works through double-specific molecules/cells, of which one is anti-S and the other anti-NS. Factor 4 is selected to be short range to avoid activation of bystander anti-S cells by spillage. All these factors are selected in concert, and result in an estimated K value of ~0.01, i.e., ~1% probability that a combining site will be anti-S, and consequently the same probability to cross-react with another NS epitope.[12]

Finally, it should be pointed out that the biology-based concept of specificity as outlined above does not enjoy general acceptance in the immunological community. The opposing view is based on two phenomena: first, a single epitope can be recognized by a number of distinguishable combining sites ('degeneracy'), and second, a set of distinguishable epitopes can be recognized by a single combining site ('mimicry'). These two interrelated phenomena suggested to proponents of the alternative view that promiscuous receptors and degenerate processes would be the leading principles of the immune system, and that without strict specificity S–NS discrimination would be impossible.[15–18] Of course, degeneracy and mimicry are facts, but the conclusion drawn from them leads to a paradox that is admitted also by proponents of the alternative view.[19] Namely, if the immune system cannot rely on the specificity of its receptors at the molecular level, how can it be so specific at the operational level?

As a matter of fact, degeneracy and mimicry can also be explained without throwing S–NS discrimination overboard.[20] One has only to appreciate that a degenerate set of binding sites has equivalent functional specificity, and that a series of 'mimotopes' exhibits the same antigenic characteristic (for which there is experimental evidence[21,22]). Consequently, a set of degenerate sites as well as a series of mimotopes is viewed by the immune system as one: if any site of the set is anti-S, all are anti-S, and if any mimotope is S the rest is also S. Thus S–NS discrimination would work by distinguishing between sets instead of individual epitopes.

'This recent debate about immunological specificity could serve as a prototype for the kind of battles fought between two camps with diagonally opposite attitudes to science', adds Dr. G. 'One camp could be called "reductionists", their goal is to extract a concept from the data, and they don't mind losing details that appear peripheral to the concept. On the other side are the "complicators" who consider every detail equally important, irrespective of whether it seems to make sense or not, as they believe that any data could become the key to solving a problem. The conflict between these two groups is unresolvable, because it is rooted in the way of thinking. But their debates remain useful, in that they call attention to problems that need a convincing solution. Since such a solution is not available for immunological specificity, all we can conclude at present is that the 130-year-old problem has not yet been settled to everybody's satisfaction.'

REFERENCES

1. Silverstein AM. *A History of Immunology*. San Diego: Academic Press; 1989.
2. Ehrlich P. *Klin. Jahrb.* 1897;**60**:199.
3. Ehrlich P. *Proc. R. Soc. London* 1900;**66**:424.
4. Landsteiner K, Lampl H. *Z. Immunitätsforsch.* 1917;**26**:258.

5. Landsteiner K, Lampl H. *Z. Immunitätsforsch.* 1917;**26**:293.

6. Talmage DW. *Science* 1959;**129**:1643.

7. Lederberg J. *Science* 1959;**129**:1649.

8. Tonegawa S. *Nature* 1983;**302**:575.

9. Griffiths GM, Berek C, Kaartinen M, Milstein C. *Nature* 1984;**312**:271.

10. Langman RE, Cohn M. *Mol. Immunol.* 1987;**24**:675.

11. Cohn M, Langman RE. *Immunol. Rev.* 1990;**115**:7.

12. Cohn M. *Cell. Immunol.* 1997;**181**:103.

13. Langman RE. *Mol. Immunol.* 2000;**37**:555.

14. Percus JK, Percus OE, Perelson AS. *Proc. Natl. Acad. Sci. USA* 1993;**90**:1691.

15. Parnes O. *Mol. Immunol.* 2004;**40**:985.

16. Cohen IR, Hershberg U, Solomon S. *Mol. Immunol.* 2004;**40**:993.

17. Dembic Z. *Scand. J. Immunol.* 2004;**60**:3.

18. Sercarz EE, Maverakis E. *Mol. Immunol.* 2004;**40**:1003.

19. Sercarz EE, Cohen IR. *Mol. Immunol.* 2004;**40**:983.

20. Cohn M. *Mol. Immunol.* 2005;**42**:651.

21. Meloen RH, Puijk WC, Sloostra JW. *J. Mol. Recognit.* 2000;**13**:352.

22. Monzavi-Karbassi B, Cunto-Amesty G, Luo P, Shamloo S, Blaszcyk-Thurin M, Kieber-Emmons T. *Int. Immunol.* 2001;**13**:1361.

Chapter 4

Monoclonal Antibodies: The Final Proof for Clonal Selection

4.1 DISCOVERY

The clonal selection theory has predicted that a single B cell and its descendants would produce one single antibody both as a cell surface receptor and in secreted form. Several pieces of data provided indirect evidence that this prediction was valid (see Section 1.1). However, a direct proof entailing the isolation and expansion of single B cells and investigation of the antibody they secrete was difficult to obtain. The major obstacle to this was the technical unfeasibility to grow B cells long term, in vitro. The idea of how to get around this problem came from César Milstein, an experienced molecular biologist and immunologist at the MRC Laboratory of Molecular Biology in Cambridge, UK, and a young German immunologist, Georges Köhler, who spent his postdoctoral fellowship in Milstein's laboratory. They set out to hybridize B cells from immunized mice with a spontaneously growing tumor cell line, and select hybrid cells that both grow infinitely and produce antibody.

The enabling technologies for the Köhler-Milstein experiment[1] were in place already, thanks mostly to somatic cell geneticists. The latter had a long-standing interest in cell hybridization, and worked out the technology of introducing drug-resistance markers into cultured cell lines and selecting hybrid cells (that complement each other in terms of drug resistance) in the presence of the drugs that killed the parental lines.[2–4] The available battery of cultured mouse myeloma and lymphoma lines[5] enabled also preliminary studies of immunoglobulin (Ig) synthesis in hybrid cell clones.[6,7]

The Köhler-Milstein study owes much of its success to the careful experimental design. As an immunogen, sheep red blood cells (SRBC) were chosen, because this enabled the detection of single antibody-forming hybrids by Jerne's hemolytic plaque assay.[8] The source of antibody-producing B cells was spleen cells from SRBC-immunized Balb/c mice. The fusion partner was P3, a plasmocytoma syngeneic with the immune spleen cells (i.e., of Balb/c origin), which was made resistant of 8-azaguanin (P3-X63-Ag8), and was thus unable to grow in selective medium (HAT[2]). Removal of non-hybridized lymphocytes was not necessary, as they died spontaneously in culture. Hybrids were cloned in soft agar, and the antibody-producing clones were easily identified by an overlay of SRBC and complement. One surprise of this study was the remarkably high

A History of Modern Immunology. http://dx.doi.org/10.1016/B978-0-12-416974-6.00004-1

frequency (~10%) of antibody-producing hybrids. This was probably due to a preferential hybridization between the P3-X63-Ag8 plasmocytoma line and antibody-producing plasmoblasts/plasma cells representing a similar state of differentiation. Another favorable aspect was the stability of hybrids: they did not show loss of chromosomes even after several months in culture.

However, these first hybrids were not truly monoclonal, as they secreted also the Ig of the fusion partner (myeloma protein MOPC 21) in addition to anti-SRBC antibody, and light chain swapping between these two Igs also occurred. This problem was taken care of by isolating non-secreting clones of the P3-X63-Ag8 line to be used as fusion partners.[9–11] The technology was improved also by the use of polyethylene glycol instead of Sendai virus to facilitate cell fusion. At this point the promise of Köhler and Milstein that 'such cultures could be valuable for medical and industrial use'[1] started to become reality.

'After Cambridge, Georges Köhler moved to the Basel Institute for Immunology', recalls Dr. G. 'The Basel youth started to whisper in advance already: "this is a very clever boy, he will get the Nobel Prize". But Georges' personality must have been a disappointment for them, because he was neither overexcited nor engaged in sparkling verbal duels; he was a quiet laboratory scientist with gray hair already at the age of 30. In addition, he was a good husband and father, who preferred to stay with his family, instead of going from one party to another. So he just did not match up with the preconceived image of a young and successful scientist. His sensitive and reserved attitude was often a disadvantage. For example, when he applied for a director position at the Max-Planck-Institute for Immunology in Freiburg, many members of the Staff Selection Board were against him, because he was "not energetic enough" for them. Finally they did not turn him down only for fear of a scandal in case he really got the Nobel Prize. And this was a wise decision, as he did receive the Prize together with César Milstein and Niels Jerne in 1984.'

'César Milstein was also a true and humble laboratory scientist, maybe this is why he teamed up with Georges Köhler so well. He possessed a broad knowledge and great experience in different areas of experimental biology, and kept working in the laboratory far beyond retirement age. He had a natural reluctance for publicity, and so he was not the one to go to big meetings and put up flashy shows.'

'The example of Köhler and Milstein must be reassuring for young scientists, because it demonstrates that science has still remained a profession in which quality is rewarded irrespective of public image and other virtualities.'

4.2 IMMUNOLOGY GOES BUSINESS

At the beginning, the reception of monoclonal antibodies (mAbs) by the immunological community was not as enthusiastic as expected. Although the unprecedented high titers monoclonals could attain impressed everybody, skeptics argued that one would have to produce a large number of mAbs before the desired specificity could be obtained, and thus the investment would be much higher than making a polyclonal antiserum. This argument originated from observations with the first anti-sheep red blood cell (SRBC) mAbs, some of which reacted with erythrocytes from a number of species, while others showed a more restricted cross-reactivity pattern, and only a few were uniquely specific for SRBC. The truth, however, was that immunologists learned the use and limitations of polyclonal sera, and were reluctant to invest extra energy into familiarizing with the new serological reagents.

But this attitude rapidly changed after the production of a number of mAbs directed against cell surface molecules that most immunologists were interested in, e.g., T-cell surface antigens and major histocompatibility complex (MHC) molecules.[12–15] In these cases, monoclonals were clearly superior to the previously available alloantisera that were usually of low titer with huge batch-to-batch variations.

The increasing popularity of mAbs represented an important impetus for a new branch of industry producing mAbs for research and diagnostic purposes. An equally important stimulus was the fact that César Milstein did not patent the hybridoma technology, and thus it was available free for start-up companies with small capital, which could not have afforded expensive licenses. The beneficial result was a sudden proliferation of small mAb companies and an explosion in the number of available mAbs. The developing policy was that researchers who needed small amounts of mAbs purchased them from the new companies, whereas those who wanted to make their own mAb could order the hybridoma from the ATCC (American Tissue Culture Collection), where most hybridomas were deposited.

'The industry was terra incognita for immunologists before' recalls Dr. G. 'The only one we knew who had to do with it was Len Herzenberg – a brilliant mind, fast like lightning, unbeatable in debates. He happened to discover the fluorescence-activated cell sorter that has become everybody's favorite toy in immunology, cell biology, medical labs, etc., and so he got involved with Becton Dickinson, the company manufacturing and commercializing the "FACS machine". Nevertheless he remained a Stanford Professor throughout. But the new mAb companies enticed many immunologists full time to the industry.'

'César Milstein's decision not to patent hybridomas was a blessing for the research community and small industry, but it annoyed those immensely who were after "big business". Some 20 years after the discovery, César complained to me bitterly that every time a grant application of his was turned down, there was a handwritten note on the side "Why didn't you patent monoclonal antibodies?" by the British Premier (the "Iron Lady") herself.'

'The success of small mAb companies raised the desire of big industry for a share, but their business model did not permit them to move a single step forward without patent protection. In the mAb arena this was problematic, because the technology was free, and the mAbs themselves were also difficult to patent, as the possibility remained open that somebody would make a different mAb with the same specificity. Therefore the industry started to patent potential target molecules to which mAbs could be made. A notorious example for this business strategy was the "Ortho patent", which claimed practically the whole T-cell surface. Of course, this broad patent could not provide very strong protection, but it was very effective in shying away other companies from immunomodulatory projects involving T cells. In essence such patents were only an obstacle to progress, and are fortunately no longer granted.'

'The most outrageous case of over-zealous patenting plans also deserves mention here, although it happened outside of immunology. This was related to the human genome sequencing project, the largest international scientific collaboration in history, the US effort of which was sponsored by the NIH (National Institutes of Health) and headed by Jim Watson, discoverer of DNA structure, and one of the three most renowned scientists on this planet. When the project approached completion, the NIH expressed its intention to patent the human genome. This happened in the late 1990s, when practically every single scientific discovery was already being patented, and so it did not come as a surprise to many. But Jim Watson objected to it by pointing out that the human genome is not an invention, it is the result of some 3000 million years of evolution, and as such it belongs to mankind. The response to his opposition was that the President of NIH (another iron lady, by the way) simply fired him from the project. Fortunately, some politicians who did not only have "iron in their heads" recognized the absurdity of this patent plan, and saved our genetic heritage from becoming private property.'

'I think these examples illustrate well the adverse effects of ruthless and uncontrolled striving for "intellectual property" as was customary in the late twentieth century.'

The big pharmacological industry really came into play when the therapeutic use of mAbs appeared to become feasible. The reason for this was that the research and developmental costs of new drugs were so high that only big, capital-strong companies could afford to produce them.

'In the 1990s, the average R&D costs of a new drug were around 150 million dollars' points out Dr. G. 'Perhaps it is interesting for colleagues in academia to learn that the preclinical (laboratory) phase of research required only a minor fraction of these costs: a project with a 10–15-membered team could be run to completion of less than 10 million. The product costs were also relatively insignificant. Although mAbs belonged to the most expensive drugs, one could get kilogram amounts, enough for a set of clinical trials, from a contract manufacturer for a few million dollars. The remaining budget, usually in excess of 100 million, was spent on clinical trials. The high costs of clinical research are not really explained by technical and organizational complexity. They rather have to do with the fact that clinical trials provide the most important efficacy and tolerability data, on which the registration of new drugs depends.'

But the way of mAbs to the clinic was not as easy as anticipated: a number of hurdles had to be overcome before their therapeutic use became reality. The first and most serious concern was that rodent antibodies proved to be strongly immunogenic in humans. This was first observed in patients who received mAbs for diagnostic purposes, and was manifested in the production of human anti-murine antibodies (HAMA).[16] Exceptions were only some immunosuppressive mAbs, e.g., anti-CD3, that inhibited all immune responses including the one against themselves. The HAMA cause rapid clearance of the therapeutic mAb and reduce its efficacy. Additionally, adverse effects ranging from allergic reactions to anaphylactic shock can occur. Although immunogenicity of xenogeneic antibodies per se was not a surprise, the observations in the praxis made the industry realize that only human mAbs could be reasonably used for therapeutic purposes. This then led to the next problems, namely, a human cell line to be used as a fusion partner for hybridoma could not be identified, and alternative methods, for example, transformation of antibody-producing human B cells with Epstein-Barr virus,[17] did not yield cell lines appropriate for industry-scale culturing. Another problem was that humans could not be intentionally immunized for ethical reasons, and thus the only cumbersome way that remained was to try to isolate B cells specific for a certain antigen, in vitro, from unprimed B-cell populations. All these difficulties finally led to the recognition that the problem of immunogenicity could not be solved by means of cell biology, and the emphasis was shifted toward molecular biological approaches.

4.3 THE TECHNOLOGY AVALANCHE: ANTIBODY ENGINEERING

The pressing need for non-immunogenic therapeutic mAbs provided a strong stimulus for the development of a set of new technologies collectively referred to as antibody engineering. The most commonly used approach was taking advantage of the ease of immunizing rodents and making hybridoma. Parts of the rodent mAbs thus generated were then stepwise replaced with homologous human immunoglobulin (Ig) sequences. Naturally, these manipulations could not have been performed on the protein itself, but they were readily doable at the DNA level, on rearranged immunoglobulin genes.[18,19]

The first generation of engineered antibodies, termed 'chimeric', was constructed by replacing the heavy (H) and light (L) chain constant (C) regions of rodent mAbs with the corresponding human domains.[20] As expected on the basis of model experiments,[21] chimerization did reduce immunogenicity substantially, but the rodent variable regions were still sufficiently foreign to induce a HAMA response. Another useful aspect of the chimerization technology was that it permitted to exchange Ig isotypes at will, and thereby control the effector function of the antibody. For example, the human $\gamma1$ CH region was chosen, when the antibody was required to induce the complement cascade and cell-mediated killing. Conversely, the relatively inactive $\gamma4$ isotype could be used in blocking antibodies and in mAbs for diagnostic imaging.

The next step in reducing immunogenicity was the exchange of framework residues in the variable (V) region of rodent mAbs, referred to as 'humanization'.

The procedure itself consisted of transferring the complementary determining regions (CDR) of an active rodent antibody onto a human VH/VL region framework (of course, at the DNA level).[22,23] The method had several variants, and was also referred to under different names, e.g., 'CDR grafting', 'reshaping', 'hyperchimerization', etc. Because the framework of V domains is a rigid β-sheet structure with the antigen-binding site formed by the six CDRs sitting on its top, the replacement of CDRs with different ones could be done without much concern about non-permissive conformational changes. Nevertheless, in some instances, conformational problems did occur, and a few additional changes in framework residues were necessary to correct them. Altogether, the humanization procedure was considered successful in reducing the immunogenicity of therapeutic mAbs to a manageable minimum. The industry was encouraged by these results, so that by the mid-1990s, 70–80 humanized mAbs were already in the R&D pipeline of different pharma and biotech companies.[24]

But the holy grail of antibody engineering was the production of 'fully human' mAbs. A rather original approach to this was the construction of transgenic mice carrying large genomic DNA fragments, called miniloci, comprised of human Ig-encoding gene segments in unrearranged germ-line configuration for both H and L chains.[25] The human Ig genes were shown to rearrange in B cells and be expressed as normal human Igs. Thus, such mice could be immunized with antigens of choice and B cells secreting human antibodies could be identified.

The technology that finally dominated the fully human mAb field was based on the construction of large libraries of antigen-binding Ig gene fragments (usually single-chain Fvs, i.e., covalently linked VH–VL pairs) displayed on the surface of bacteriophages.[26–28] The libraries could then be panned on antigen bound to a solid surface, and binding phages isolated. Of the appropriate binders full antibodies could be constructed by using an earlier method developed for chimerization. The phage display technology also permitted the improvement of antibody affinity by mimicking the physiological process of somatic hypermutation, in vitro.[29] Meanwhile different advanced forms of antibody libraries exist, including, for example, synthetic combinatorial libraries with exchangeable CDR cassettes.[30,31]

'Antibody engineering was the first example to demonstrate very effectively what biotechnology is capable of doing' adds Dr. G. 'Interestingly, the most active participant of this field, Greg Winter, worked at the very same place, the MRC Laboratory of Molecular Biology in Cambridge UK, where Milstein and Köhler had discovered monoclonal antibodies more than a decade earlier. But, in contrast to César Milstein, Greg Winter obeyed the command of the time and patented his technologies, probably to the great satisfaction of the "Iron Lady".'

'What remains to be discussed briefly is the issue of immunogenicity from an immunologist's angle of view. Two important points have to be made in this context. First, it should be remembered that Igs are polymorphic, several allotypes of them exist in the human population, and the injection of a mAb with a particular allotype induces antibody response in recipients having different allotypes. Thus anti-allotype responses are expected in at least some of the mAb-treated patients. Exchange of the allotypic amino acid residues to "consensus" residues may or may not solve this problem. Second, the antibody repertoire is generated somatically by a process including random changes in CDR3s and additional somatic mutations after antigen encounter, i.e., the repertoire is individualized. The host develops self-tolerance to its own antibody repertoire, which could only cover an external antibody by chance. Thus, the possibility of anti-idiotypic responses to the somatically varied parts of external antibodies can never be completely excluded. Consequently, the construction of an antibody that would totally lack immunogenicity for humans is theoretically impossible. This, however, is not meant to discourage antibody therapy. By now there are several examples of mAbs with impressive therapeutic effect, and the present mAb constructions are certainly safe enough to be used without much concern.'

REFERENCES

1. Köhler GK, Milstein C. *Nature* 1975;**256**:495.
2. Littlefield JW. *Science* 1964;**145**:709.
3. Harris H, Watkins JF. *Nature* 1965;**205**:640.
4. Chu EH, Brimer P, Jacobson KB, Merriam EV. *Genetics* 1969;**62**:359.
5. Horibata K, Harris AW. *Exp. Cell Res.* 1970;**60**:61.
6. Cotton RG, Milstein C. *Nature* 1973;**244**:42.
7. Schwaber J, Cohen EP. *Proc. Natl. Acad. Sci. USA* 1974;**71**:2203.
8. Jerne NK, Nordin AA. *Science* 1963;**140**:405.
9. Köhler GK, Howe SC, Milstein C. *Eur. J. Immunol.* 1976;**6**:292.
10. Köhler GK, Milstein C. *Eur. J. Immunol.* 1976;**6**:511.
11. Kearney JF, Radbruch A, Liesegang B, Rajewsky K. *J. Immunol.* 1979;**123**:1548.
12. Oi VT, Jones PP, Goding JW, Herzenberg LA, Herzenberg LA. *Curr. Top. Microbiol. Immunol.* 1978;**81**:115.
13. Ledbetter JA, Herzenberg LA. *Immunol. Rev.* 1979;**47**:63.
14. Lemke H, Hämmerling GJ, Hämmerling U. *Immunol. Rev.* 1979;**47**:175.
15. Hogarth PM, Potter TA, Cornell FN, McLachlan R, IFC McKenzie. *J. Immunol.* 1980;**125**:1618.
16. Lind P, Lechner P, Hausman B, Smola MG, Koeltringer P, Steindorfer P, Cesnik H, Passl R, Eber O. *Antibod. Immunoconj. Radiopharm.* 1991;**4**:811.
17. Kozbor D, Steinitz M, Klein G, Koskimies S, Mäkelä O. *Scand. J. Immunol.* 1979;**10**:187.
18. Neuberger MS, Williams GT, Fox RO. *Nature* 1984;**312**:604.
19. Neuberger MS, Williams GT, Mitchell EB, Jouhal SS, Flanagan JG, Rabbits TH. *Nature* 1985;**314**:268.
20. Morrison SL, Johnson MJ, Herzenberg LA, Oi VT. *Proc. Natl. Acad. Sci. USA* 1984;**81**:6851.
21 Brüggemann M, Winter G, Waldmann H, Neuberger MS. *J. Exp. Med.* 1989;**170**:2153.
22. Jones PT, Dear PH, Foote J, Neuberger MS, Winter G. *Nature* 1986;**321**:522.
23. Riechmann L, Clark M, Waldmann H, Winter G. *Nature* 1988;**332**:323.
24. Emery SC, Adair JR. *Exp. Opin. Invest. Drugs* 1994;**3**:241.
25. Taylor LD, Carmack CE, Schramm SR, Mashayekh R, Higgins KM, Kuo CC, Woodhouse C, Kay RM, Lonberg N. *Nucl. Acids Res.* 1992;**20**:6287.

26. Ward ES, Güssow D, Griffiths AD, Jones PT, Winter G. *Nature* 1989;**341**:544.

27. Huse WD, Sastry L, Iverson SA, Kang AS, Alting-Mees M, Burton DR, Benkovic SJ, Lerner RA. *Science* 1989;**246**:1275.

28. Clackson T, Hoogenboom HR, Griffiths AD, Winter G. *Nature* 1991;**352**:624.

29. Chowdhury PS, Pastan I. *Nat. Biotech.* 1999;**17**:568.

30. Knappik A, Honegger A, Pack P, Fischer M, Wellnhofer G, Hoess A, Wölle J, Plückthun A, Virnekäs B. *J. Mol. Biol.* 2000;**296**:57.

31. Söderlind E, Strandberg L, Jirholt P, Kobayashi N, Alexeiva V, Äberg AM, Nilsson A, Jansson B, Ohlin M, Wingren C, Danielsson L, Carlsson R, Borrebaeck CAK. *Nat. Biotech.* 2000;**18**:852.

Chapter 5

The First Victory of Molecular Biology: Mechanisms of the Generation of Antibody Diversity

5.1 THEORETICAL TREATMENT OF THE PROBLEM

Already the widely used abbreviation GOD (generation of diversity) illustrates the position of this problem in the value system of immunologists, and also the mystery surrounding it. As discussed before (Chapter 3), the puzzle dates back to Landsteiner's hapten studies showing that antibodies are not only formed against pathogenic microorganisms or their toxic products, but can also be raised against small organic compounds that had never existed in nature. This finding implied that the antibody repertoire must be enormously large, and this, in turn, led to the question of how such a variability could be generated. The question was then re-raised in connection with Burnet's clonal selection theory, and two diametrically opposing hypotheses were offered for explanation.

According to the 'germ-line' theory championed by Talmage,[1,2] the antibody repertoire is not as large as it seems, because the combinatorial distribution of epitopes on antigens permits the recognition of a vast number of antigens by a limited number of antibodies, say about 5000. Consequently, the genome can manage to encode all antibodies required for protection of the host.

The 'somatic mutation' concept, first proposed by Lederberg,[3] rejected the germ-line explanation, first, because certain observations such as the change of antibody quality during the course of immune response (affinity maturation) suggested that antibodies and thus the genes encoding them can change somatically, and second, because it was difficult to envisage how a large number of similar, and probably tandemly arranged genes could be maintained in the genome (the selective pressure on each single antibody gene would be too weak to account for its preservation). Therefore, it was proposed that the specificity repertoire should be generated by somatic mutations of a few antibody genes.

'These two concepts divided immunologists into two competing camps fighting against each other for the "truth" that nobody knew.' comments Dr. G. 'Competition is, of course, a normal constituent of behavior that occurs everywhere from politics

A History of Modern Immunology. http://dx.doi.org/10.1016/B978-0-12-416974-6.00005-3

to sports, and back in history, from medieval religious debates to tribal wars in the Stone Age, and most commonly in the animal kingdom (where it actually belongs). Although some consider it as an important driving force of development, it has also some shortcomings, especially in science. The specific problem here is that the rules of logic demand a clear discrimination between the competing views, and thus, each is forced to take up an extreme position, in order to avoid the critique of being wishy-washy conceptual tinkering. However, nature does not favor extremes, indeed she is wishy-washy as much as evolution is a tinkerer, and therefore, both views are bound to be wrong at least partially from the very beginning. And as we will see later that this was exactly the case for the germ-line and somatic mutation theories.'

The good thing about fights is that they tend to recede when no decision is achievable, and this happened also to the debate between the adherents of the above two theories. And at this point, Jerne came up with a new theory on the somatic generation of antibody diversity.[4] It appeared in 1971, on the first page of the first volume of *European Journal of Immunology*, and no journal could have wished a better advertisement for its launching. This theory had all typical 'Jernean' attributes. First, it sounded so clear and intuitively appealing that most immunologists imagined to recognize their own thinking in it. Second, it had elements of a brilliant foresight. Third, it dealt exclusively with antibodies (as also his previous and subsequent theory) without much attention of their cellular origin. And finally, certain facts that were not central to his thinking were boldly omitted.

Jerne, like everybody else at that time, was puzzled by the unexpectedly high frequency of alloreactive cells responding to a single allelic major histocompatibility complex haplotype, in vivo,[5] in the graft-versus-host reaction, and also in vitro,[6] in the mixed lymphocyte reaction. The measured frequencies were in the order of 1–2%, and this seemed to contradict the clonal selection theory, because the latter would require that an animal possesses at least 10^4 or 10^5 different clones, i.e., the clonal frequency to a single antigen should be two to three orders of magnitude lower. Note that we are dealing in these cases with T-cell responses, not antibody responses. Yet, Jerne proposed that *antibody* V-genes encoded in the germ-line must recognize allelic variants of histocompatibility antigens. This jump in his logic was partially justified by the contemporary belief that the antigen receptor of T cells was immunoglobulin.

He then made some efforts to explain how these V genes are maintained in the genome by natural selection. One of his arguments was that since antigen-specific cells must arise before they encounter foreign antigens, the selective pressure cannot be foreign antigens, it must be self antigens of the animal. Although the idea in this formulation is incorrect, what it implies is that because the germ-line V genes serve as substrates for random mutations, natural selection acting on the final mutated product cannot know what the original substrate was. But the consequence of this is that the germ-line repertoire may as well be random. To avoid this obvious flaw, which is actually a common weakness of all somatic mutation theories, Jerne made the somewhat far-fetched proposition that the recognition of histocompatibility antigens by complementary V-gene products may be essential for the morphogenesis of all metazoa. And because histocompatibility genes and antibody V genes segregate independently, the latter cannot know what histo-compatibility alleles they will be associated with in an individual. Consequently, the V-gene repertoire must cover all allelic variants of histocompatibility anti-gens of the species, and thus the two gene sets, i.e., histocompatibility alleles and V-genes, maintain each other by a kind of balanced evolution.

Jerne then sent the precursors of antigen-sensitive cells into the thymus. Being fascinated by the high rate of lymphocyte proliferation and death in the thymus, he considered the thymus to be a mutant-breeding organ. He proposed that the V-gene set specific for self-histocompatibility alleles must mutate to avoid elimination by self-tolerance, and such mutants will then form the anti-body repertoire. In contrast, the V-genes encoding specificities for other his-tocompatibility alleles absent from the individual will remain unmutated, and these will be responsible for the high frequency of alloreactive cells.

What are the merits of this hypothesis? First of all, the recognition that the generation of diversity occurs in the central lymphoid organs, even though the mechanism is not only somatic mutation. However, nobody could have sus-pected at that time what the actual mechanisms were. Second, because Jerne's thinking was preoccupied with T cells, the theory came very close to reality as far as the T-cell repertoire is concerned.

The major flaw of the theory is that it is not applicable to the B-cell antibody repertoire at all.

5.2 THE EXPERIMENTAL SOLUTION

Fortunately, Jerne was thinking about the problem of GOD also from the experi-mental point of view, and realized very early that it cannot be solved at the pro-tein level, to the disappointment of some immunochemists at the Basel Institute.

'If one wants to study genes, one should look at the DNA' he used to empha-size. Thus, he attracted a young and very well-trained molecular biologist, Susumu Tonegawa, to the Institute to work on the problem.

Tonegawa proved to be the right person for this task, he not only worked well, but also with an obsession, so that he only emerged from his lab for short meals, and then disappeared again.

'I often saw his wife sitting late at night in the lobby of the Institute with an offended face, and waiting for him' recalls Dr. G. 'This usually indicated that Susumu forgot to go home for several nights in a row.'

By 1974, Tonegawa's work started to yield results, and when he first reported[7] that there were too few V-genes to account for a germ-line encoded diversity, but too many for somatic mutations, panic broke out in both camps. But finally,

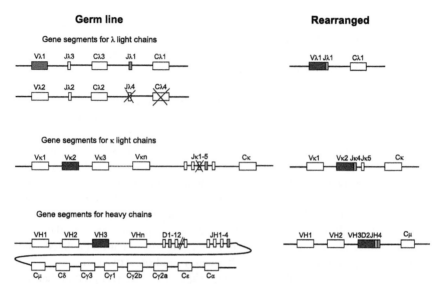

FIGURE 5.1   Genetic organization of light and heavy chain gene families in germ-line configuration and after rearrangement. The Vλ1 segment rearranges preferentially to Jλ3Cλ3 and Jλ1Cλ1, and the Vλ2 segment to Jλ2Cλ2; the Jλ4Cλ4 pair is defective. One rearrangement per gene family is shown as an example (shaded gene segments). L segments coding for signal peptides are omitted, and the multisegment organization of CH genes is not shown. Based on Reference 8. (Adapted by permission from Macmillan Publishers Ltd: *Nature* **302** issue 5909 © 1983.)

positive thinking took the lead, and because there were still >300 *V*-genes in the genome, and somatic mutations of antibody genes were also shown to occur, they comforted themselves by stating that everybody was 'a little right'.

Subsequently, Tonegawa unravelled GOD's secrets almost single-handedly. The results are now an obligatory part of every immunology textbook, and their essence (reviewed by Tonegawa[8]) is shown in Fig. 5.1. Each immunoglobulin chain is encoded in the germ-line in three or four separate DNA segments, namely (in 5′ to 3′ direction), *V* (variable), *J* (joining) and *C* (constant) for light (L) chains, and *V*, *D* (diversity), *J*, and *C* for heavy (H) chains. Each *V*-gene segment encodes the majority of the V region, in the case of the L chain, all three complementary determining regions, CDR1, 2 and 3, and three of the four framework regions, FR1, 2, 3, whereas most of FR4 is encoded in the *J* segment. The genetic composition of H-chain encoding segments is similar, except that the additional *D* segment encodes CDR3. The constant region of L chains is encoded in a single *C* gene, in contrast, the C_H genes consist of multiple exons corresponding to structural domains of the C_H region.

In mice the genes encoding λ, and κ L chains and H chains, respectively, are unlinked (reside in different chromosomes) and the organization of the corresponding gene families is somewhat different (Fig. 5.1). The simplest is the λ gene family consisting of two *V*λ segments and four pairs of *J* and *C* segments corresponding to the three λ subtypes (one *J–C* pair is defective). The κ L-chain gene family consists of 90–300 different *V* segments, a cluster of five *J* segments (one of which is defective) and a single *C* segment. The gene family for H chains contains a cluster of 100–200 different *V* segments, and separate clusters of 12 *D*, and four *J* segments, followed by a cluster of eight *C* segments each encoding a separate H-chain isotype (in the order μ, δ, γ3, γ1, γ2b, γ2a, ε, α).

During B-cell ontogeny in the bone marrow, various combinations of *V* and *J* or *V, D*, and *J* segments are joined together to form a single continuous *VJ* (L chains) or *VDJ* (H chain) gene by a process termed rearrangement (Fig. 5.1). The intervening DNA sequences are excised. This process could, in principle, generate a large number of joining variants, namely, 2 *Vλ*, × 3 *Jλ* – 6 λL chains, 300 *Vκ* × 4 *Jκ* = 1200 κL chains, i.e., altogether 1206 L chain sequences, and 200 V_H, × 12 *D* × 4 J_H = 9600 H chain sequences, although in reality, some of these combinations may occur rarely or not at all. Furthermore, the joining of segments is imprecise, resulting in additional junctional site diversities at the V_L–J_L, V_H–*D* and *D*–J_H junctions. Insertions can also occur at the V_H–*D* and *D*–J_H junctions. A rough estimate of the total junctional diversity is ~10^2 for L chains and ~10^{10} for the H chains (ten codons, ten amino acids per position). Thus the total number of H+L pairs with different amino acid sequences is (~$10^3 × 10^4 × 10^2 × 10^{10}$) ~$10^{19}$, an astronomical number. Superimposed on this diversity are high-frequency somatic mutations after antigen encounter[9] that occur throughout the *VJ* and *VDJ* segments.

Immunoglobulin gene rearrangement occurs only once per chromosome, i.e., twice per diploid cell, and due to the imprecise joining, most cells will contain none or at most one productively rearranged H and L chain gene. Cells without functionally rearranged immunoglobulin genes will die. Thus the combinatorial GOD functions with a high proportion of waste, but ensures thereby that in most cases one cell will express only one antibody (i.e., allelic exclusion of H chains and isotype exclusion of L chains; although additional mechanisms for this may also exist[10]).

The rearranged *VJ* and *VDJ* sequences are then transcribed together with the adjacent *C* segment, and the non-coding spacer in between is removed during mRNA processing. Thus the first complete H chain to be synthesized is μ defining IgM, the isotype that appears first in B-cell development. During isotype-switch, the same *VDJ* sequence is joined with another C_H segment (δ, γ, ε, or α), which requires additional sequence reorganization either at the DNA level or during mRNA processing.

5.3 WHAT DID WE LEARN FROM THE MECHANISMS OF GOD?

First of all, one cannot but admire the ingenuity of evolution in figuring out how a high degree of diversity can be generated from relatively few germ-line genes. Of the actual mechanisms, germ-line diversity and mutational diversity were predicted, but the somatic rearrangement mechanism was beyond the imagination of most of us, because genes were at that time considered to be constant, changeable only by recombination or random somatic mutations. Thus the existence of a sophisticated DNA-tailoring mechanism that allows gene fusions and changes on the same chromosome was entirely unexpected.

The most important biological message of Tonegawa's studies is that there are mechanisms designed to generate diversity by joining a randomly selected gene segment out of a series of many with another randomly selected member of another series. In addition, the three gene families studied (λ, κ, H) have revealed slightly different strategies to achieve the same goal, giving a 'work in progress' type of picture of the evolutionary process. Moreover, these are not the only mechanisms that have evolved in nature to serve the same purpose. For example, in chicken, the GOD mechanism is completely different. Here, there is a single functional immunoglobulin gene, and a series of pseudogenes, and diversity is generated by a high rate of gene conversion, i.e., by borrowing short sequences from the pseudogenes and building them into the single functional one.[11] The fact that nature experimented so much around this problem strongly suggests that there must have been a pressing evolutionary need for antibody diversity.

However, the nature of the evolutionary force was not easy to understand. Obviously it was not natural selection, because the latter could only work on existing germ-line genes, but not on their non-inheritable somatic variants.

'The explanation for this enigma came from another Susumu namely, Susumu Ohno, who was also at the Basel Institute at that time' interposes Dr. G. 'Ohno belonged to the great Japanese school of formal genetics, and his famous book Evolution by gene duplication was known by almost everybody. Indeed, I learned more about evolution from this enjoyable and idea-rich book than throughout my entire studies. Ohno was a quiet and polite man, who impressed with a well-balanced personality, although his appearance was somewhat unusual with his huge moustache, the kind that only herdsmen in the Hungarian plains wear for the sake of the tourists.'

As an evolutionary driving force for the somatic generation of antibody diversity, Ohno introduced the concept of 'Promethean evolution', or the evolution of foresight.[12] He has pointed out that natural selection has only hindsight, in that it can only favor already-existing mutants under given environmental conditions, and thus provide a selective advantage for the population as a whole, but never for every member of a population. In contrast, the antibody diversity of every individual is large enough to deal with all sorts of molecules, some of which have never existed in nature, and thus the immune system appears to have evolved in anticipation of future needs. The necessity for this Promethean foresight lies in the huge difference between the generation times of pathogenic microorganisms and their vertebrate hosts, which allows the pathogens to change much faster by mutation than a germ-line-encoded defense system of vertebrates could do. For example, an antiviral antibody selected on the basis of past efficacy would be useless, because some of the quickly arising new mutant viruses would certainly escape recognition. And by the time a successful antibody gene-mutant is passed on to the next generation, the virus has already mutated >10 000 times, thus the winner in the mutational race will always be the microorganism. Under these conditions vertebrates had no other choice than to produce new specificities somatically, excluding thereby the factor of generation time from the race.

Of course, the germ-line-encoded *V* genes remain under the control of natural selection, and therefore they must represent specificities of more durable usefulness, for example those against certain stable features of common pathogens, such as bacterial polysaccharides.[13] But during ontogeny each individual can modify randomly these heritable genes to generate a wide variety of specificities. These new specificities are no longer bound to the past: some of them can recognize antigens never encountered before. Thus the ability of the immune system to cope with the future is linked to its proven ability of coping in the past and present. This evolutionary solution must have been obligatory at a certain stage of phylogeny, in order to protect long-lived organisms from short-lived microorganisms.

Ohno thinks that the evolution of human intelligence has also depended on a Promethean mechanism, which allows the development of random interneuronal connections, and thus prepares the nervous system to respond to stimuli not encountered in the past. The grand scheme of Promethean evolution, according to Ohno, is to transfer the benefit of genetic polymorphism from the population as a whole to every single member of the population.

Of course, this concept, attractive as it may sound, remains a hypothesis, which can neither be proven nor refuted (as all good hypotheses). It has served as a useful guideline for the thinking of immunologists for some time, and will probably remain so until new insights necessitate a conceptual change.

As the above concept illustrates, Ohno has been a highly original thinker, and sometimes he went even to extravagance. For example, once he circulated a manuscript, in which he described the transformation of DNA coding sequences into music, and vice versa.[14] The world of life-sciences that had become very reasonable (i.e., business-like) by that time, was scandalized, and Ohno must have had a hard time getting the paper published. Fortunately, there were still a few 'relicts' left, who did not shy away from extravagance, and one of them was Jan Klein, the Editor-in-Chief of *Immunogenetics*. Klein gave the manuscript to Dr. G for review, because he knew that G was a pianist, and could thus look into the musical part as well.

'I agreed with Ohno in that the "gene-music" was very sad and lonely, and so it was probably not incidental that it showed homologies to Chopin's Nocturnes, the most sad and lonely cycle in the music-literature' comments Dr. G. 'For the average reader, all this rather original paper has shown is that meaningful sequences of different nature can be translated into each other, particularly when they also share certain patterns or motifs. What exactly Ohno's message has been, however, remains a mystery, because the paper lacks discussion and conclusions. But even if it had just been a foolish idea, it is always better when the wise plays a fool than the other way around.'

From a twenty-first century perspective, we are less surprised about somatic variations of genes, because we now know that the total number of structural genes in vertebrates is usually smaller than the number of proteins needed for living. For example, humans have ~30 000 genes and ~100 000 proteins, i.e., at average each gene should encode >3 different proteins, and this is only possible if somatic variation of genes and/or transcripts is the rule rather than the exception. Thus, the 'grand scheme' may be either that there is a limit on the number of genes to be carried in a genome, or that somatic variation provides more advantage than maintaining a 1:1 gene to protein ratio (or perhaps both).

Altogether, it is not exaggerating to say that Tonegawa's discovery has been among the most informative and revealing ones in the history of immunology. Thus, it would have really been very surprising if he had not been awarded with the Nobel Prize for it.

'Tonegawa's success was not only the luck of the prepared mind but also that of the trained experimentalist' points out Dr. G. 'This is the success of the one, who is not satisfied with peeping into secrets, but also takes the trouble of cracking them. For Goddess Fortuna does not want voyeurs, she prefers the one, who grabs her (and sometimes the young, innocent one, whom she can easily seduce).'

5.4 A BAROQUE EMBELLISHMENT OF ANTIBODY DIVERSITY: THE IDIOTYPE NETWORK

What we shall try to follow-up here is how the diversity of antibodies has become intellectually equivalent to the diversity of antigens, and how this twist of thinking has led to the most controversial and mystic piece of immunological concept: the idiotype network theory.

It all started with the discovery that immunization with antigen–antibody complexes resulted in antibodies specific for the antibody part of the complex, and not reacting with other immunoglobulins.[15,16] Thus, such antiantibodies appeared to recognize 'private' determinants on another antibody that were associated with the antigen-specificity of the latter, i.e., these determinants were probably located at the antigen-combining site. To distinguish from other antigenic sites on immunoglobulins, e.g., allotypes, these new determinants were termed idiotypes.[17] Although the structure of immunoglobulins was not yet completely elucidated at that time, it was clear that idiotypes arose as a result of amino acid variability in the V-region, and thus the unavoidable consequence of generating antibody diversity seemed to be the creation of a perhaps comparably large idiotype diversity. The question was then raised how self–non-self discrimination could deal with such a huge variability of immunoglobulins? Namely, if every idiotype were considered by the immune system to be a self antigen, clonal deletion would have to eliminate the total B-cell compartment.[18] However, because such a proposition would have been absurd, and because anti-antibody formation was usually observed only in autoimmune diseases,[19–23] the consensus was reached that idiotypes under normal physiological conditions may not be immunogenic. Nevertheless, the dilemma remained, and it shattered the belief in certain postulates of the clonal selection theory in many immunologists' minds. The community was thus well prepared for a new paradigm, which could encompass the phenomenon of idiotypy, and resolve the conceptual problems associated with it.

Time was, therefore, ripe for Jerne to present his new theory about idiotype networks.[24] One of the secrets behind the universal and enthusiastic acceptance of Jerne's concepts in immunology has always been good timing: he was capable of sensing the conceptual needs of immunologists very precisely, and he responded to these needs at a time point when they became most pressing. This is why he launched his natural selection theory of immunity,[25] when the instructionistic views became clearly untenable, and came up with the somatic generation of immune recognition concept,[4] when the phenomenon of alloreactivity has puzzled virtually every immunologist, and seemed to threaten the validity of the clonal selection theory.

It is not known what inspired Jerne to think in terms of networks. One can only note that the general idea of networks emerged around that time from the work of the new and successful computer industry, and the term itself started to establish itself as a 'buzzword' in contemporary Western societies. Another possible influence might have been the formal analogy between the immune system and the nervous system, namely, that both are capable of 'learning' and have 'memory' (although the actual processes described by these terms are completely different for the two systems), and the nervous system is indeed a network. Altogether, network was a popular idea at that time, and most of us understood it as a system consisting of a large number of interconnected units, which, beyond a certain degree of complexity, starts to develop its own patterns of behavior that are superimposed on, and not directly related to, the behavior of its units. The implication of this view is that networks cannot be understood solely on the basis of knowledge about their elements, and thus, studying networks demands development of a higher order of logic, i.e., this is an enterprise for those only, who can take the intellectual challenge to reach the status of the initiate. Probably this is why so many bright and imaginative immunologists fell in with the morbid charm of the idiotype network theory, while the majority of the community accepted it for its mysticism that demanded faith, and thus automatically relieved from the obligation of further thinking.

But let us now recapitulate the theory itself, which will not be easy, because it has never been satisfactorily formulated as Jerne himself admits.[26] The essence of the theory, as laid down in a series of four publications,[24,26–28] is the following. All formulations of the concept are based on certain 'axioms', the first of which is the a priori statement that the immune system is 'complete',[29] i.e., it can recognize any foreign (or self) epitope it is presented with. The second axiom follows from the 'completeness' thesis, namely that the repertoire of the combining site-associated idiotypic determinants (idiotopes) has to be complete too, and consequently, each idiotope will find its complementary an anti-idiotype. Of course, an anti-idiotype expresses its own idiotype, and the latter would in turn be recognized by another anti-idiotype, and so on. Thus, idiotypes and anti-idiotypes would create an endless web of interactions, and this could provide a means of regulating the immune system. It has remained unclear how this regulation works in detail, but the minimal requirement for regulation would be that the network should mediate stimulatory, as well as inhibitory, signals.

The most explicit part of the theory describes how Jerne envisages self–non-self discrimination in the network context. As a first step, he rejects the opinion that antibody V genes have evolved under the selective pressure of pathogenic microorganisms, by saying that 'I have never liked this facile idea'. What he proposes instead is that germ-line V genes encode antibodies that recognize self antigens of the species. This seems to be a recurrent theme in his thinking, as it was already present in his previous theory on somatic generation of antibody diversity.[23] It is interesting to note why he thinks so: his argument is that he sees no other way to generate millions of antibody specificities out of a few V genes while avoiding anti-self. Thus, he appears to believe that mutations away from anti-self would necessarily generate anti-non-self. For those anti-self V genes that may be expressed unmutated, he proposes that 'evolution has favored' the emergence of anti-idiotypic V genes, and the products of the latter would suppress anti-self reactivity. Eventually anti-idiotypic antibodies to anti-self should make up the majority of normal immunoglobulins in his view. And if occasionally another anti-self specificity arises by mutation, this would, upon binding to the self antigen, evoke the production of an anti-idiotype, which would suppress the self-reactive idiotype. The question of how the system would provide protection against pathogens is easily settled by referring to the completeness of the repertoire, which ensures that viruses and bacteria can never escape.

It is beyond the scope of this book to give a detailed critical assessment of the network theory. The reader is referred to publications by Cohn and Langman,[30–33] as they were the only authors who raised written criticism against the idiotype network concept over the period of more than a decade, when it was in vogue. However, because their counter-arguments are sometimes almost as complicated as the theory itself, it would be interesting to ask an average immunologist's opinion about this concept. The choice fell on Dr. G, who was on site at the birth of the theory, and was thus confronted with it very early. It is his turn now to tell us his impressions.

'I am afraid, I am not the right person to be asked for this, because I have never worked on idiotypes, nor have I incorporated the network idea into my thinking. The first time I came across it was in 1974 in Basel, at a short seminar given by Jeff Hoffmann, a young Canadian network enthusiast, a mathematician by training, if I remember correctly. This was a seminar with a single slide, in which an idiotype and an anti-idiotype were pictured, and two arrows pointing in opposite directions, one representing stimulation and the other suppression. Because the seminar was correspondingly short, I did not really understand what the message was, although, judged by its reception, it must have been an important one. Since it was immediately clear to me that I would not be able to envisage how this works, I decided that I was not intelligent enough to grasp its essence, and stopped thinking about it. But I can still remember what my problems were with the concept from the very beginning.'

'First of all, where is the network? The necessarily large number of units to be interlinked is there, these are lymphocytes, but the wiring is missing. Direct cell contacts between the idiotype and anti-idiotype bearing partner cells would not work, because they would hardly have a chance to meet each other, particularly in a "complete" repertoire. If one assumes that circulating antibodies substitute for the wiring, one must endow them with different messenger properties. However, antibodies are not functional messengers, they are targeting devices for immune effector functions, thus the only message they can convey is: "Kill it!" Although stimulatory antibodies also exist in rare instances, when they happen to mimic a stimulatory ligand for a receptor, but as a rule, antibodies induce either complement-dependent lysis or antibody-dependent cellular cytotoxicity both leading to death of the targeted cell. Thus idiotype suppression is easy to envisage, but how does the stimulatory pathway work? In addition, how does the antibody know what to do, stimulate or suppress?'

'Second, if circulating antibodies are idiotypes and anti-idiotypes, they should interact, i.e., bind to each other. This would lead to an enormous extent of immune-complex formation, eventually resulting in the elimination of all immunoglobulins from the circulation. Thus, as far as I could see, the outcome of an idiotype network can only be disaster.'

'Third, I have an intuitive objection against ideas, e.g., that the immune system is "self-referential", it has its own "internal life", in which the appearance of a foreign antigen means nothing more than a temporary "perturbation". Such a system bears a frightening resemblance to big empires or international firms in their late stage of decadence, when their citizens or employees only care about internal communication, and forget about the existence of the outside world, until the latter takes its vengeance. In a biological world, the immune system is measured by its success in protecting the host from invaders, and not by its sophisticated internal life. I personally would not like to have an immune system that wastes too much energy on unnecessary networking, and feels perturbed, when an antigen comes by from outside. In fact, the same principle applies to the nervous system, a real network: namely, it is measured by the adequacy of its motory output that follows after the processing of a sensory input, because this is the only selectable quality for which evolution can reward or punish. I am aware that my arguments lack scientific subtlety. But they do address some simple basic principles, and I would have difficulties in accepting ideas that are not compatible with them.'

'Of course, if necessary, I could also raise some more scientific-sounding criticism, particularly concerning the lack of acceptable evolutionary arguments for the existence of the network. But I will refrain from doing so, because, as you pointed out, Mel Cohn and Rod Langman[30–33] had done this long ago, and in great enough detail.'

Indeed, criticism alone, no matter how hard, was not sufficient to shatter the popularity of the network among its adherents. The reason why the theory slowly faded away was that it turned out to be extremely difficult to obtain conclusive experimental evidence for the existence of an idiotype network. Although several laboratories reported on successful manipulation of antibody responses by injection of anti-idiotypic antibodies[34–39] this did not constitute formal evidence for the network. What would have been necessary to demonstrate, was that natural antibodies in the same, unimmunized animal comprise a web of idiotypic and anti-idiotypic antibodies, and this was technically almost impossible to achieve. Therefore, the most prominent network researchers, such as Pierre-Andre Cazenave, Jacques Urbain, Klaus Rajewsky, and many others, became disappointed after a while, and moved out of the field. Finally even the most steadfast ones, such as Antonio Coutinho, who considered himself to be Jerne's spiritual son, gave up the network pursuit. Interestingly, however, the belief remained firm deep inside, and there are still several colleagues who would give their life's scientific achievement for a single piece of conclusive evidence for the idiotype network.

Thus, the idea was die-hard, and so it is not surprising that, after its failure in basic immunology, it was still lingering on for a long while in applied immunology. One potential application was the so-called idiotypic vaccines. The idea here was that micro-organism-based vaccines could be substituted with anti-idiotypic antibodies that mimic the antigen (being the 'internal image' of antigen). Indeed, this has been shown to be the case for a number of anti-idiotypic antibodies. Proponents of this approach argued that, from a safety point of view, idiotypic vaccines should be preferred over, e.g., attenuated pathogens, and this is certainly true. However, nowadays virtually any recombinant protein can be expressed and produced in large amounts, and this fact renders the above argument, as well as idiotypic vaccines, obsolete.

Subsequently, the network idea entered the field of autoimmune diseases. For example, it has been reported that vaccination with T cells or with peptides of the T-cell antigen receptor (TCR) provides a therapeutic benefit in experimental autoimmune encephalitis models, and this effect has been ascribed to the induction of an anti-idiotype network.[40,41]

'Because these studies implied that TCRs should be immunogenic, I decided, for my own curiosity, to address this question in an appropriate experimental model' tells Dr. G. 'The results have clearly demonstrated T helper cell tolerance to TCRs, at least to their germ-line encoded sequences.[42] Although immunization with synthetic TCR peptides sometimes induced a T helper cell response, this happened only when the immunizing peptide did not correspond to any naturally occurring peptide produced upon degradation of the TCR protein, in vivo. Thus, the immunogenic TCR peptides have turned out to be non-self antigens, since they never occur in vivo. The T cells induced by such peptides fail to cross-react with naturally occurring TCR peptides, and consequently cannot engage in network interactions. Based on these results, I have concluded that TCR networks are unlikely to exist, unless junctional diversity in the third hypervariable region renders some TCRs immunogenic. But the approach of TCR vaccination was removed from the list of potential therapies for a different reason, namely, because it caused in some cases disease exacerbation, instead of remission.[43']

This is how far the idiotype network concept spread around in immunology. But taken its strong emotional impact, it could recur any time, or as Av Mitchison used to put it: 'we never know when the network sticks up its ugly head again'. Perhaps the most embarrassing aspect of this story is that the question initially asked by the discoverers of idiotypes, namely, how the immune system tolerates the potentially huge number of idiotypes, has remained unanswered, with or without network.

'Undoubtedly, the idiotype network was Jerne's most popular idea, although not his best one' comments Dr. G. 'It was even believed by many, in particular by doctors in the clinic with interest in immunology, that the Nobel Prize was awarded to Niels Jerne for the network theory. An often heard argument was at that time: "the network must be true, otherwise Jerne would not have received Nobel Prize for it". To avoid further misunderstanding, it may be worth discussing here briefly the history of Jerne's Nobel Prize. As it is known, the prize in 1984 was shared by Cesar Milstein and Georges Köhler for the discovery of monoclonal antibodies, and Niels Jerne for his theoretical contributions that made this discovery possible. Taking this explanation at face value, one cannot but conclude that Jerne was awarded for Burnet's clonal selection theory, because this was the only concept that predicted monoclonal antibodies. However, Burnet had already received the prize for immunological tolerance (that he actually did not discover), and the clonal selection theory could not have been considered for the prize until it became proven by the existence of monoclonal antibodies. And here was also Niels Jerne, whose life achievement including his theories as well as the plaque-forming cell assay[44] that permitted the study of immune responses at the single cell level was, as a whole, worth a Nobel Prize. Thus, the Nobel Committee made a political decision, the result of which was that it did the right thing, but for the wrong reason. I wish this happened sometimes also in real politics!'

REFERENCES

1. Talmage DW. *Science* 1959;**129**:1643.
2. Hood L, Talmage DW. *Science* 1970;**168**:325.
3. Lederberg J. *Science* 1959;**129**:1649.
4. Jerne NK. *Eur. J. Immunol.* 1971;**1**:1.

5. Simonsen M. *Cold Spring Harbor Symp. Quant. Biol.* 1967;**32**:517.

6. Wilson DB, Nowell PC. *J. Exp. Med.* 1970;**131**:391.

7. Tonegawa S, Steinberg C, Dube S, Bernardini A. *Proc. Natl. Acad. Sci. USA* 1974;**71**:4027.

8. Tonegawa S. *Nature* 1983;**302**:575.

9. Griffiths GM, Berek C, Kaartinen M, Milstein C. *Nature* 1984;**312**:271.

10. Wabl M, Steinberg C. *Proc. Natl. Acad. Sci. USA* 1982;**79**:6976.

11. Reynaud CA, Anquez V, Grimal H, Weill JC. CA Reynaud, A Dahan, V Anquez, JC Weill, Cell 59: 171(1989). *Cell* 1987;**48**:379.

12. Ohno S. *Perspect. Biol. Med.* 1976;**19**:527.

13. Langman RE, Cohn M. *Mol. Immunol.* 1987;**24**:675.

14. Ohno S, Ohno M. *Immunogenetics* 1986;**24**:71.

15. Oudin J, Michel M. *C.R. Hebd. Seances Acad. Sci.* 1963;**257**:805.

16. Gell PGH, Kelus A. *Nature (London)* 1964;**201**:687.

17. Oudin J. *Proc. R. Soc. London, Ser. B.* 1966;**166**:207.

18. Gell PGH, Kelus A. *Adv. Immunol.* 1967;**6**:476.

19. Milgrom F, Dubiski S. *Nature (London)* 1957;**179**:1351.

20. Zanetti M, Bigazzi P. *Eur. J. Immunol.* 1981;**11**:187.

21. Abdou NI, Wall H, Lindsley HB, Halsey JF, Suzuki T. *J. Clin. Invest.* 1981;**67**:1297.

22. Neilson EG, Phillips SN. *J. Exp. Med.* 1982;**155**:179.

23. Cohen PL, Eisenberg RA. *J. Exp. Med.* 1982;**156**:173.

24. Jerne NK. *Ann. Immunol. (Inst. Pasteur)* 1974;**125C**:373.

25. Jerne NK. *Proc. Natl. Acad. Sci. USA* 1955;**41**:849.

26. Jerne NK. *Immunol. Rev.* 1984;**79**:5.

27. Jerne NK. *The Harvey Lectures Ser.* 1976;**70**:93.

28. Jerne NK. *EMBO J.* 1985;**4**:847.

29. Coutinho A. *Ann. Immunol. (Inst. Pasteur)* 1980;**131D**:235.

30. Cohn M. *Cell. Immunol.* 1981;**61**:425.

31. Cohn M. *Ann. Inst. Pasteur.* 1986;**137C**:64.

32. Langman RE, Cohn M. *Immunol. Today* 1986;**7**:100.

33. Cohn M. In: Capra JD, editor. *Idiotypy & Medicine*. New York: Acad. Press; 1986. p. 321.

34. Cosenza H, Köhler H. *Science* 1972;**176**:1027.

35. Hart DA, Wang A, Pawlak LL, Nisonoff A. *J. Exp. Med.* 1972;**135**:1293.

36. Cazenave PA. *Proc. Natl. Acad. Sci. USA* 1977;**74**:5122.

37. Urbain J, Wikler M, Franssen JD, Collignon C. *Proc. Natl. Acad. Sci. USA* 1977;**74**:5126.

38. Fernandez C, Möller G. *Proc. Natl. Acad. Sci. USA* 1979;**76**:5944.

39. Rajewsky K, Takemori T. *Ann. Rev. Immunol.* 1983;**1**:569.

40. Lider O, Reshef T, Beraud E, Ben-Nun A, Cohen IR. *Science* 1988;**239**:181.

41. Vandenbark AA, Hashim G, Offner H. *Nature (London)* 1989;**341**:541.

42. Falcioni F, Vidovic D, Ward ES, Bolin D, Singh G, Shah H, Ober B, Nagy ZA. *J. Exp. Med.* 1995;**182**:249.

43. Desquenne-Clark L, Esch TR, Otvos Jr L, Heber-Katz E. *Proc. Natl. Acad. Sci. USA* 1991;**88**:7219.

44. Jerne NK, Nordin AA. *Science* 1963;**140**:405.

Chapter 6

The Major Histocompatibility Complex

During the 1970s and 1980s immunology became focussed very strongly on cellular immunity. It appeared as if the field had strived to compensate for the earlier neglect of cell-mediated immunity, and this succeeded too well, so that cellular studies over-dominated in these two decades almost as much as serology used to do in the 'dark ages'. The bulk of research undertaken in this period was into two major areas, namely T-cell biology, and the genetics and biology of the major histocompatibility complex (MHC). Both areas were full of surprise, and the speed at which our understanding accumulated was quite variable. For example, T-cell studies yielded an early insight into important biological aspects of antigen recognition, while the identification of the T-cell antigen receptor itself took an almost embarrassingly long time. Studies of the MHC were limited at the beginning to transplantation, later they were considered as part of immunology, but as soon as T-cell studies hinted at an immunological function for MHC, they became so prolific that they branched out as a separate discipline under the name 'immunogenetics'. Nevertheless, the final understanding of how MHC molecules present antigen to T cells had to await the X-ray crystallographic studies of the 1990s.

An inherent didactic problem about discussing T cells and MHC is that one cannot be understood without the other, and yet the complexity of each topic per se necessitates dealing with them separately. And if one decides for a rather artificial separation of the two, the next question is which of them to discuss first. Finally, the only more or less reasonable approach left is to follow the chronological order and start with the MHC, as its history had begun long before T cells became known.

6.1 MHC CLASS I

6.1.1 Discovery

In one of his rather journalistic reviews,[1] Jan Klein called the MHC 'the master trickster', mostly because the phenomena that permitted its discovery turned out later to be irrelevant to its true biological function, and in addition, many genes mapped to it on the basis of phenotypic traits have proven to be illusions. Thus,

A History of Modern Immunology. http://dx.doi.org/10.1016/B978-0-12-416974-6.00006-5

Klein certainly had a point, although it is unlikely that the discovery and characterization of MHC would have been more error-prone than that of any other genetic system. This appearance was probably created by the fact that the MHC was a favorite object of investigation due to its high antigenic 'visibility' for several disciplines besides genetics, e.g., transplantation, tumor biology, and immunology, and thus enjoyed (or suffered) more publicity than other gene systems.

The first MHC-associated phenomenon was transplant rejection that was observed at least a century before the discovery of the MHC itself. The replacement of damaged or missing tissues or organs with healthy ones had been a long-standing dream of surgeons, and pragmatic-minded as they have always been, they had tried over and again to transplant tissues from the early nineteenth century onward, rather than tolerating unfulfilled dreams for too long. But they soon had to realize that only autologous tissues can be transplanted with success, whereas tissue grafts from different individuals of the same species (allografts) usually failed, and the exchange of grafts between different species (xenografts) was virtually impossible. Thus there seemed to exist some biological mechanisms to preserve individuality, the nature of which, however, remained a mystery. Subsequently, tumor biologists entered the scene involuntarily, as they observed rejection of transplantable tumors in experimental animals. They were the first to work out the major rules of transplantation, among others, that the success of grafting was dependent on a close genetic relationship between donor and recipient, and that a second graft of the same origin was rejected faster than the first one. Perhaps even more importantly, they established that the same set of rules governs the transplantation of both tumors and normal tissues.

The discovery of MHC as the genetic basis for graft rejection was another consequence of the strong immunogenicity of the molecules it encodes. In 1936, Peter Gorer immunized mice with erythrocytes of other mouse strains, and obtained specific antisera reacting with what he thought to be blood group antigens,[2] but in reality they were class I MHC antigens. Meanwhile it has become clear that erythrocytes express only small, residual amounts of MHC molecules after expulsion of their nuclei, yet the dominating specificity in these sera was anti-MHC. In his subsequent studies, Peter Gorer identified a hemagglutinating antibody, whose formation was associated with tumor rejection.[3] It thus appeared as if blood group antigens had been responsible for tumor rejection, and he termed the antigen involved antigen II.

At about the same time, George Snell joined the Jackson Laboratory at Bar Harbor, Main, to study the genetic basis of host response to transplanted tumors. The Jackson Laboratory was founded shortly before by Clarence Little, with the aim of identifying genetic factors that control the susceptibility and resistance to transplanted tumors, using genetically homogeneous inbred mouse strains. Snell, among other contributions, developed an ingenious method for the production of mouse strains that were genetically identical except for the locus controlling resistance to tumors. The procedure was as follows: he took an inbred strain 's' sensitive to a tumor cell line derived from the same strain, crossed it with a resistant strain 'r', and backcrossed the resulting (s × r) F1 hybrids to the sensitive strain 's'. The backcrosses were then intercrossed and segregated with respect to tumor resistance into 'ss', 'sr', and 'rr' individuals, of which only the 'rr' animals survived after inoculation with the tumor, because for the other two groups the tumor was 'self'. The surviving resistant 'rr' mice were backcrossed again to strain 's', and intercrossed to yield the next generation of 'rr' segregants. The procedure was then repeated several times (there is a precise mathematics behind this method to calculate the number of backcrosses required). The final result of this breeding-selecting strategy was a mouse strain that carried the homozygous resistance gene in an 'isolated' form, because most if not all the remaining 'background' genes were from the sensitive strain.[4] He termed the strains thus produced 'congeneic resistant'. Snell's work led to the discovery of a locus primarily responsible for tumor rejection, and he termed this H (for histocompatibility).[5] It was then established in a collaborative study that Peter Gorer's antigen II was indeed controlled by Snell's H locus[6] (mapped in the ninth linkage group, now known to be chromosome 17). Hence the term *H-2*, the genetic designation of the mouse MHC ever since.

More than four decades later, when the biological significance of MHC appeared to be clear enough, George Snell was awarded with the Nobel Prize for his discovery. Unfortunately, Peter Gorer did not live to receive the Prize.

'My meeting with George Snell has remained vivid in my memory' recalls Dr. G.

' It happened in 1980, after he received the award in Stockholm, and on his way back home he made a stop-over in Tübingen to visit Jan Klein's Immunogenetics Department. I even held his Nobel Medal in my hand, while thinking that this was probably the closest I could ever get to a Nobel Prize, and time has proven me right' he adds sarcastically.

'Klein prepared a festive speech for this occasion, in which he tried to point out how certain events, he called these "binary decisions", in Snell's life had led to the prize-winning discovery. But the text could not conceal his anger about the fact that the prize for his pet project was already given. George Snell remained unimpressed by both Klein's address and his emotions. He was in his late seventies, far beyond all vanities, indeed so far that I had to assume he had never really cared about them altogether. In my eyes, George Snell was the best personification of a great old scientist, he was humble, quiet, serious, not very talkative, but every word he said testified wisdom. He travelled together with his wife, who was another unique personality: lively, open, natural, warm-hearted, and completely free from the mannerism that ladies in her age and social status often have. It was moving to see how much youthful love was reflected in the interaction between Dr. and Mrs. Snell. I think I have never met a more charming old couple than the Snells.'

6.1.2 Class I MHC Molecules

The example of the Snell–Gorer collaboration, i.e., the combination of genetics with serology set the standard for MHC studies for a long time. But the analysis of *H-2* locus turned out to be much more difficult than expected for the following reasons: first, most congeneic strains produced by Snell[5,7] rejected skin grafts of each other, indicating an unusually high number of alleles (polymorphism) at this locus. And the degree of polymorphism observed in inbred mice was still an underestimate, as studies of wild mice by Pavol Ivanyi[8] and Jan Klein[9] identified a number of additional independent H-2 haplotypes. Second, the discovery of recombination[10,11] between antigenic factors revealed that *H-2* was in fact not a single locus, it encompassed a minimum of two but possibly more genes. Third, the serological analysis showed an extremely complex picture of antigenicity.

The antisera used for MHC serology were raised by alloimmunization, e.g., by injection of lymphoid cells of one congeneic strain into another. The sera were then tested against lymphoid cells of a panel of standard and recombinant mouse strains by complement-dependent cytotoxicity, and absorption analysis. The reaction pattern obtained with a particular selected antiserum was termed an 'H-2 specificity'. By contemporary terminology, this would correspond to an antigenic determinant or epitope, or a small group of epitopes. The problem was that it was impossible to determine at that time how many distinct molecules these specificities were distributed to. As so often in science, also here, there were two opposing trends at work. On the one side were the complicators, who were delighted by the discovery of every new specificity, because complexity was their element of life. Their preferred view was that each specificity represented a separate gene product, and they created increasingly complex genetic maps of *H-2*. On the opposite side were the reductionists, who would have preferred to find rules that would permit a simpler interpretation of the system, even at the expense of losing some details. Initially the complicators had the upper hand, and thus the number of specificities was constantly growing, but a reasonable interpretation of the data was missing until after 1970. Finally, with the improvement of serological definition of antigens, thanks mostly to the work of Peter Démant and George Snell,[12,13] Snell[14] was able to propose that certain unique, 'private' H-2 specificities could be arranged into two distinct allelic series, whereas the remaining, broadly crossreactive 'public' specificities were most likely expressed on molecules encoded at different locations within the *H-2* complex.[15] This interpretation was facilitated by studies of other *H-2*-associated traits, notably *Ss-Slp*[16] that genetically separated the two H-2 antigenic series (and coded for a protein that later turned out to be the C4 component of complement[17,18]). All these results allowed Don Shreffler to formulate a 'duplication model' of *H-2* proposing that there are genes on both sides of the *S*-region (encoding *Ss-Slp*) that descended from a common ancestral gene, and the genes in the *K* region (left of *S*) and *D* region (right of *S*) have diverged sufficiently so that their products are serologically distinct, but are also homologous enough to allow for common 'public' determinants on the molecules they encode.[19]

Perhaps the term 'region' deserves further explanation, because it has always appeared confusing for many immunologists. 'Region' is a cautious genetic term that denotes a segment of DNA containing a marker locus, and defined by a recombination on each side. Because the length of this segment is not known precisely, it may or may not comprise more genes in addition to the marker locus. In everyday use, the term 'region' has often been equated with the marker locus, and sometimes this is, indeed, the case, but the term itself leaves the possibility open for additional loci to be identified.

The duplication model has been proven to be essentially correct by biochemical studies from Stanley Nathenson's laboratory.[20] The *H-2* products isolated by immunoprecipitation from detergent solubilized membranes were shown to be glycoproteins with approximate molecular weight of 45 000. They are non-covalently associated with another small polypeptide (MW ~12 000), β_2-microglobulin,[21] encoded outside the MHC (in chromosome 2[22]). Two distinct polypeptides carrying *K*- or *D*-region-associated specificities could be separated from each other, and in *H-2* heterozygotes four polypeptide chains were found, two H-2K and two H-2D molecules. These molecules were referred to as 'classical' H-2 antigens, later on class I MHC molecules, and by the most recent 'lazy' terminology simply MHC-I. Subsequent studies have confirmed that the *K*-region contains only one gene encoding the H-2K molecule, however, the *D*-region encompasses two loci, one coding for H-2D, and the other for a less polymorphic class I molecule, termed H-2L.[23]

But the complicators were unhappy with this model, and waited for the next opportunity to challenge it. This came when it was reported from several different laboratories that certain tumor cell lines express 'alien' H-2 specificities normally present only on allelic class I molecules supposed to be absent from the *H-2* haplotype of the tumor.[24–26] These data were interpreted to indicate that genes encoding different, assumedly allelic forms of MHC class I molecules are present in every *H-2* haplotype, but they are normally repressed so that only one gene set is expressed. However, under exceptional circumstances, such as malignant transformation, the silent genes become derepressed and their products expressed.[27] This hypothetical mechanism attracted substantial attention, mostly because of its potential medical significance. Finally, a new, alternative interpretation of *H-2* polymorphism was formulated on the basis of alien specificities, proposing that polymorphism is the consequence of the segregation of polymorphic regulatory genes that mimic the Mendelian inheritance of structural *H-2* genes.[28] This view was later rendered untenable by the molecular biological characterization of the *H-2* complex.[29] In retrospect, the finding of alien specificities was probably just one manifestation of the numerous genetic aberrations that tumor cell lines are known to carry.

The H-2 serology must have provided a useful guide in the studies of Jean Dausset and his colleagues in Paris, who found leukocyte-specific iso(allo)antibodies in the blood of transfusion patients, and using these antibodies discovered an antigenic system termed HLA (human leukocyte antigen) that bore similarities to H-2 antigens in mice.[30,31] Indeed, the *HLA* gene system has turned out to be the human MHC that encodes three class I molecules, HLA-A, -B, and -C, homologous to H-2K, -D, and -L, respectively, in mice.

Dausset himself was a hematologist with considerable administrative responsibility as Director of the National Blood Transfusion Center. Yet he maintained a broad medical-scientific interest ranging from technical aspects of blood transfusion through serodiagnostics, hematological diseases, blood group antigens, allergology and oncology to organ transplantation, and published an immense number of papers on these most diverse topics. His serological studies of HLA antigens, besides their scientific value, provided also the conceptual and technical basis for the contemporary tissue typing procedure, the most important prerequisite of successful tissue and organ transplantation.[32] For the discovery of the HLA system, Jean Dausset shared the Nobel Prize with George Snell in 1980.

6.1.3 Class I MHC-Associated Traits and Their Relationship

Although almost everybody in the field assumed that the serologically and biochemically detected class I molecules were identical with the histocompatibility antigens causing transplant rejection, direct evidence to prove their unity was missing. Perhaps the strongest evidence pointing in this direction was that certain mutations in class I regions resulted in serologically detectable alterations of the respective class I molecule, as well as in reciprocal skin graft rejection with the parental strain.[33] However, other mutations did not affect serology, while causing graft rejection,[34] and this finding again raised the possibility that the two traits might be controlled by separate gene loci. Another evidence supporting unity was that the injection of purified class I molecules presensitized for an accelerated graft rejection,[35] but it could not be excluded with certainty that the preparations were contaminated with other proteins, and the latter might have been responsible for the sensitization.

Similar arguments applied to the target antigens in cell-mediated lympholysis (CML). It has been repeatedly demonstrated that in mixed lymphocyte cultures between two *H-2* disparate strains, cytotoxic (killer) cells are generated that lyse target cells sharing class I regions with the stimulating strain.[36–38] Thus the CML cultures appeared to represent an in vitro correlate for graft rejection. Although it was demonstrated that antisera directed against H-2K or H-2D antigens specifically blocked killing,[39] it was virtually impossible to exclude the possibility that undetected antibodies in the sera, directed against closely linked gene products, were responsible for the blocking. The uncertainty was further increased by some findings demonstrating weak CML or complete lack of CML in certain strain combinations,[38,40] the reasons for which were not understood at that time.

Thus the rigorous interpretation of experimental results taken together with contradicting data seemed to favor the view of the complicators, and made the notion that all three traits, i.e., transplant rejection, serological antigens, and CML target antigens were the manifestations of one and the same set of molecules, appear as mere reductionism. Finally, the unity of class I-associated traits could only assert itself as a majority opinion based on overwhelming indirect evidence.

'The level of understanding as outlined above was reached around the mid-1970s, i.e., 40 years after the discovery of the MHC' adds Dr. G. 'For young scientists of the twenty-first century, this seems an incomprehensibly long time. How would they proceed? They would clone the gene of interest, or preferably, fish out its sequence from the mouse genome library, synthesize it, transfect it into cells syngeneic to the test strain, and show that the transfected cells would then be rejected and killed in CML. The whole project would be completed within 6 months. I think one could hardly find a better example to illustrate the breath-taking development of biological sciences in the past two to three decades.'

6.1.4 Participants of MHC Research in the Classic Era

Although the previous chapters covered the major proceedings of MHC research in this early, heroic period in sufficient detail, the description fell somewhat short in dealing with the contributors to the field. Therefore, I would ask Dr. G, whether he has anything to say about the authors, whose work I referred to in the text.

'For sure!' he replies, 'I met the majority of them, some were even my friends.'

'An interesting group of people was, for example, the 'Czechoslovakian legion', including the Ivanyi brothers, Pavol and Juraj, Peter Démant, Jan Klein, and also others not listed in the References. They had all originated from the same "nest", Milan Hašek's famous Institute of Experimental Biology and Genetics in Prague that was one of the very few places in the Eastern Block where internationally acknowledged science was conducted. Obviously, Hašek was not only an outstanding scientist, he also had eyes for recognizing talent, and thus managed to attract excellent people. I should point out here that doing genetic research in the East required quite some courage, because genetics was considered to be a politically incorrect topic at that time. Indeed, until the mid-1960s, ideologists of the system regarded the gene as a decadent capitalistic fiction. It is thus not surprising that the small island of sanity in Prague could not withstand the waves of the surrounding ocean of nonsense too long, and the members of the institute were finally scattered around the Western world, Pavol Ivanyi and Peter Démant moved to the Netherlands, Juraj Ivanyi to England, and Jan Klein to Texas and subsequently to Germany. The "Czechoslovakians", when they got together, formed a very cheerful assembly, with the good old East-European sense of humor and delight in living. The only deviant was Jan Klein, whom one could not call cheerful with the best will. His mere physique was already frightening, because, in contrast to his name ("klein" translates to "small"), he was almost seven feet tall, and he must have weighted at least 350 pounds. At an immunology meeting, somebody wrote on the elevator warning plate "for 4 persons only" the very apt remark: "or one Jan Klein". Moreover, Klein was not a mild giant, he often had brutal outbreaks of fury, thus working with him required good nerves. I think his problem was that he put himself under too much pressure, and did the same to his coworkers, without ever realizing that he could have achieved much more with a more relaxed managerial style.'

Stanley Nathenson's claim to fame was twofold, first, the discovery of class I MHC molecules, and second, to be the most illustrious example for the statement: "one can do science even in the Bronx". Those, who have ever seen the neighborhood of the Albert Einstein College, Stanley's workplace, would immediately understand what this statement implies. But I think this is not quite fair, as pleasant locations offering too much diversion could also become deleterious for scientific productivity. Thus, I can imagine that doing science at Stanford or Marseille-Luminy could also be sometimes difficult. Furthermore, I believe Stanley never cared about this aspect. He was a humble man with great strength of character, and kept making valuable contributions until the late 1990s.

'Don Shreffler was a leading figure of the scene in the 1970s, who mastered the skill of transforming stress into creative energy. But his move from Ann Arbor, Michigan to St. Louis turned out to be an unhappy choice. He lost momentum there, and died young.'

'I also met Fritz Bach a couple of times, who was a lively man with a Bohemian character, corresponding to his Viennese origin. Of his former coworkers, I often met Dolores Schendel, presently Professor of Hematology in Munich, with whom I had some collaborative work around the turn of the millennium.'

'Markus Nabholz, Tommy Meo, and Vincenzo Miggiano formed the core of the transplantation immunology team at the Basel Institute, with which I shared laboratory for a while. Markus was particularly supportive during my early, disoriented stumblings at the Institute. He was Swiss, and as most young, benevolent intellectuals at that time, somewhat left-oriented politically. Therefore he felt some indignation at my slightly rightish views, instead of appreciating the fact that we both were in opposition to our own political system. Tommy and Vincenzo came from Italy, from Ceppellini's empire. Tommy was a very talented young scientist, the identification of the Ss-Slp protein, and the chromosomal mapping of immunoglobulin light and heavy chain genes being just examples of his contributions. Later he moved to Munich, where Gert Riethmüller made efforts to establish a truly international team of immunology, and subsequently he joined the immunology scene in Paris. He stayed there until his untimely death. Vincenzo was a typical Ceppellini victim. He was sent by Ceppellini to the US to learn somatic cell genetics, and after his return he was told that he would by no means be doing somatic cell genetics. Being a sensitive person, he could never recover from this disappointment.'

'I could continue the narrative until the exhaustion of your list, but I think the remaining participants can be dealt with more appropriately in subsequent chapters.'

6.2 MHC CLASS II

6.2.1 Immune Response Genes

The path of discovery of MHC class II was even more crooked and adventurous than that of class I. It began with observations back in the 1940s indicating that the capacity to form antibodies against certain antigens was inheritable. Some random-bred experimental animals were found to be high and others low responders to the same antigen, and selective breeding resulted after several generations in uniform high- and low-responder populations.

But studies of the hypothetical immune response (Ir) genes started to gain momentum only 20 years later, when Michael Sela entered the field. Around 1960, it was clear that the induction of antibody responses requires proteins, either as the immunogen itself, or as a carrier to render small non-protein moieties antigenic. Thus, proteins appeared to be the sine qua non for antibody responses, and Sela might have wondered why it was so. His approach to the problem was to test out the lower limits of protein antigenicity, and for this purpose he synthesized linear copolymers consisting of only two to four amino acids.[41] In these polymers, for example, Glu-Ala, Glu-Lys-Tyr, or Glu-Ala-Tyr, the ratio of amino acids was constant, but the actual sequence of the polymers was random. To gain an idea about the relevance of three-dimensional structure for antigenicity, he produced branched copolymers, in which, for example, short random Tyr-Glu sequences were attached to a poly-Ala–poly-Lys backbone. To avoid misunderstanding by the modern-time reader, I have to briefly deal with the abbreviations used for these copolymers, which deviate from the presently accepted single letter code of amino acids. For example, the widely used abbreviations for the four copolymers listed above were: GA, GLT, GAT, and (T,G)-A–L, which would mean Gly-Ala, Gly-Leu-Thr, Gly-Ala-Thr, and (Thr-Gly)-Ala-Leu by the present single letter code. The correct abbreviation of the polymers by the single letter code would be EA, EKY, EAY, and (Y,E)-A–K. Since the copolymers were the most popular antigens in immunology research for almost three decades, the entire immunology literature of this period used this misleading system of abbreviations.

'It is hard to imagine that Michael Sela, when he designed these copolymers, could have foreseen the enormous impact they would make on immunology', reflects Dr. G. 'Even though he was a man of huge mental power, who spoke a dozen languages, in addition to the scientific knowledge that he stored in his mind. But on whatever ground, he certainly made the right choice, because the copolymers proved to become the most powerful tools in gaining new, unexpected information about the immune system, and as the icing on the cake, one copolymer consisting of Ala, Lys, Glu and Tyr turned out some 30 years later to be effective in the treatment of relapsing–remitting multiple sclerosis[42,43] and is now, under the tradename "Copaxone", part of the standard care of the disease. Thus, I consider Michael Sela to be a truly successful scientist, and a successful person altogether, not really on account of his administrative career as Director of the Weizmann Institute, in Rehovot, Israel, but because of his mental-physical integrity that permitted him to remain a robust and ageless man even in his seventies, when I met him last time, and I am quite sure that he is still with us in good health.'

The first simple, artificial antigen to be used in genetic studies was dinitrophenyl coupled to poly-L-lysine (DNP-PLL). Baruj Benacerraf and his colleagues were able to show that random-bred guinea pigs mounted either high or low antibody response to this antigen, and breeding experiments indicated that the response was controlled by a single autosomal gene, and that high responsiveness was dominant.[44,45] The availability of two inbred guinea pig strains, strain 2 and 13, gave further impetus to these studies, and enabled the demonstration of Ir-gene control of immune responses to several random amino acid copolymers.[46] At this point, of course, nobody could suspect where these gene were located.

The first revealing mapping studies were performed by Hugh McDevitt, who used Michael Sela's branched copolymers (Tyr,Glu)-Ala–Lys, and the related polymer (His,Glu)-Ala–Lys in two inbred mouse strains, C57 and CBA, and found that C57 was a high responder to (Tyr,Glu)-Ala–Lys and low responder to (His,Glu)-Ala–Lys, whereas CBA showed the opposite pattern of responsiveness.[47] The dominant autosomal gene controlling these responses was defined in crosses of the above two strains, and was termed 'immune response-1' (Ir-1).[48] The logical assumption at this point was that Ir-1 should be associated with immunoglobulin (Ig) genes, but McDevitt found no linkage to Ig heavy chain allotypes.[49] The mouse model proved to be the superior choice for these studies, because of the availability of a series of congeneic mouse strains with different H-2 haplotypes developed by George Snell. McDevitt and Chinitz took advantage of these strains and were able to demonstrate that the immune responsiveness was correlated with their MHC (H-2) haplotype.[50] Subsequently, the MHC-linkage of Ir genes was also confirmed in the guinea pig model.[51] This finding was a real 'big bang' that opened up a new world in front of immunologists' eyes, because it pointed, for the first time, to a true immunological function of the MHC. For the idea that the MHC would have evolved merely to make the lives of transplant surgeons miserable did not satisfy anybody. Finally, by the analysis of responsiveness in intra-H-2 recombinant strains, McDevitt et al.[52] were able to map Ir-1 to the interval between the H-2K and Ss loci. Because several recombinant strains positioned Ir-1 to the right of H-2K and to the left of *Ss*, these studies defined a new H-2 region, now known as I region, between the K and S regions.

'Hugh McDevitt has been a person who hated self-advertisement, or "selling" of his scientific achievements' comments Dr. G. 'Thus, he usually presented his discovery with a humorous understatement. In his talks he always emphasized the fortunate coincidences that enabled his discovery, such as the availability of Michael Sela's copolymers, and his choice of the particular copolymers to be used in the mouse strains available for him. He also did not conceal that the initial choice of mouse strains was simply dictated by the fact that no other inbred strains were available at the Medical Research Institute at Mill Hill, where he started his studies. His choice of mouse strains, of course, dramatically improved, when he moved to Stanford University. He usually concluded his talk by saying: "Irish science needs Irish luck", by which he might have hinted to the Irish origin of his family. What I liked most about Hugh' continues Dr. G, 'was his outspokenness: he never cared to wrap his thoughts into mystic or political veils as many others do, and this provided him with many friends, and perhaps even more enemies.'

The discovery of MHC control of immune responses triggered an avalanche of Ir-gene studies, so that within a couple of years more than 20 different *H-2*-linked immune responses were reported. An interesting observation emerging from these studies was that almost each of the 20 or so antigens tested showed a different pattern of responsiveness, when tested on a panel of mouse strains carrying independent *H-2* haplotypes. This indicated a high degree of polymorphism in Ir genes, either due to multiple genetic loci, or multiple alleles, or both. The expectation of most immunologists was that multiple distinct Ir-gene loci should exist, each determining the response to one particular antigen, because such a model seemed to explain the data better than multiple alleles at a single locus or at a few loci. Somewhat disappointing for this concept was, however, that no genetic recombination was found that would have separated the Ir genes described. Thus one had to assume either that the number of Ir genes was smaller than expected, or that they were very tightly clustered.

The first supportive data for the expectation that multiple Ir genes might exist came from studies of the immune responses to the IgG_{2a} myeloma protein, MOPC 173, and to the enzyme lactate dehydrogenase B (LDH-B).[53,54] Mouse strains of the *H-2^b* haplotype were high responders, whereas *H-2^a* mice were low responders to these antigens. One out of several recombinants between these two haplotypes, namely *H-2^{h4}* [strain B10.A(4R)], remained a high responder, although it carried the low-responder allele at the *Ir-1* locus. The formal genetic interpretation of these data was that the crossover in this strain on the right of the *Ir-1* locus resulted in the introduction of the high-responder allele from the *H-2^b* parent, and thus the locus controlling these two responses must be separate from, and localized on the right of *Ir-1*. This interpretation was correct, although the evidence was not very firm, as it was based on a single recombinant. These findings divided the I region into two subregions, termed Ir-1A and Ir-1B, and later simply I-A and I-B. Subsequently, three additional immune responses were mapped to the I-B region. The pattern of responsiveness to one antigen was identical[55] and to the other two antithetical[56,57] in comparison to the anti-MOPC 173 and anti-LDH-B responses. Importantly, the mapping of these responses was again based on the very same recombinant mouse strain B10.A(4R).

Later, when the genetic subdivision of the I region was further refined to include the I-C and I-E subregions between I-B and S, a new, interesting type of Ir-gene control was discovered. It was again Benacerraf and colleagues[58,59] who demonstrated that in the responses to Glu-Lys-Tyr (GLT) and Glu-Lys-Phe (GLΦ) two non-responder strains can complement each other so that the F1 hybrids become responder. By the use of intra-H-2 recombinant strains, the two complementing genes were mapped to the I-A and the I-C/E subregions, respectively.

As this short account illustrates, within 10 years, the Ir-gene studies have yielded a data mass of respectable size and complexity. These studies were instrumental in assigning a new, truly biological function to the MHC, and helped to define new genetic loci and regions within it. At the same time, however, they also raised new questions, such as: What are Ir genes, and how do they exert their effect? As we will see later, additional 5–8 years were required to obtain satisfactory answers to these questions.

Since the MHC had remained for three decades an extensively studied gene cluster without function, the discovery of its involvement in immune responses was considered to be a significant achievement, worth a Nobel Prize. Thus, the third scientist awarded in 1980 for MHC research beside George Snell and Jean Dausset was Baruj Benacerraf.

But Dr. G seems to be keen on making a comment again, so I give him the word.

'This time I do not intend to give a personal account of Benacerraf. I could not even do so, because I have never really met him, except having seen him once at a meeting. His appearance was that of a conservative gentleman, quite in contrast to most immunologists, who preferred the look of a hippy or at best an artist at that time. What I found conspicuous about him was his intensity of listening to the speaker, whose topic was obviously of great interest for him. I haven't met too many people in my life, who could listen like this. But I would rather try to assess his scientific output, which will not be easy, because he was extremely active, particularly between 1960 and the mid-1980s, and tackled practically all exciting topics of immunology. In this period, probably not a single issue of the *Journal of Experimental Medicine* appeared without at least one paper from Benacerraf. The Department of Pathology at Harvard Medical School that he chaired was well known to be one of the top locations in the world of immunology. He usually reported very intriguing data resulting from complicated experimental setups that the average immunologist could not even understand. To present a Benacerraf paper at a journal club was, therefore, a task that hardly anybody was able to master. Indeed, only Mel Cohn shouldered this occasionally at the Basel Institute. Benacerraf's working style was obviously to cover as many topics of his interest as possible, instead of following up every single observation to its final clarification. This explains why some of his findings had remained puzzles until someone else found out what they meant. For example, he had discovered the carrier effect, but Mitchison was the one, who found out later that it was the result of cell–cell collaboration (see Section 1.3). Similarly, the single gene control of immune response was Benacerraf's discovery, but it was McDevitt, who showed the association of Ir genes with the MHC. In fact, the Nobel Prize for this finding should have been awarded to both of them. The same pattern could also be observed later: e.g., Benacerraf and his colleagues[60] had discovered the requirement for I region identity in T–B-cell collaboration, but its mechanism was only understood later, after the discovery of MHC restriction by Zinkernagel and Doherty.[61] Altogether, the way Benacerraf made science resembled the work of a fisher, who casts out a huge net and collects all the fish that got stuck in it, instead of taking a harpoon and going for the big fish only. But this comparison does not quite hold, because in Benacerraf's net there was usually only big fish. Therefore, I assume he must have had a particular talent and/or intuition that permitted him to distinguish between important and unimportant.'

'I should perhaps remark here that many immunologists envied Benacerraf for his working style. According to contemporary gossips, he could only afford to act so, because he was a wealthy man, the owner of a bank (or a chain of banks), so whenever a project of his was not funded, he just financed it out of his own pocket. Admittedly, I have never checked this gossip for validity, but recently an Oriental man has told me that "Benacerraf" is an Arabic word and its meaning is money changer. Thus, on a "nomen est omen" basis, there might have been a grain of truth in the gossip.'

6.2.2 Stimulation in the Mixed Lymphocyte Reaction

One of the most useful artifacts ever produced by immunology research is the mixed leukocyte reaction (MLR). It is based on the observation that normal peripheral blood leukocytes from two different donors, when mixed together, stimulate each other to proliferate.[62] The incorporation of ^{3}H-thymidine into DNA was introduced as a quantitative assay to measure the proliferation of cells responding in MLR.[63] The reaction was then rendered one-way by treating one of the cell populations with mitomycin C or X-irradiation that inhibits DNA synthesis, but does not impair the capability of these (stimulator) cells to induce proliferation of the other (responder) cell population.[64] The MLR was the first cellular immune reaction in the history of immunology that could be induced in vitro, and was thus a technical breakthrough of utmost importance. It was subsequently used as an experimental model in a vast number of immunological studies.

Naturally, the first question to be addressed by the use of MLR was concerned with the nature of antigens that stimulate the proliferative response. It soon became clear that the stimulating antigens were associated with the MHC both in mouse and human,[65,66] but uncertainties remained about the localization of the relevant genes within the complex. Finally, Fritz Bach and colleagues,[67] who played a pioneering role in MLR research, and subsequently Tommy Meo and colleagues[68,69] were the ones to establish a major (although not exclusive) role of I-region associated genes in MLR stimulation, by the use of pairs of new congeneic, *H-2*-recombinant mouse strains as responders and stimulators, respectively. The major findings reported in these studies were the following.

Strongest stimulation was observed in combinations of whole I-region disparity with or without additional differences in other regions. Within the I region, the I-A subregion seemed to contain most stimulatory genes, whereas products of the C/E subregions were less stimulatory, and the I-B subregion appeared to be silent. Disparities in class I regions K and D were found to exert only minimal stimulatory effect.

Thus, one could have concluded that the I region was responsible for MLR stimulation, had there not been a couple of notable exceptions to this rule. One was the H-2^{ba} mutation that was found to stimulate strong MLR as well as CML (cell-mediated lympholysis: cytotoxic T-cell response to class I antigens),[70] and thus it appeared as if a combined stimulation with both K and I region gene products would have taken place. Since at that time there was no other way to determine whether the mutation affected a gene in the K region or the I region or both, the mystery remained unresolved. It took another 5–8 years to understand that the mutation affected only the *H-2K* gene, but the mutant wild-type MLR combinations address a special T-cell subpopulation that is capable of both proliferating and developing into cytotoxic T cells.[71,72] The next puzzle was even more difficult to solve. It was the finding of a mixed leukocyte stimulating (*Mls*) locus by Hilliard Festenstein that stimulated strong MLR but no CML, and thus behaved as a bona fide I region gene, but it was not linked to the MHC.[73] Fifteen years later it has turned out that this response is mechanistically different from MLR: namely, the Mls gene product induces proliferation by crosslinking certain T-cell receptors with MHC class II molecules.[74,75] Thus the exceptions, serious as they might have seemed, finally failed to invalidate the statement that the I region is primarily responsible for stimulation in MLR.

Studies of the graft-versus-host reaction (GVHR) performed also in the early 1970s have revealed that the genetic disparities that induce this reaction are remarkably similar to the genetic requirements of MLR stimulation, and both are mapped to the I region.[76,77] It was therefore hypothesized that there were genes in the I region coding for 'lymphocyte activating determinants' (Lads) responsible for stimulation in both MLR and GVHR. Although direct evidence to prove the identity of MLR-Lads and GVHR-Lads was not available, the community surprisingly accepted this hypothesis without objection.

Thus, at this point there were two, virtually different sets of genes mapped to the I region, *Ir* genes and *Lad*-s, but their molecular products were unknown, and consequently, their relationship also remained a mystery.

6.2.3 MHC Class II (Ia) Antigens

Up to the early 1970s, all known I-region-associated traits were assayed by specific lymphocyte responses (antibody response to certain antigens, mixed lymphocyte, and graft-versus-host reactions), and based on this fact, they appeared to be lymphocyte-defined, in contrast to the class I gene products that could be detected by serological methods. But this appearance was short-lived.

In 1973, Chella David and his colleagues[78–80] reported on antibodies that were raised by reciprocal immunizations using two mouse strains A.TL with H-2 haplotype composition K^s I^k S^k D^d and A.TH with K^s I^s S^s D^d. In this historically important strain combination the K and D antigens were identical, and therefore, in principle the antibodies were supposed to recognize allelic products of the I and S regions. The alloantibodies were cytotoxic in the presence of complement on a subset of lymphoid cells of the donor strain, and also crossreacted with lymphoid cells from a number of different strains. Analysis of these sera on H-2 recombinant strains localized the genes controlling the detected antigens between the K and S regions, in other words, to the I region. This was thus the first demonstration of serologically detected, I-region-associated (Ia) antigens, or by modern terminology, MHC class II antigens. Almost simultaneously, Hauptfeld et al.[81,82] also identified Ia antigens using antisera produced by cross-immunization of two strains B10.AQR and B10.T(6R) that, similarly to the A.TL-A.TH combination, differed only at the I and S regions.

'The discovery of Ia antigens raised even more attention among immunologists than that of class I antigens', recalls Dr. G. 'This is probably explained by the purportedly higher immunological significance of the I region than of the class I regions, the latter being considered at that time to be involved only in the non-physiological situation of transplant rejection. It is thus not surprising that the discoverers, in particular Chella David, Don Shreffler and Jan Klein, became famous almost overnight in immunology circles. And as it often happens, great discoveries tend to react on the discoverer. Apparently this happened to Chella David, who – according to Jan Klein – was a nonchalant, womanizing young man before, but "the I region completely changed him" – as Jan used to put it. I could not witness this metamorphosis, because I met Chella years later. All I can state for certain is that a decade after the discovery he was a very nice guy; and he still liked women.'

The tissue distribution of Ia antigens also seemed to underscore their immunological significance: whereas class I 'transplantation' antigens were detected ubiquitously, in practically every organ, the expression of Ia antigens was restricted to the lymphoreticular tissue.[79] Initially there were some debates about the type of Ia-expressing cells, in particular, whether T or B cells or both would be Ia-positive. Later on it has been demonstrated that all B cells express Ia antigens stably, at high levels, whereas only a small subset of T cells show weak Ia expression. A variable degree of expression was detected on cells of the macrophage–monocyte lineage.

Subsequently, the study of Ia antigens took up a course very similar to that of MHC class I serology. Antibodies with more restricted specificity were produced, and antigens (or epitopes) Ia.1…n were determined, some of which proved to be private, present only in a given H-2 haplotype, and others public, shared among several haplotypes. All these were expected on the basis of class I serology. But the mapping efforts to localize these antigens within the I region led to some surprises.

First, the overwhelming majority of Ia specificities turned out to reside in the I-A subregion.

Second, a B10.A(4R) anti-B10.A(2R) serum detected antigens, the genes for which did not localize in the expected subregion. This strain combination was unique, in that it showed a one-way immune reactivity: MLR and antibody response were obtained only in the 4R anti 2R-direction, but not vice versa. Since this combination was key to define the I-B subregion, the antiserum was expected to detect antigens encoded in this subregion. This was, however, not the case. The strain distribution of reactivity with this serum indicated that the antigen(s) mapped between the I-B and S regions, defining thereby a new subregion that was designated, using the next available capital letter, I-C.[83]

Third, although new recombination sites within the I region were identified in the course of these studies, Ia antigens could only be conclusively mapped to the I-A and I-C subregions suggesting that the number of expressed Ia molecules may be small, perhaps not more than two.

'For the reader who is interested in more detail, I can recommend a review by David and Shreffler[84] that contains all relevant facts and references', adds Dr. G. 'Although some of the discussed findings have become outdated by now, the fair, balanced and careful interpretation of experimental data renders this paper exemplary, and a good reading even 35 years after its appearance. To my opinion, this is perhaps the best review ever written on the H-2 complex.'

6.2.4 Biochemical Characterization of Class II MHC Molecules

The initial characterization of murine class II (Ia) molecules was the achievement of Susan Cullen[85] in Stanley Nathenson's laboratory. She used anti-Ia antisera to precipitate radiolabeled cell membrane molecules from lymphoid cells, and detected peaks of 30 000 and 61 000 apparent molecular weight by SDS polyacrylamide gel electrophoresis. Reduction converted the whole precipitated material into a 28 000–30 000 molecular weight form. Appropriate controls confirmed that these molecules were glycoproteins associated with the cell membrane, they were clearly distinct from class I molecules, and were indeed the products of genes localized in the I-region. Furthermore, sequential precipitation experiments with antibodies directed against different Ia specificities revealed that at least two separable Ia molecules, controlled by different I-subregions, were present in the antigen preparations.

Subsequent studies have shown that class II molecules are built up of two non-covalently associated subunits, a 33 000 mw α and a 28 000 mw β chain, both spanning the cell membrane. All these characteristics set them apart from the single chain 45 000 mw membrane spanning class I molecule that is non-covalently associated with β_2 microglobulin, the latter not being associated with the cell membrane. However, with further progress in the chemical character-ization of MHC molecules, similarities between class I and class II molecules also became apparent. For example, the extracellular part of the class I molecule was shown to comprise an amino-terminal (membrane-distal) domain without disulfide bridge, and two disulfide-bonded domains, plus β_2 microglobulin contributing a third disulfide-bonded domain.[86] Of the class II subunits, the α chain has two extracellular domains, the membrane-proximal one is disulfide-bonded, and the amino-terminal one is not, whereas the β chain comprises two disulfide-bonded domains.[87] Thus both classes of MHC molecule have four extracellular domains, three of which are disulfide-bonded. Moreover, the membrane-proximal domains of both class I and II, as well as β_2 microglobulin have been shown to exhibit homologies to each other and to immunoglobu-lin domains.[88,89] Thus, all MHC molecules comprise two membrane-proximal, immunoglobulin-like domains, and two additional domains of comparable size, i.e., they are rather similar in their tertiary and quaternary structures, suggesting that they must have evolved to fulfill similar functions.

The biochemical studies provided also some important feedback to the genetics of MHC. For example, sequential immunoprecipitation studies sug-gested that certain Ia specificities were borne by different molecules encoded in different subregions.[85,90,91] These studies led to the subdivision of the I-C subregion, part of which was then designated I-E. But some doubts remained about the separability of these subregions, and therefore, many authors used the uncommitted designation of I-E/C subregion. Later, Cullen and her coworkers[92] demonstrated that the subdivision was not fully substantiated by the data, and she recommended to retain the term I-E, and drop the I-E/C designation.

Most informative were the biochemical studies performed by a brilliant postdoctoral fellow, Patricia Jones,[93] in McDevitt's laboratory. She used two-dimensional gel electrophoresis for the study of Ia molecules, a method that enabled distinction between the cytoplasmic and cell membrane forms of class II chains. By combining this method with sophisticated genetics, she has shown that while the gene encoding the α chain of the class II molecule E resides in the I-E subregion, the Eβ chain is encoded in the I-A subregion. These two sub-regions were thought at that time to be separated from each other by two inter-vening subregions, I-B and I-J. Thus, the two chains were the products of two clearly distinct, complementing genes. (In the case of the other class II molecule AαAβ, a genetic separation of chains was not possible, for lack of intra-I-A recombinants.) The entire I region appeared to code for only four class II chains, Aα, Aβ, Eβ, and Eα. The remaining subregions, notably I-B, I-J, and I-C, did not seem to encode class II chains. Further, she has shown that mice carrying

H-2 haplotypes *b* and *s* fail to produce Eα chains, possibly due to a defect in the corresponding gene, and the relevant β chains, Eβ^b, and Eβ^s, respectively, although produced normally, remain in the cytoplasm. But these chains can be expressed on the cell surface in F1 hybrids with another haplotype (e.g., *H-2^k*) that produces Eα chains. Thus, intracytoplasmic association of the α and β chain turned out to be a prerequisite for cell membrane expression. Such a functional complementation of *Eβ* and *Eα* genes was shown to occur also in *cis* configuration, i.e., when the two genes were on the same chromosome, in appropriate recombinant strains. The gene complementations identified by these studies are shown schematically in Fig. 6.1.

These findings readily explained the mysterious immunological behavior of some recombinant strains, such as the ominous B10.A(4R). This strain turned out to carry a functional *Eβ^k* gene together with a defective *Eα* gene, the latter from the *H-2^b* parental strain, and thus fails to express E molecules on the cell surface. Therefore it behaves as a loss mutant compared to the closely related

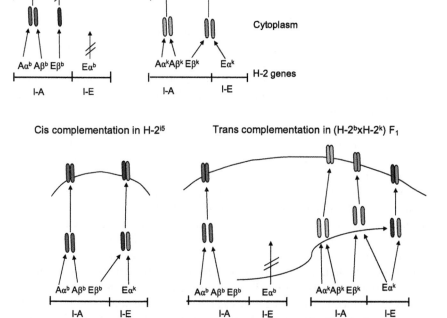

FIGURE 6.1   Gene complementation in the expression of the EβEα class II molecule. The *H-2^b* haplotype carries a defective *Eα* gene, and thus cannot produce the Eα chain. The Eβ chain although produced, remains in the cytoplasm. In *cis* and *trans* complementations, the Eα chain is contributed by the *H-2^k* haplotype. Based on Reference 93.

B10.A(2R) strain that does express the Eβ^{k}Eα molecule. This results in a one-way immune reactivity (4R → 2R) between these strains. As we will discuss later, the demonstration of *Eβ-Eα* gene complementation provided also the first important clue to the understanding of Ir genes. Interestingly, there are further *H-2* haplotypes, i.e., *f, q,* and some wild-mice-derived haplotypes, in which the expression of both Eα and Eβ is defective, suggesting that a single class II molecule (the AαAβ heterodimer) is sufficient for survival, whereas the EαEβ heterodimer may be dispensable. The finding that several different molecular defects in both *Eβ* and *Eα* genes account for the failure of E-molecule expression[94–98] in different strains supports this conclusion.

'Pat Jones' results brought a quantum leap in our understanding of the I region', recalls Dr. G. 'From then on, the superscript letters at I-subregions were no longer merely abstract allele designations, but gained a mechanistic meaning, because we learned which alleles code for a protein, and which of them are defective. This new knowledge was essential in designing experiments to test the immunological functions of the I region. Little wonder that Pat was offered a tenure position at Stanford University for this work. She was also the one who discovered most molecular defects leading to a failure of E-molecule expression,[95–97] while some of these mechanisms were clarified by Diane Mathis,[94] another rising star among female immunologists.'

The characterization of human class II MHC lagged somewhat behind the murine studies. This was typically the case in the pre-molecular biology era, when the collection of inbred mouse strains represented the most powerful tool for such studies. But the situation changed dramatically upon the entry of molecular biology into the field around 1980. From then on, the study of human MHC took over the lead so that finally the HLA complex has become characterized in much more detail than the MHC of any other species.

Not too surprisingly, human class II molecules have turned out to bear many similarities with their murine equivalents.[98,99] They were shown to be composed of two non-covalently associated glycoprotein chains with molecular weights similar to those of murine class II α and β chains. The extracellular part of molecules exhibited the same four-domain build-up as all other known MHC molecules. The membrane proximal domains of both chains were found to be Ig-like, showing sequence homology not only to Ig constant region domains, but also to each other, to Ig-like domains in class I molecules, and to β$_2$ microglobulin.[100] A difference between the two species was found in the number of expressed class II molecules: whereas mice have two of them, I-A and I-E, humans express three different class II molecules, initially designated HLA-DR, -DC, and -SB, and subsequently HLA-DR, -DQ, and -DP. Homologies to murine class II molecules were also observed, most significantly between I-E and HLA-DR: in both molecules a monomorphic α chain is associated with a polymorphic β chain, and sequence homologies are strong, particularly between the α chains. Interestingly, while in mice the I-E molecule appears to be dispensable, i.e., several mouse strains fail to express it, HLA-DR in humans is a dominant molecule accounting for about 75% of all cell-surface expressed class II, and a selective defect of DR-expression has never been reported. Thus, I-E-type molecules had made a spectacular evolutionary 'career' on their way from mouse to human. On the contrary, HLA-DQ, the human homologue of the more successful murine I-A, plays only a subordinate role compared to HLA-DR.

6.2.5 What are Immune Response Genes in Reality?

The discovery of class II MHC (Ia) antigens certainly represented an important milestone in understanding the I region. For example, it became immediately clear – even in the absence of direct evidence – that the so-called Lad-s that stimulate in mixed lymphocyte reaction and graft-versus-host reaction were in fact the class II antigens themselves. However, the puzzle of *Ir* genes was not so easy to crack, for at least two major reasons.

First, although some I-subregions, e.g., I-A, contained both *Ia* and *Ir* genes, only *Ir* but not *Ia* genes were mapped to the I-B subregion, and the opposite was the case for the I-C subregion. Thus, there was no clear correlation between these two sets of gene. Second, there was a controversy about the cellular site of expression between *Ir* and *Ia* genes. Although *Ir* genes appeared to control the level of antibody responses, this applied only to T-dependent responses, suggesting that the *Ir* genes were expressed in T cells. Indeed the virtual anti-gen-specificity of *Ir* genes led Benacerraf and McDevitt[101] to believe, at least initially, that these genes would code for the antigen receptor of T cells. Thus, while Ia antigens were shown to be expressed primarily in B cells and mono-cytes, the Ir-gene product was assumed to be in T cells.

But some observations pointed in the opposite direction. Notably, the immune responses to Glu-Lys-Tyr (GLT), and Glu-Lys-Phe (GLΦ) polymers were con-trolled by two complementing *Ir* genes in the I-A and I-E subregion,[102,103] and this correlated perfectly with the gene complementation required for the cell surface expression of the I-E molecule (the EαEβ heterodimer).[93] For exam-ple, mice of the *H-2^b* haplotype are non-responders to GLT, because they fail to express I-E molecules on the cell surface (see in Fig 6.1); *H-2^k* mice are also non-responders, because they express the Eβ^{k}Eα^k heterodimer that cannot participate in the response. However, in the F$_1$ hybrids, the Eβ^{b}Eα^k molecule, not expressed by either parental strain appears on the cell surface, and the Eβ^b allelic form of the β chain conveys responsiveness to GLT. Of course, the *H-2^{i5}* recombinant haplotype [strain B10.A(5R)], in which the expression of Eβ^{b}Eα^k molecule results from *cis*-complementation (Fig. 6.1), is also a responder. Thus, in these instances the products of *Ir* genes appeared to be identical with the α and β chain of the I-E molecule.

Initially, the readout used in all Ir-gene studies was the titer of antibodies produced in response to the test antigens. Although this was a robust and reli-able assay, it was clear for everybody in the field that it measured a down-stream consequence of Ir-gene control, since these genes were not expected to act directly on B cells. The obvious goal of subsequent studies was then to determine the cellular site of Ir-gene action, for which a cellular assay was urgently needed that was subject to the same Ir-gene control as the antibody response. This requirement was met by the antigen-specific T-cell proliferation assay, first introduced by Rosenthal and Shevach[104] for guinea pigs, followed by two different versions for the mouse, one using T-cell-enriched peritoneal exudate cells described by Schwartz and coworkers,[105] and the other antigen-primed lymph node cells developed by Corradin and colleagues.[106] In this assay, T cells from immunized animals were co-cultured with antigen-presenting cells (APC) and the priming antigen, and the secondary, antigen-specific proliferative response of T cells was measured by ^{3}H-thymidine incorporation. The MHC-dependent responder status of T cells in this assay correlated with the level antibody response in the same strain to the same antigen indicating identical Ir-gene control[104,101] of both responses. The important technical and conceptual breakthrough brought by the T-cell proliferation assay was the fact that it reduced the potential sites of Ir-gene action to two cells, namely, the T helper cell and the APC, and it also allowed the question of which cell type expresses these mysterious genes to be addressed experimentally.

The answer came soon, and it was unequivocal in both guinea pig and mouse models: it was the APC (at that time referred to as 'the macrophage') and not the T cell that was found to express *Ir* genes.[107–110] In 1973, this finding was entirely unexpected, because – according to the opinion held by the majority – *Ir* genes were supposed to code for the T-cell antigen receptor. But this view changed radically with the discovery of MHC restriction[111] in 1974. The new fact that T cells only recognize foreign antigen together with self MHC molecules, and, in particular, that helper T cells use exclusively class II molecules for antigen recognition,[112] suggested that the Ir-gene phenomenon might be a special case of class II MHC restriction. This idea gained further support from the data of biochemical studies by Jones et al.[93] that represented the first clear case, in which Ir-gene products and class II (Ia) antigens appeared to be identical. Thus, by the end of the 1970s, practically everybody expected that Ir-gene products and Ia antigens were two different facets of the same thing, although direct evidence to prove this was not yet available.

At this point, the chronicler can afford the luxury of putting down his pen and relaxing, because he has a witness statement, from Dr. G, of course, who used to participate actively in this area of research.

'I was lucky enough to enter the *Ir*-gene arena early in 1980', commences Dr. G, 'when all conceptual and technical conditions seemed to be in place to settle the remaining outstanding issues. But my interest was not as pragmatic: I just enjoyed the complexity of this field, which provided enough mental challenge to keep one going. In addition, the fact that it required a sound background of mouse genetics that most colleagues coming from a medical background missed gave a feeling of exclusivity. The major question at that time was, how to relate *Ir* and

Ia genes and their products. A simple and straightforward assumption was that if the products of Ir genes were Ia antigens, then the Ir-gene-controlled response of T cells should be inhibitable with anti-Ia antibodies. Of course, the idea was not new, there were even published studies in this direction already, from the labs of Ethan Shevach[113] and Ron Schwartz[114] at the NIH. However, in these early studies, polyclonal anti-Ia sera were used, and thus, it remained uncertain whether the inhibitory components of the sera were really directed against Ia antigens, or alternatively, against some closely linked putative Ir-gene products. Fortunately, we lived in the era of monoclonal antibodies, the use of which could circumvent this problem, and shortly before, a whole bunch of anti-MHC monoclonals had been published by Hilmar Lemke and the Hämmerling brothers.[115] I knew the Hämmerling brothers very well, they were as different as only brothers could be: Günther was aggressive and extroverted, whereas Uli was quiet and reticent. But they were similar in being locality-bound: Uli could not live outside Manhattan (he hardly ever crossed the Hudson or East River), and Günther felt the same about Heidelberg. This is all they shared, in addition, of course, to the monoclonal antibodies. A request to them for monoclonals was easy, because they distributed their hybridoma freely in the community, particularly after Günther's workplace, the German Cancer Research Center, had denied him the permission to open his own antibody company.'

'Thus, we set out to study T-cell responses to two amino acid copolymers à la Michael Sela, namely to Glu-Ala controlled by an *Ir* gene in the I-A subregion, and to Glu-Lys-Tyr controlled by two complementing genes in the I-A and I-E subregion. The results were as simple as the experimental question, nonetheless important: the response to Glu-Ala was selectively inhibited with monoclonals specific for the I-A (AαAβ) molecule, whereas the anti-Glu-Lys-Tyr response was inhibited by an I-E (EαEβ)-specific antibody.[116] The Benacerraf group rushed almost a year after us to publish similar findings.[117] (Actually, I felt the successful competition with them more satisfying than the results themselves.) Simultaneously, Ethan Lerner, a postdoc in Charlie Janeway's lab at Yale, produced a monoclonal antibody recognizing several allelic forms of the Eβ chain, and demonstrated specific inhibition by this antibody of T-cell responses to two different antigens under double (I-A and I-E) *Ir*-gene control.[118] Thus, *Ir*-gene control by the I-A subregion translated mechanistically into MHC restriction by the AαAβ molecule, whereas the response was controlled by two complementing *Ir* genes into restriction by the EαEβ molecule.'

'The next question that sprang immediately to mind was: what about the responses controlled by genes in the I-B subregion? We looked at one of them, the T-cell response to lactate dehydrogenase B (LDH-B), in great detail, and found that it was inhibited with I-A-specific monoclonal antibodies, i.e., it was I-A restricted.[119] As I shall explain later, the I-B subregion itself turned out to be a formal genetic artifact. All these data have provided convincing evidence that the two known class II MHC molecules, AαAβ and EαEβ, are indeed the long sought-for *Ir*-gene products.'

'But these results, straightforward as they seemed, revealed also an intriguing aspect of *Ir*-gene control. We took note of this upon testing a large number of different mouse strains for *Ir*-gene-controlled T-cell responses. For these experiments, we used Jan Klein's strain collection, which was the largest in the world, as he generated many new strains carrying wild-mice-derived *H-2* haplotypes, to be able to assess the degree of MHC polymorphism, a pet project of his. The surprising observation was that the responses to Glu-Ala and LDH-B were *always* I-A restricted in altogether 42 responder haplotypes expressing many different allelic forms of the I-A and I-E molecule.[119] Thus, only I-A molecules were used in these responses, and *all* allelic forms of the I-E molecule were completely excluded, even in strains where no I-A-restricted response was detected. The latter were complete non-responders. This finding was predicted by the *Ir*-gene phenomenon itself, because the responses could not have been mapped to the I-A subregion, if they had oscillated between the I-A and I-E molecule in different strains. Nevertheless, this degree of "faithfulness" to one of the two possible class II types was staggering to see. More or less the same applied to the I-E restricted response to Glu-Lys-Tyr: here we found ten responder haplotypes out of 32 tested, and in eight of them the response was I-E restricted, although in two strains I-A restricted response was detected.[119] However, the two "misfit" haplotypes carried defective *Eα* and *Eβ* genes, and thus in these strains the *I-A* genes must have evolutionarily adapted to compensate for the lack of the I-E molecule.'

'Thus, two different kinds of constraint could be identified in *Ir*-gene-controlled responses: first, one of the two possible class II types was completely excluded, and second, of the remaining class II type some allelic forms mediated a response and others did not. Of course, we were aware that both constraints had to do somehow with the limited immunogenicity of the test antigens, because in responses to more complex antigens both class II types were functional, and non-responsiveness did not occur.[120] But a mechanistic explanation for the selective 'I-A-ness' or 'I-E-ness' of *Ir*-gene-controlled responses remained difficult to provide for a long time.'

'In retrospect, the finding that *Ir* and *Ia* genes are identical qualifies as demystification rather than discovery, because it implies that *Ir* genes as distinct, mysterious entities do not exist. In a way this is analogous to saying that witches don't exist: it is self-evident today, but would have been a bold, progressive statement in the Middle Ages. Another implication of this finding is that since all helper T-cell responses are class II restricted, they are also *Ir*-gene controlled. This formulation, although correct, would do injustice to *Ir*-gene studies of the preceding 15 years by making them appear as a collection of odd phenomenology. However, the real issue here was not the response, but the absence of it. Unresponsiveness established itself as a distinctive feature of *Ir*-gene controlled responses as opposed to "common" helper T-cell responses, it was MHC-associated, was of biological-medical significance, and its mechanisms remained unknown. Therefore, subsequent studies focussed on unravelling these mechanisms.'

6.2.6 Mechanisms of MHC-Controlled Unresponsiveness

The last and most difficult question that Ir-gene studies owed an answer to was: how could MHC-controlled unresponsiveness arise? In fact, the problem of unresponsiveness turned out to be a general one, not limited to T helper (Th) cell responses. For example, it was observed that mice infected with different viruses mounted cytotoxic T lymphocyte (Tc) responses in which only one of the class I molecules, either K or D, was active.[121–125] Thus, the failure of certain MHC molecules to participate in T-cell response to a given antigen, i.e., the Ir-gene phenomenon itself, seemed to apply to both class I and class II MHC. The only difference between the two types of response was that in class I-restricted antiviral responses phenotypic non-responders did not occur (either the K or the D molecule was always active), probably because viral proteins had more immunogenic epitopes than the amino acid copolymers used in classical Ir-gene studies. For this reason, and because Th cell responses were more amenable to experimental manipulations than Tc responses, subsequent studies into the mechanism of unresponsiveness utilized predominantly Th-cell response models.

As discussed in the previous section, by the early 1980s it had become well established that, first, *Ir* genes were expressed in the antigen-presenting cells (APC) and not in T cells, second, they indeed coded for class II MHC molecules (Ia antigens), and third, they seemed to affect the response of Th cells directly. Unresponsiveness was therefore understood as a failure of interaction between the antigen receptor of Th cells, the antigen, and class II MHC molecules of APC (although it was unknown how these three components would come together). At that time the most important outstanding questions appeared to be: first, the cellular site of the Ir-gene defect (i.e., the APC, the T cell, or both?), and second, the possible mechanism(s) by which unresponsiveness could arise.

Because class II molecules were detected on the surface of APC but not on most T cells, it was tempting to speculate that the defect should also lie in the APC. However, a simple explanation, e.g., a 'defective' class II molecule in non-responders, was impossible to provide, because any particular class II molecule that appeared defective with respect to one antigen was perfectly capable of mediating responses to other antigens. Thus the defect seemed to lie in the specific antigen–MHC combination, and not in the MHC molecule itself. This appeared as a perfect mystery for most immunologists at that time.

'The one who first addressed this problem experimentally was Ethan Shevach, the Einstein of *Ir*-gene studies', points out Dr. G. 'He used the old "in-house" model of the NIH, the immune response of strain 2 and strain 13 guinea pigs that had also permitted the discovery of Ir genes by Benacerraf a decade earlier. In Ethan's studies,[108,126] strain (2x13)F₁ hybrid guinea pigs were immunized with an antigen for which one parental strain was responder (R) and the other non-responder (NR). Immune T cells from the (RxNR)F₁ animals were then shown to give a secondary response, *in vitro*, only when the antigen was presented by APC ("macrophages") of the R parent, but failed to respond to the same antigen on APC from the NR parent. Since in these experiments the T cells were kept identical, whereas the APC varied, the authors concluded that the decision about responsiveness must have occurred at the level of the APC, and consequently, the cellular site of the Ir-gene defect was the APC. A few years later Barcinski and Rosenthal[127] presented a further refined version of this model. These authors demonstrated that strain 2 and strain 13 guinea pigs reacted to two different antigenic determinants (epitopes, by present terminology) of pork insulin, namely, strain 2 responded to an epitope in the A chain of insulin, and strain 13 to another epitope in the B chain. Insulin-primed $(2x13)F_1$ T cells responded to intact insulin presented by either parental APC, but the response was directed selectively to the A-chain epitope together with strain 2 APC, and to the B chain epitope presented by stain 13 APC. They concluded that different MHC molecules selected different epitopes of the same antigen for presentation to T cells, and the concept formulated on the basis of these results was termed "determinant selection". According to this hypothesis, the MHC molecule physically interacts with the epitope, and the interaction has a certain degree of specificity. When the interaction cannot take place, unrespon-siveness ensues.'

'The determinant selection hypothesis proposed a completely novel mecha-nism – a specific interaction between MHC and antigen – that was beyond the imagination of most immunologists at that time, and thus it was a bold concept', continues Dr. G. 'Moreover, it turned out to be true many years later. The only problem with it was that it became instantaneously the "official" concept of the NIH, and as such a political rather than scientific issue. This was most obvious from the methods by which the concept was propagated: it was usually presented as the ultimate truth, alternative possibilities were de-emphasized or omitted, and it was repeated as many times as required for being hammered into the heads of immunologists.'

'Here I must emphasize that conclusive results and ideas are, as a rule, accepted unanimously by the community. Thus the use of the above-mentioned methods is warranted only when something is unclear. And this was exactly the case for the determinant selection hypothesis. The results of F_1 experiments could also be explained in a different way, namely that unresponsiveness arises because of the lack of T cells capable of recognizing the antigen together with the non-responder MHC molecule. This latter hypothesis was referred to as "holes in the T-cell repertoire".'

'Although it has been shown by several groups that there is nothing wrong genetically with non-responder T cells,[128–133] the development of the T-cell rep-ertoire is a somatic process, which provides ample opportunities for "holes" to arise. There are at least two mechanisms that can be envisaged to punch such holes. First, the adjustment of the T-cell repertoire for complementarity to self MHC during ontogeny in the thymus, referred to as "positive selection". In this process T-cell clones specific for certain epitopes may not be selected to enter the repertoire, because their receptors do not possess sufficient complementar-ity to self MHC. The result will be antigen-specific, and MHC-dependent holes. By this mechanism, responsiveness will be dominant, as most Ir-gene-controlled responses are, because $(RxNR)F_1$ animals will have the repertoire of both parents. Second, the deletion of autoreactive T cell clones by self tolerance (referred to as "negative selection") can also induce unresponsiveness to antigenic epitopes that incidentally resemble self. This mechanism could allow for dominant, and in some instances recessive responsiveness. Examples for the latter have also been reported.'[134,135]

'Of course, the "determinant selection" and the "holes in the repertoire" hypotheses are not mutually exclusive, they both could cause unresponsiveness within the same individual (a schematic representation of the two hypotheses is given in Fig. 6.2). But the point to emphasize here is that the latter concept can account completely for MHC-linked unresponsiveness, even if the non-responder MHC were capable of presenting the antigen. Thus the autocracy of determinant selection seemed to be shaking.'

'It would be a mistake to believe that NIH scientists would have overlooked the alternative interpretation. They were too brilliant for that. Indeed, one of them, Ron Schwartz, a major proponent of determinant selection, was the one who first formulated a clonal deletion model for unresponsiveness.[136] And yet, they supported determinant selection unanimously in the public. This situation made me realize that, despite all advantages, it could sometimes be difficult to be an NIH scientist.'

'The question was then, which of the two proposed mechanisms was at work in reality. It was clear to me that asking the $(RxNR)F_1$ experimental model to provide an answer would be like trying to solve a single equation with two unknowns. To achieve a clear-cut distinction between the two mechanisms an experimental system was needed, in which the T cells had not been exposed during their ontogeny

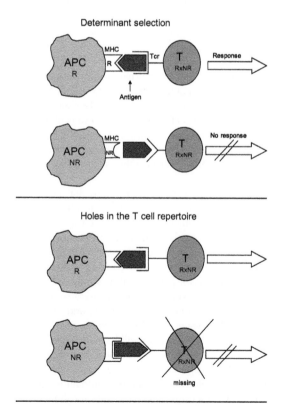

FIGURE 6.2   Schematic representation of the two competing hypotheses to explain MHC-linked unresponsiveness. Based on References 108, 126, 142.

to the MHC of APC. In other words, a fully artificial system, where T cells and APC differ in MHC (are allogeneic). Because T cells give a strong mixed leukocyte reaction (MLR) to allogeneic APC without any added antigen, these alloreactive cells had first to be removed from the cell mixture. The method of choice to achieve this was a treatment of MLR cultures with bromodeoxyuridine and light that causes DNA crosslinking in proliferating cells, and thereby kills them or at least prevents their further division.[137] After removal of alloreactivity, the remaining cells can be primed, in vitro, with antigen presented on the same allogeneic APC, and the primed cells will specifically recognize the combination of antigen plus allogeneic MHC of APC, i.e., they are "allorestricted".[137,138] We adapted this system to amino acid copolymer antigens, and were able to show that non-responder APC could induce responses of allogeneic T cells, and these responses were inhibited by monoclonal antibodies against the non-responder MHC on APC.[139,140] These experiments provided therefore formal evidence against a failure of antigen presentation by non-responder MHC, and by exclusion, favored the "holes in the repertoire" hypothesis. It was reassuring to see that Ethan Shevach in the NIH, using the same experimental system obtained analogous results to ours in the guinea pig model.[141]

'But results obtained from a fully artificial system should be interpreted with caution. This applies also to allo-restricted T cells, despite the fact that their existence was clearly demonstrated by their response to antigen plus allogeneic APC, and by the lack of response to the allogeneic APC alone or to the same antigen plus syngeneic APC. Clones of such T cells could also be produced. Nevertheless, the existence of allo-restricted cells made no immunological sense. It was also peculiar that their induction seemed to be contingent on a preceding MLR: in the presence of syngeneic APC, T cells could not be primed at all, in vitro. It is therefore possible that allo-restricted cells might represent a special subset of allo-reactive cells. Finally, the only valid point our experiments could make was that a complete failure of non-responder MHC molecules to present the antigen probably does not exist.'

'Of course, this self-criticism does not imply that the "holes in the repertoire" hypothesis was wrong. Indeed, there is at least one well-documented case for this mechanism in the literature.'[142]

'Amidst the big *Ir*-gene debate, one day I received, to my surprise, an invitation from the NIH to be a speaker in their special seminar series', recalls Dr. G. 'This was an honor that hardly any colleague had in Europe. Besides, this was probably the best remunerated scientific seminar in the world ($750 plus travel and accommodation for a 1-hour talk). I was all excited about the opportunity to get to know the "opposite camp". At that time, the Immunology Branch of the National Institute of Allergy and Infectious Diseases was headed by Bill Paul, and it comprised a number of distinct groups headed by Jay Berzofski, Richard Hodes, Gene Shearer, Ethan Shevach, Ron Schwartz, and Al Singer. A "recent acquisition" was, in addition, Ron Germain, who had come here from Harvard, after the crash of the suppressor T-cell "business", for a sabbatical year to learn molecular biology, and then he stayed on. The NIH team received me very friendly, so that I had not at all the feeling to venture into the "grizzly bear's cave". They had nothing bear-like, on the contrary, most of them looked quite familiar to me, particularly Ethan Shevach, whose stature and moustache would have made him fit in any East-Hungarian town, say Debrecen, better than in Bethesda, Maryland.'

'My "special seminar" was a success, but much less the personal discussions, in which any one of the NIH immunologists proved to be at least ten times brighter than myself. As an excuse, I may mention that I was not used to such verbal fireworks. All NIH scientists – as expected – were of one mind when it came to determinant selection. The individual differences among them were more temperamental than conceptual: for example, the most flexible ones were Ethan Shevach and Al Singer, the brightest minds to my appreciation, Ron Germain was aggressive-dogmatic, and Ron Schwartz, with his non-confrontational attitude, wished that everybody were a little right. Finally, I am afraid we could not convince each other.'

'What perplexed me most in the discussions with NIH scientists was that I could never be quite sure how much of what they said was science and how much politics. But this talking style was probably a consequence of their social situation: they held well-paid, safe, life-long government positions, they did not need to compete for research grants, and they were pretty well off, owning big houses and luxury cars, at a time when most immunologists were just poor Bohemians. Apparently, for so much advantage one could even take some politics into account.'

'At this point, the Ir-gene debate was back to square one, and stayed there for a while. I must admit, I still refused to believe in determinant selection, and favored the holes in the repertoire concept. There was only one set of data that worried me, namely the selective restriction of response to a given antigen to either I-A or I-E molecules in many different MHC haplotypes,[143,144] or the "-A-ness" or "I-E-ness" of a response, as I liked to refer to it. This phenomenon was not derived from some fancy in vitro system, it was observed after in vivo immunization of mice, and thus was likely to reflect biological reality. The problem with it was that it was extremely difficult to envisage, how exactly the same holes could arise in the T-cell repertoire of mice with different I-A and I-E molecules, respectively. Much easier was to assume that all I-A molecules had similar strategies to select an antigenic epitope, and this was different from the strategies of I-E molecules. In other words, determinant selection was the easier way to interpret these data.'

'My uneasy feelings were further strengthened by a paper of Rock and Benacerraf[145] a couple of years later. These authors demonstrated that the response of Th cells (T-cell hybridoma in their experimental system) to the copolymer Glu-Ala-Tyr (GAT) plus I-A^d was inhibited by the structurally related copolymer Glu-Tyr (GT), to which the T cells did not respond. The inhibition was specific, in that other I-A^d-restricted responses were not affected, it was unique to GT as other similar copolymers were not inhibitory, and it was reversible by increased amounts of GAT. The site of competition between the two copolymers appeared to be the APC. The results were interpreted to indicate a specific interaction between the antigen/competitor and the class II molecule, I-A^d. But this point was not proven conclusively, partly because the competitor, GT, was itself a "weird" antigen that had previously been shown to induce preferentially suppressor T cells.[146] It was also possible that GT presented on the APC, instead of competing with GAT, provided some kind of shut-down signal directly to the T-cell receptor. This latter concern was addressed, although not really eliminated in a follow-up paper.[147] Finally, the one who solved the problem with a wave of his hand was Emil Unanue, a sensitive and talented little Latin-American man, who devoted most of his career to studying macrophages; a second Eli Metchnikoff, so to say. Unanue realized that the experimental systems to prove determinant selection had one component too many, and this was the T cell. As the question was whether a specific interaction between epitopes and MHC existed or not, he decided to study exactly this. In their published study,[148] Unanue and coworkers used a T-cell epitope, peptide 46-61 of hen-egg lysozyme (HEL) that was known to be immunogenic in mice expressing the I-A^k molecule, but failed to induce a response in mice with I-A^d. Using detergent solubilized purified class II molecules, they were able to show that peptide HEL (46-61) binds specifically to I-A^k at low µM affinity, whereas no binding to I-A^d could be detected. With his known modesty, Unanue concluded that "perhaps the affinity of the interaction between *Ia* and peptide would dictate the *Ir* gene responder status". Certainly, his data and those of the following "peptide revolution" provided sufficient support for this conclusion.'

'The evidence for specific peptide–MHC interaction marked the end of the *Ir*-gene era. From the mid-1980s on, nobody talked about *Ir* genes or determinant selection anymore, because these terms were translated into binding affinities between peptides and MHC molecules. The debate between proponents of determinant selection and holes in the repertoire also subsided. Evidence was available that both mechanisms can cause unresponsiveness, and the issue was over-discussed anyway. The relative contribution of determinant selection and holes in the repertoire to unresponsiveness was estimated to be 70% and 30%, respectively.[149] Therefore the consensus of the majority has been that peptide–MHC interactions play a dominant role, although some investigators, for example Polly Matzinger,[142] think that holes caused by self tolerance are equally important. Thus, like many other polarizing debates in science, this one has also ended up as a drawn game', concludes Dr. G.

6.3 SORTING OUT THE GENETICS OF MHC

6.3.1 The Era of Formal Genetics

Until about 1980, formal genetics had been the only possible approach to MHC research. One consequence of this was that the overwhelming majority of studies were done in mice, the best model species of mammalian genetics. Indeed, MHC research was considered for some time to be equal to studying the H-2 complex, the murine MHC. Of course, the mouse model was ideal for these studies, because of the availability of H-2 homozygous inbred, congeneic, and recombinant strains.

A summary of how our knowledge about the H-2 complex expanded over a period of almost 30 years of formal genetics is given in Table 6.1. The discoveries listed in the table are described in detail in Sections 6.1 and 6.2.

TABLE 6.1 Characterization of the H-2 Complex by Formal Genetics

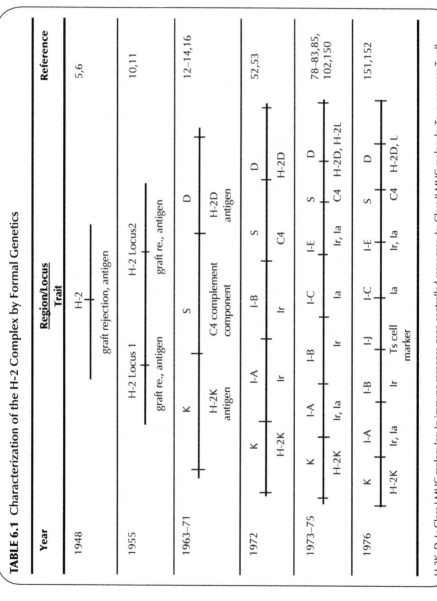

Year	Region/Locus Trait						Reference
1948	H-2 graft rejection, antigen						5,6
1955	H-2 Locus 1 graft re., antigen		H-2 Locus2 graft re., antigen				10,11
1963–71	K H-2K antigen	S C4 complement component		D H-2D antigen			12–14,16
1972	K H-2K	I-A Ir	I-B Ir	S C4	D H-2D		52,53
1973–75	K H-2K	I-A Ir, Ia	I-B Ir	I-C Ia	I-E Ir, Ia	S C4	D H-2D, H-2L	78–83,85, 102,150
1976	K H-2K	I-A Ir, Ia	I-B Ir	I-J Ts cell marker	I-C Ia	I-E Ir, Ia	S C4	D H-2D, L	151,152

H-2K, D, L: Class I MHC molecules; Ir: immune response-gene controlled responses; Ia: Class II MHC molecule; Ts: suppressor T cell.

By a quick glance at the table, one can establish that the development was rather slow, but taken the long time required for the production of new inbred strains, this is not surprising. Toward the end of the formal genetics era, an expansion of the field, and a concomitant increase of the recombinant strain collection took place. A consequence of this was that the 1970s witnessed a literal burst of new H-2 regions and subregions, of which the table only lists the most persistent ones, i.e., the ones that were relatively well established. But the full picture was much more complex: in fact, the collection of registered regions of H-2 and the adjacent Qa, and Tla complexes (encoding so called 'non-classical' MHC molecules) used up all letters of the alphabet from A through V, with the exception of O and P. Most of these regions proved to be short lived: they could either not be confirmed, or the findings could be explained also without the need of a new region. Thus it was not quite unfounded that Jan Klein[153] called this interpretation of the H-2 complex 'madman's alphabet'.

At this point, I am curious how Dr. G would explain this unprecedented proliferation of H-2 regions.

'I think the increased number of investigators and mouse strains is just one facet of the problem. The conceptual drive behind this development was the idea that the MHC was in fact not histocompatibility but rather an immunity complex, encoding a diverse array of traits, including the T-cell antigen receptor, T suppressor cell function, complement, etc., all of which having to do with the immune response. It was felt that the efficiency of immune response was the selective pressure that had kept all these loci together. Another, almost equally important aspect was that MHC studies came full in trend, and so everybody knew that the identification of a new H-2 region ensured a safe publication in a relatively high-impact scientific journal. Therefore, all biological and pathological phenomena on earth were tested for MHC association. This could be done easily by testing the selected phenomenon in a series of H-2 disparate mouse strains that were already available commercially at that time. The investigation of new and sometimes very complex biological phenomena combined with wishful thinking can perhaps be made responsible for the creation of most illusory H-2 regions.'

However, even if one disregarded the 'short lived' H-2 regions, the 'established' 1976 stand of H-2 (see in Table 6.1) appeared too complicated by the early 1980s, in particular in the I region. The problem was that new data on the nature of class II molecules and *Ir* genes came in conflict with the assigned I subregions, and these controversies necessitated a new interpretation of the genetic composition of MHC.

6.3.2 A Simplified Interpretation of MHC Based on Biochemical and Functional Studies

The new interpretation of MHC has been based on the thesis that each single MHC locus is pleiomorphic, i.e., it controls a series of different biological traits.[154] In other words, the MHC molecule (class I or class II) encoded by a particular locus is responsible single-handedly for all phenomena associated with this locus, such as graft rejection, cell-mediated lymphocytotoxicity (CML), mixed lymphocyte reaction (MLR), control of antibody response (Ir gene effect), and restriction of T-cell specificity.

As far as class I loci are concerned, this view gained acceptance already in the 1970s, even in the absence of direct evidence. Thus, almost everybody in the field agreed that all class-I-associated functions, i.e., rapid allograft rejection, strong CML, weak MLR, and restriction of cytotoxic T-cell specificity are carried out by the 45 kDa class I molecules (H-2K, D, and L) encoded in the K and D regions.

However, the case of class II regions (i.e., I subregions) proved to be more troublesome. Here, the concept that class II molecules (*Ia* antigens) were responsible for all I-region-associated traits did not seem to apply in certain instances. For example, the I-B subregion was known to be responsible for the *Ir*-gene control of several immune responses while it did not encode *Ia* antigens, and the opposite was true for the I-C subregion (see in Table 6.1). Thus, in these subregions *Ir* and *Ia* genes appeared to exist and function separate from one another, which can obviously not be the case, if they were identical. The I-J subregion posed another problem, as it appeared to encode a cell surface marker on suppressor T cells, but neither *Ia* nor *Ir* genes were demonstrable in this region. In contrast, the I-A and I-E subregions contained both *Ia* and *Ir* genes, thus supporting the thesis of unity.

'In face of these contradictions one had to assume that either the thesis was not applicable to class II, or there was something wrong about the assignment of certain I subregions', recalls Dr. G. 'Of these two alternatives only the latter made sense to me, because it was testable experimentally. So we decided to reinvestigate the traits encoded by the "aberrant" I subregions, and the results were surprising enough to be recapitulated here.'

The *I-B subregion* was originally defined on the basis of the strain distribution of responsiveness to two antigens, the IgG$_{2a}$ myeloma protein MOPC173,[53] and the enzyme porcine lactate dehydrogenase B (LDH-B),[54] as already mentioned in Section 6.2.1. The mapping of these responses was based on the finding that the *H-2^a* haplotype (e.g., strain B10.A) confers low, and the *H-2^b* haplotype (e.g., B10) high responsiveness, and two reciprocal recombinant haplotypes derived from *H-2^{a}xH-2^b* crosses, namely *H-2^{h4}* [B10.A(4R)] and *H-2^{i5}* [B10.A(5R)] both confer high responsiveness. By formal genetic interpretation, this pattern of responsiveness is only possible, if the gene(s) controlling these responses is located in the interval between the two recombination sites as shown in Fig. 6.3. Because this interval is marked by a recombination on each side and it may contain more than one gene locus, it appeared fully justified to consider it a separate I subregion.

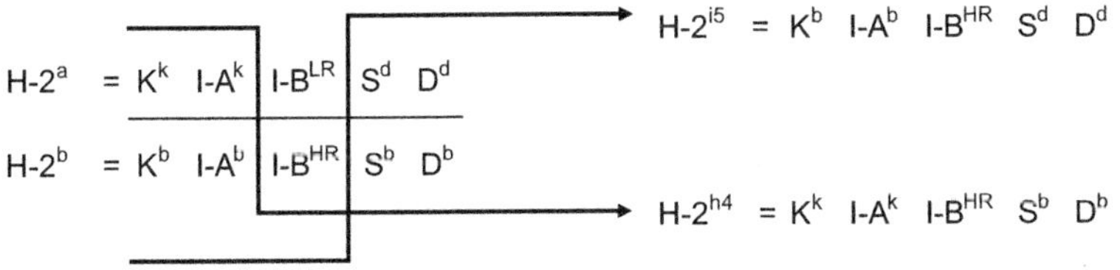

$$H\text{-}2^{i5} = K^b \quad I\text{-}A^b \quad I\text{-}B^{HR} \quad S^d \quad D^d$$

$$H\text{-}2^a = K^k \quad I\text{-}A^k \quad I\text{-}B^{LR} \quad S^d \quad D^d$$

$$H\text{-}2^b = K^b \quad I\text{-}A^b \quad I\text{-}B^{HR} \quad S^b \quad D^b$$

$$H\text{-}2^{h4} = K^k \quad I\text{-}A^k \quad I\text{-}B^{HR} \quad S^b \quad D^b$$

FIGURE 6.3   Formal genetic definition of the I-B subregion. The arrows indicate how two recombinant haplotypes $H\text{-}2^{i5}$ and $H\text{-}2^{h4}$ could have arisen from $H\text{-}2^a$ and $H\text{-}2^b$ parents. HR and LR indicate high and low responsiveness to MOPC 173 and LDH-B (see text). To explain the pattern of responsiveness, a separate I-B subregion had to be postulated between the two recombination sites. Based on Reference 154.

'In 1980, we had two major advantages over the investigators, who defined the I-B subregion eight years earlier', points out Dr. G. 'First, we knew that the entire I region encoded only four expressed class II chains, $A\alpha$, $A\beta$, $E\beta$ in the I-A subregion, and $E\alpha$ in the I-E subregion, and that the $E\alpha$ $E\beta$ molecule was not expressed on the cell surface in several mouse strains due to genetic defects (see Section 6.2.4 for explanation). Second, we were in the position of studying T-cell responses to these antigens, for which no assay existed in 1972, when the I-B subregion was defined (based on antibody response). The strain distribution pattern of responsiveness turned out to be the same in both T-cell and antibody response, confirming that we were dealing with the same type of *Ir*-gene control. The first surprise came when we found that the T-cell response to both MOPC 173 and LDH-B was I-A ($A\alpha$ $A\beta$)-restricted in all responder strains,[143,155] raising the question of how the I-B subregion could be involved in these responses. The key to this puzzle was provided by the observation that all mouse strains expressing the $A\alpha^k A\beta^k$ (A^k) molecule together with the $E\alpha^k E\beta^k$ (E^k) molecule (e.g., B10.A) were non-responders, but in strain B10.A(4R) where A^k is expressed in the absence of any E molecule, an A^k-restricted response was detected. Thus, it appeared that the E^k molecule somehow interfered with the response channeled through the A^k molecule. We have then found that the E^k molecule induces T cells that inhibit the A^k-restricted T-cell response to the same antigen[155] We referred to the inhibitory cells as suppressor T (Ts) cells by the fashion of the time, but based on their demonstrated failure to produce their own growth factors, they may also qualify nowadays as regulatory T cells (Treg). When these cells were removed, or the E^k molecule was blocked with antibody, the non-responder strains were turned into responder. These results have clearly demonstrated that the unresponsiveness of $A^k + E^k$-expressing mouse strains is for immunoregulatory rather than genetic reasons, i.e., it is explained without postulating an I-B subregion.'

'There were three additional immune responses, whose control mapped to the I-B region, namely the antibody response to TNP-MSA (trinitrophenyl-mouse serum albumin conjugate),[55] to staphylococcal nuclease,[56] and the delayed-type hypersensitivity (DTH) response to oxazolone.[57] Unfortunately, we could not study them, because we were unable to induce a proliferative T-cell response to these antigens. But the pattern of responsiveness to TNP-MSA was like that to LDH-B and MOPC173, suggesting that a similar type of immunoregulatory mechanism may operate here. To the other two antigens, $A^k + E^k$-expressing strains were high responders, whereas B.10A(4R), without E molecules on the cell surface, was low responder suggesting that the T-cell responses should be E^k-restricted. Thus, finally, all responses could be explained without the need for I-B region, and consequently, this region was likely to be an illusion.'

The *I-C subregion* was defined on the basis of serological studies demonstrating that certain Ia determinants mapped in the interval between the I-B and S regions.[83] In addition, this subregion appeared to code for a variety of traits, such as histocompatibility antigen,[156] *Ir* and *Is* (immune suppression) genes,[157] MLR determinants,[158] and MLR suppressor factor.[159] Further serological analysis revealed, however, that some Ia determinants originally assigned to the I-C subregion were indeed controlled by the I-A and the newly defined I-E subregion. It was then shown that the Ia determinants defining the I-C and I-E subregions localized on the same molecule.[160] Furthermore, the mapping data for *Ir* genes were also consistent with a localization in the I-E subregion. The difficulties to separate these two subregions led to the uncommitted temporary designation of I-E/C, but finally most investigators referred to this subregion simply as I-E.

'Although it was not quite clear why I-C was dropped and I-E retained, and not the other way around', adds Dr. G, 'it was predictable that the I-C subregion was going to fall slowly into oblivion. Therefore, we decided not to do too much work around it. We tested only one I-C-associated trait, namely, histocompatibility, by generating cytotoxic T lymphocyte (Tc) response in the purportedly I-C disparate strain combination B10.AM anti-B10.A(1R). By analyzing the specificity of CTLs, we have found that they do not recognize any I-C-associated histocompatibility, instead, they detect minor histocompatibility antigens encoded by loci not linked to the MHC.[161] The explanation for this specificity is that the B10.AM line is not fully B10-congeneic, it has retained "contaminating" minor histocompatibility genes from its original C3H background. Thus, this study just accelerated the disappearance of the I-C subregion from the H-2 chart.'

The *I-J subregion* owed its (temporary) existence to an alloantiserum, [B10.T(6R)x B10.D2]F$_1$ anti-B10.AQR, that reacted with B10.A(5R), but not with B10.A(3R) suppressor T (Ts) cells. The target of this antisera was assumed to be an alloantigen with at least two allelic forms, one expressed in 5R and the other in 3R Ts cells, and encoded in a locus flanked by the recombination sites in these two strains, i.e., between I-B and I-C.[151,152] This newly defined section of MHC was termed I-J subregion.

'Because this discovery came at a time when Ts cells were very much in vogue, it attracted enormous attention from the immunological community', comments Dr. G. 'The discoverers, Don Murphy and Tomio Tada (later the father of Japanese immunology) became famous overnight, and everybody was waiting for further exciting developments. Numerous attempts were then made to isolate and characterize the I-J molecule, but they all failed despite the fact that meanwhile monoclonal antibodies against I-J determinants were also raised.'[162]

'I personally was reluctant to join I-J research, because it appeared too risky to me. Yet, I was interested in finding out whether the map position of genes controlling I-J determinants was correct or not. It was reasonable to assume that I-J, similarly to other loci between the I-A and I-E subregions, might be the reflection of some kind of interaction between products of the latter two subregions, i.e., the I-J subregion might only be virtual. Indeed, we were able to produce data supporting this interpretation by using a rather complex experimental system.[163] But the final blow was delivered by molecular biology: no gene was found in the region reserved for I-J, and there was no DNA sequence difference between B10.A(3R) and B10.A(5R) in this region.[164] Thus, the I-J determinants, whatever they may be, are definitely not encoded in the MHC. Of course, this is not meant to say that they do not exist, because monoclonal antibodies cannot be raised against an illusion. But their nature has remained a mystery ever since. My personal guess would be that they may represent the product of some contaminating polymorphic gene from the original background, retained after production of the B10 congeneic lines. This possibility is inherent to the strategy of generating such lines (explained in Section 6.1.1.) that resembles diluting whisky with water: no matter how much you dilute, some whisky will always remain.'

The disappearance of problematic I subregions from the H-2 chart permitted a simple and straightforward interpretation of the MHC.[154] According to this, the H-2 complex comprises three class I loci, K, D, and L, each encoding a 45-kDa class I molecule, and four class II loci $A\beta$, $A\alpha$, $E\beta$, and $E\alpha$, coding for the corresponding subunits of the two class II molecules. Because no additional functional genes were assumed to map to the MHC, the 'region' designation became superfluous. Only one locus coding for a non-MHC molecule, namely $C4$ encoding a complement component remained within the MHC, between $E\alpha$ and D (in the former S region), but its map position was assumed to be incidental. It could be considered as an "entrapped" locus that remained in the middle of MHC, because of the selective pressure for maintaining the latter as a single block.

One final question that I would like to address for sake of the interested reader: how did the scientific community receive the new interpretation of MHC?

'The overwhelming majority of immunologists loved it, because it made intuitive sense, and was easy to understand', replies Dr. G. 'Exceptions were perhaps some of the "complicators", who might have resented our turning of the H-2 complex into H-2 simplex. There were also some colleagues who remained skeptical. They argued that the evidence for the new interpretation was not much more conclusive than the one on which the assignment of regions was based, and decided to wait for further evidence from molecular biology. And they did not have to wait too long.'

6.3.3 Molecular Biology has the Last Word: The Organization of MHC at the DNA Level

Tonegawa's spectacular success in discovering the structure and rearrangement of immunoglobulin genes (Section 5.2) marked the beginning of a new era in immunology. Although it took some time for most immunologists to familiarize themselves with the new facts and to learn the language of new genetics, by the end of the 1970s it was clear for everybody that the outstanding 'big questions' would most likely be solved by means of molecular biology. It appeared therefore imperative for many scientists to learn this powerful new technology.

'We had practically no choice other than learning nucleic acid technology, or else give up the ambition of contributing to the field significantly', recalls Dr. G. 'But this was a non-trivial undertaking, because the technology itself had a huge amount of built-in science, most of which was unknown for the average immunologist. Colleagues with a background in biochemistry made the shift with relatively little effort, and thus it was not surprising that the two biggest protein chemistry "factories" in the field, namely Lee Hood's group at Caltech, Pasadena, and Jack Strominger's Biochemistry Department at Harvard (known to collect the largest amount of grant money in the state of Massachusetts) were the first to be retooled for molecular biology. Of course the leap was bigger from serology or cellular immunology, and colleagues who were specialized in these areas had to struggle a lot more in order to keep pace with the development. But there was no way to get around it: the pressure was so high that even "living classics", for example Hugh McDevitt at the age of over 50, had to take the time and trouble to attend a course of molecular biology.'

Obviously, the genetic organization of MHC, a problem tailored ideally for molecular biology, was the first to be tackled. Several competing groups started working on this project simultaneously, and so it was predictable that only the biggest groups could win the race: indeed, the first HLA class I gene was cloned at Strominger's lab,[165] and the first H-2 class I gene by Lee Hood's group.[166]

'The first authors on these two papers, Hidde Ploegh and Michael Steinmetz, were young fellows just having had their PhD completed, but their demonstrated hands-on skills in molecular biology made them instantaneously the most wanted scientists in the field, who could get any position they wished', comments Dr. G. 'Their only problem was how to sort out the offers they had received. Hidde, after some hesitation, accepted a tenure professorship in his home country, the Netherlands, where he was treated like a God. But this did not satisfy him, and so he returned to Boston for more of a challenge. Michael did not go home to Germany, because his former supervisor was of the opinion that one molecular biologist was enough for the country (he meant, of course, himself). Thus, after his postdoctoral fellowship with Lee Hood, he decided for a tenure position at the Basel Institute for Immunology (nota bene, a position that was non-existent for common mortals). Later he made an impressive career as a research manager and financer in the pharmacological industry.'

Although the cloning of the first MHC genes was an important event from the historical point of view, in reality, it was just the notorious small pebble that triggered the avalanche, namely, the following heroic technical efforts that resulted finally in the full molecular map of the MHC region in mice and human. The cloning of the entire MHC, encompassing a DNA stretch of about 3500 kilobases (kb) in human,[167] and 2000 kb in mice[168] was the largest-scale molecular biological operation in history till then, in which the most modern weapons, e.g., chromosome walking by using overlapping large (30–50 kb) DNA fragments cloned into cosmid vectors,[168] and sophisticated electrophoretic techniques (pulsed-field gel, orthogonal-field alteration gel) for the separation of DNA fragments,[167,169] were deployed. The project took several years, and is considered to be an important precursor of the whole genome sequencing efforts almost 20 years later.

Some of the individual findings along the course of this work confirmed earlier expectations. For example, MHC genes were found to comprise a number of exons that corresponded exactly to the structural domains of proteins they encoded.[170,171] Confirmed and extended was also the earlier finding that both class I and class II MHC genes exhibit strong homology to immunoglobulin genes suggesting a common origin.[166,172] The homologous sequences corresponded to the membrane proximal extracellular domains of MHC chains (and β2 microglobulin), and the constant region domains of immunoglobulins.[172,173] But no homology to immunoglobulin variable regions was noted, and as expected, MHC genes did not undergo somatic rearrangement,[166] in contrast to immunoglobulin genes. And finally, in the molecular map of the H-2 I region there was no sign of I-B and I-J subregions,[174] as predicted on the basis of functional studies.[154]

Perhaps the most surprising aspect of these studies was that the number of identified MHC genes exceeded by far the number of known MHC proteins. This was most conspicuous in the case of class I genes. For example, in mice as many as 36 distinct class I genes were identified,[29] 12 times the number of expressed class I molecules. However, many of the extra genes turned out to be defective (pseudogenes), and others mapped outside the telomeric end of H-2, to the adjacent Qa-Tla region.[169] In human, the telomeric end of the HLA complex contained a smaller number of class-I-like genes that were not homologous to Qa-Tla genes and encoded so-called class IB molecules,[167] whose function was later shown to be different from that of class I proper. The class II region contained a less impressive number of extra genes, some of which were pseudogenes and others were later shown to be members of the antigen processing and presentation machinery.

The up-to-date, somewhat-simplified gen maps of murine and human MHC are depicted in Figure 6.4. The genetic organization of MHC is clearly analogous in these two species, with the single difference that H-2K, the HLA-A homologue, lies on the centromeric end of the complex, probably as a result of a translocation. This translocation accounts for at least some of the size difference

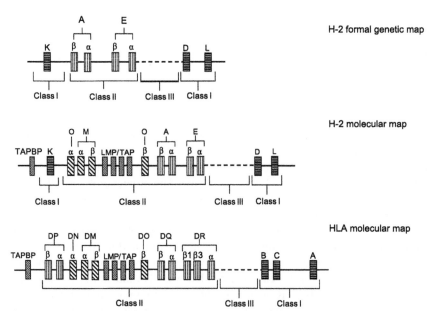

H-2 formal genetic map

H-2 molecular map

HLA molecular map

FIGURE 6.4 Genetic organization of the murine (H-2) and human (HLA) MHC. Class I (horizontal lines) and class II (vertical lines) genes encode the corresponding MHC molecules. In the class III region are genes not related to MHC proper(complement components, TNF, 21-Hydroxylase; not shown). The class II-like genes O, M, DM, DN, DO (slant lines) encode regulators of peptide binding to class II molecules. Genes TAPBP, LMP, TAP (dotted patterns) encode molecules involved in antigen processing. Pseudogenes, and class IB genes are omitted, genetic distances are not shown. Centromeres are on the left hand side. Based on References 167, 168, 174, 154, 175–180.

between the two complexes (2000 kb in mouse and 3500 kb in human), as the class I region in mouse is only about one-third that of human.[167,168] The map of the murine H-2 complex corresponds to a large extent to the one proposed previously[154] on the basis of biochemical and functional studies (see in Fig. 6.4). The class II region shows species-specific differences. Whereas the murine H-2 contains only four functional genes ($A\beta$, $A\alpha$, $E\beta$, $E\alpha$) encoding the chains of the two expressed class II molecules (I-A and I-E), the human HLA contains seven expressed genes encoding the α and β chains of the three class II molecules, DR, DQ, and DP. The I-E homologue DR is encoded in three genes of which $DR\alpha$ is practically monomorphic as is $E\alpha$ in mice, $DR\beta1$ is highly polymorphic as is the murine $E\beta$, and the second expressed $DR\beta$ gene (e.g., $DR\beta3$ shown in Fig. 6.1) has limited polymorphism and encodes another β chain detected serologically as a 'supertypic' specificity.[175] The DR α chain associates with both β chains, thus humans express two different DR molecules per haplotype. The additional class-II-like genes, namely, M and O in mice, and DM, DN, and DO in human, encode regulators of peptide binding to class II molecules.[176] Genes LMP and TAP in the class II region, as well as $TAPBP$ at the centromeric end are unrelated to either class I or class II, they encode molecules involved in antigen processing.[177,178] In the region denoted class III there are genes whose products are functionally unrelated to MHC proper, such as complement components (C4A, C4B, C2, Bf), tumor necrosis factor α and β[179,180] and the enzyme 21-hydroxylase involved in steroid synthesis.

'By and large, the molecular biology studies confirmed the latest genetic maps of MHC proposed on the basis of biochemical and functional analysis', thinks Dr. G. 'There were, however, important differences. First of all, the evidence provided at the DNA level was undisputable, it could be regarded as final. Furthermore, several new MHC-associated genes with previously unsuspected functions were discovered. And finally, these studies brought the level of understanding of the human MHC up to that of the murine MHC, or even above, which would not have been possible without molecular biology.'

REFERENCES

1. Klein J, Figueroa F, Nagy ZA. *Ann. Rev. Immunol.* 1983;**1**:119.
2. Gorer PA. *Br. J. Exp. Pathol.* 1936;**17**:42.
3. Gorer PA. *J. Pathol. Bacteriol.* 1937;**44**:691.
4. Snell GD, Jackson RB. *J. Natl. Cancer. Inst.* 1958;**21**:843.
5. Snell GD. *J. Genet.* 1948;**49**:87.
6. Gorer PA, Lyman S, Snell GD. *Proc. Roy. Soc. Ser. B* 1948;**135**:499.
7. Snell GD. *J. Natl. Cancer. Inst.* 1958;**21**:843.
8. Ivanyi P, Démant P, Vojtiskova M, Ivanyi D. *Transplant. Proc.* 1969;**1**:365.
9. Klein J. *Science* 1970;**168**:1362.
10. Amos DB, Gorer PA, Mikulska ZB. *Proc. Roy. Soc. Ser. B* 1955;**144**:369.
11. Allen SL. *Genetics* 1955;**40**:627.
12. Démant P, Cherry M, Snell GD. *Transplantation* 1971;**2**:238.
13. Snell GD, Démant P, Cherry M. *Transplantation* 1971;**11**:210.
14. Snell GD, Cherry M, Démant P. *Transplant. Proc.* 1971;**3**:183.
15. Shreffler DC. In: Aminoff D, editor. *Blood and Tissue Antigens.* New York: Acad. Press; 1970. p. 85.
16. Shreffler DC, Owen RD. *Genetics* 1963;**48**:9.
17. Lachman PJ, Grennan D, Martin A, Démant P. *Nature* 1975;**258**:242.
18. Meo T, Krasteff T, Shreffler DC. *Proc. Natl. Acad. Sci. USA* 1975;**72**:4536.
19. Shreffler DC, David CS, Passmore HC, Klein J. *Transplant. Proc.* 1971;**3**:176.
20. Nathenson SG, Cullen SE. *Biochim. Biophys. Acta* 1974;**344**:1.
21. Poulik DM, Reisfeld RA. *Contemp. Top. Mol. Immunol.* 1976;**4**:157.
22. Michaelson J. *Immunogeneitcs* 1981;**13**:167.
23. Lemonnier P, Neauport-Sautes C, Kourilsky FM, Démant P. *Immunogenetics* 1975;**2**:517.
24. Martin WJ, Ebsen E, Cotten G, Rice JM. *Brit. J. Cancer 28* 1973;**48**(Suppl.1).
25. Invernizzi G, Parmiani G. *Nature* 1975;**254**:713.
26. Garrido F, Schirrmacher V, Festenstein H. *Nature* 1976;**259**:228.
27. Festenstein H. In: Cudkowicz G, Landy M, Shearer GM, editors. *Natural Resistance Systems Against Foreign Cells, Tumours and Microbes.* New York: Acad. Press; 1978.
28. Bodmer WF. *Transplant. Proc.* 1973;**5**:1471.
29. Steinmetz M, Winoto A, Minard K, Hood L. *Cell* 1982;**28**:489.

30. Dausset J, Rapaport FT, Colombani J, Feingold N. *Transplantation* 1965;**3**:701.

31. Davies DA, Manstone AJ, Viza DC, Colombani J, Dausset J. *Transplantation* 1968;**6**:571.

32. Dausset J. *Vox Sang.* 1969;**16**:263.

33. Klein J, Egorov IK. *J. Immunol.* 1973;**111**:976.

34. Bailey DW, Snell GD, Cherry M. *Proc. Symp. Immunogenet. H-2 Syst.* 1970:155.

35. Nathenson SG. *Ann. Rev. Genet.* 1970;**4**:69.

36. Abbasi K, Démant P, Festenstein H. J Holmes B Huber, M Rychlikova, *Transplant. Proc.* 1973;**5**:1329.

37. Sorensen SF, Hawkes SP. *Transplant. Proc.* 1973;**5**:1361.

38. Schendel DJ, Alter BJ, Bach FH. *Transplant. Proc.* 1973;**5**:1651.

39. Nabholz M, Vives J, Young HM, Meo T, Miggiano V, Rijnbeck A, Shreffler DC. *Eur. J. Immunol.* 1974;**4**:378.

40. Démant P. *Transplant. Rev.* 1973;**15**:164.

41. Katchalski E, Sela M. *Adv. Protein Chem.* 1958;**13**:243.

42. Bornstein MB, Miller A, Slagle S, Weitzman M, Crystal H, Drexler E, Keilson M, Merriam A, Wassertheil-Smoller S, Spada V, et al. *N. Engl. J. Med.* 1987;**317**:408.

43. Johnson KP, Brooks BR, Cohen JA, Ford CC, Goldstein J, Lisak RP, Myers LW, Panitch HS, Rose JW, Schiffer RB. *Neurology* 1995;**45**:1268.

44. Levine BB, Ojeda A, Benacerraf B. *J. Exp. Med.* 1963;**118**:953.

45. Levine BB, Benacerraf B. *Science* 1965;**147**:517.

46. Bluestein HG, Green I, Benacerraf B, Exp J. *Med* 1971;**134**:458.

47. McDevitt HO, Sela M. *J. Exp. Med.* 1965;**122**:517.

48. McDevitt HO, Sela M. *J. Exp. Med.* 1967;**126**:969.

49. McDevitt HO. *J. Immunol.* 1968;**100**:485.

50. McDevitt HO, Chinitz A. *Science* 1969;**163**:1207.

51. Ellman L, Green I, Martin WJ, Benacerraf B. *Proc. Natl. Acad. Sci. USA* 1970;**66**:322.

52. McDevitt HO, Deak DB, Shreffler DC, Klein J, Stimpfling JH, Snell GD. *J. Exp. Med.* 1972;**135**:1259.

53. Lieberman R, Paul WE, Humphrey W, Stimpfling JH. *J. Exp. Med.* 1972;**136**:1231.

54. Melchers I, Rajewsky K, Shreffler DC. *Eur. J. Immunol.* 1973;**3**:754.

55. Urba WJ, Hildemann WH. *Immunogenet.* 1978;**6**:433.

56. Lozner EC, Sachs DH, Shearer GM. *J. Exp. Med.* 1974;**139**:1204.

57. Fachet J, Ando I. *Eur. J. Immunol.* 1977;**7**:223.

58. Dorf ME, Benacerraf B. *Proc. Natl. Acad. Sci. USA* 1975;**72**:3671.

59. Schwartz RH, Dorf ME, Benacerraf B, Paul WE. *J. Exp. Med.* 1976;**143**:897.

60. Katz DH, Hamaoka T, Dorf ME, Maurer PH, Benacerraf B. *J. Exp. Med.* 1973;**138**:734.

61. Zinkernagel RM, Doherty PC. *Nature* 1974;**248**:701.

62. Hirschhorn K, Bach FH, Kolodny RL, Firschein IL, Hashem N. *Science* 1963;**142**:1185.

63. Bain B, Vas MR, Lowenstein L. *Fed. Proc. Fed. Amer. Soc. Exp. Biol.* 1963;**22**:428.

64. Bach FH, Voynow NK. *Science* 1966;**153**:545.

65. Dutton RW. *J. Exp. Med.* 1966;**123**:665.

66. Amos DB, Bach FH. *J. Exp. Med.* 1968;**128**:623.

67. Bach FH, Widmer MB, Segall M, Bach ML, Klein J. *Science* 1972;**176**:1024.

68. Meo T, Vives J, Miggiano V, Shreffler DC. *Transplant. Proc.* 1973;**5**:377.

69. Meo T, Vives J, Rijnbeck AM, Miggiano VC, Nabholz M, Shreffler DC. *Transplant. Proc.* 1973;**5**:1339.

70. Widmer MB, Alter BJ, Bach FH, Bach ML. *Nature New Biol.* 1973;**242**:239.

71. Burakoff SJ, Finberg R, Glimcher L, Lemonnier F, Benacerraf B, Cantor H. *J. Exp. Med.* 1978;**148**:1414.

72. Nagy ZA, Kusnierczyk P, Klein J. *Eur. J. Immunol.* 1981;**11**:167.

73. Festenstein H. *Transplant. Rev.* 1973;**15**:62.

74. Kappler JW, Staerz U, White J, Marrack PC. *Nature* 1988;**332**:35.

75. MacDonald HR, Schneider R, Lees RK, Howe RC, Acha-Orbea H, Festenstein H, Zinkernagel RM, Hengartner H. *Nature* 1988;**332**:40.

76. Livnat S, Klein J. *Nature New Biol.* 1973;**243**:42.

77. Oppltová L, Démant P. *Transplant. Proc.* 1973;**5**:1367.

78. David CS, Shreffler DC, Frelinger JA, *Genetics* 1973;**74**:58.

79. David CS, Shreffler DC, Frelinger JA. *Proc. Natl. Acad. Sci. USA* 1973;**70**:2509.

80. David CS, Frelinger JA, Shreffler DC. *Transplant. Proc.* 1973;**5**:1815.

81. Hauptfeld V, Klein D, Klein J. *Science* 1973;**181**:167.

82. Hauptfeld V, Klein D, Klein J. *Transplant. Proc.* 1973;**5**:1811.

83. David CS, Shreffler DC. *Transplantation* 1974;**18**:313.

84. David CS, Shreffler DC. *Adv. Immunol.* 1975;**20**:125.

85. Cullen SE, David CS, Shreffler DC, Nathenson SG. *Proc. Natl. Acad. Sci. USA* 1974;**71**:648.

86. Nathenson SG, Ewenstein BM, Uehara H, Martinko JM, Coligan JE, Kindt TJ. In: Ferrone S, Reisfeld R, editors. *Current Trends in Histocompatibility.* ;**Vol. 1**New York: Plenum Press; 1979.

87. Uhr JW, Capra JD, Vitetta ES, Cook RG. *Science* 1979;**206**:292.

88. Orr HT, Lancet D, Robb RJ, Lopez de Castro JA, Strominger JL. *Nature* 1979;**282**:266.

89. Larhammar D, Schenning LS, Gustafsson K, Wiman K, Claesson L, Rask L, Peterson PA. *Proc. Natl. Acad. Sci. USA* 1982;**79**:3687.

90. Delovitch TL, Murphy DB, McDevitt HO. *J. Exp. Med.* 1977;**146**:1549.

91. Shreffler DC, David CS, Cullen SE, Frelinger JA, Niederhuber JE. *Cold Spring Harbor Symp. Quant. Biol* 1977;**41**:477.

92. Cullen SE, Shreffler DC, Kindle CS, David CS. *Immunogenet.* 1980;**11**:535.

93. Jones PP, Murphy DB, McDevitt HO. *J. Exp. Med.* 1978;**148**:925.

94. Mathis DJ, Benoist C, Williams II VE, Kanter M, McDevitt HO. *Proc. Natl. Acad. Sci. USA* 1983;**80**:273.

95. Tacchini-Cottier FM, Jones PP. *J. Immunol.* 1988;**141**:3647.

96. Vu TH, Tacchini-Cottier FM, Day CE, Begovich AB, Jones PP. *J. Immunol.* 1988;**141**:3654.

97. Vu TH, Begovich AB, Tacchini-Cottier FM, Jones PP. *J. Immunol.* 1989;**142**:2936.

98. Korman AJ, Boss JM, Spies T, Sorrentino R, Okada K, Strominger JL. *Immunol. Rev.* 1985;**85**:45.

99. Travers P, Blundell TL, Sternberg MJ, Bodmer WF. *Nature* 1984;**310**:235.

100. Korman AJ, Auffray C, Schamboeck A, Strominger JL. *Proc. Natl. Acad. Sci. USA* 1982;**79**:6013.

101. Benacerraf B, McDevitt HO. *Science* 1972;**175**:273.

102. Dorf ME, Benacerraf B. *Proc. Natl. Acad. Sci. USA* 1975;**72**:3671.

103. Schwartz RH, Dorf ME, Benacerraf B, Paul WE. *J. Exp. Med.* 1976;**143**:897.

104. Rosenthal AS, Shevach EM. *J. Exp. Med.* 1973;**138**:1194.

105. Schwartz RH, Jackson L, Paul WE. *J. Immunol.* 1975;**115**:1330.

106. Corradin G, Etlinger HM, Chiller JM. *J. Immunol.* 1977;**119**:1048.

107. Schwartz RH, Paul WE. *J. Exp. Med.* 1976;**143**:529.

108. Shevach EM, Rosenthal AS. *J. Exp. Med.* 1973;**138**:1213.

109. Schwartz RH, Yano A, Stimpfling JH, Paul WE. *J. Exp. Med.* 1979;**149**:40.
110. Longo DL, Schwartz RH. *J. Exp. Med.* 1980;**151**:1452.
111. Zinkernagel RM, Doherty PC. *Nature* 1974;**248**:701.
112. Erb P, Feldmann M. *J. Exp. Med.* 1975;**142**:460.
113. Shevach EM, Paul WE, Green I. *J. Exp. Med.* 1972;**136**:1207.
114. Schwartz RH, David CS, Dorf ME, Benacerraf B, Paul WE. *Proc. Natl. Acad. Sci. USA* 1978;**75**:2387.
115. Lemke H, Hämmerling GJ, Hämmerling U. *Immunol. Rev.* 1979;**47**:175.
116. Baxevanis CN, Wernet D, Nagy ZA, Maurer PH, Klein J. *Immunogenet.* 1980;**11**:617.
117. Nepom JT, Benacerraf B, Germain RN. *J. Immunol.* 1981;**127**:31.
118. Lerner EA, Matis LA, Janeway CA, Jones PP, Schwartz RH, Murphy DB. *J. Exp. Med.* 1980;**152**:1085.
119. Nagy ZA, Baxevanis CN, Ishii N, Klein J. *Immunol. Rev.* 1981;**60**:59.
120. Marusic M, Nagy ZA, Koszinowski U, Klein J. *Immunogenet.* 1982;**16**:471.
121. Blank JJ, Freedman HA, Lilly F. *Nature* 1976;**260**:250.
122. Gomard E, Duprez V, Reme J, Colombani MJ, Levy JP. *J. Exp. Med.* 1977;**146**:909.
123. Doherty PC, Biddison WE, Bennink JR, Knowles BB. *J. Exp. Med.* 1978;**148**:534.
124. Zinkernagel RM, Althage A, Cooper S, Kreeb G, Klein P, Sefton B, Flaherty L, Stimpfling JH, Shreffler DC, Klein J. *J. Exp. Med.* 1978;**148**:592.
125. Müllbacher A, Blanden RV. *Immunogenet.* 1979;**7**:551.
126. Shevach EM, Green I, Paul WE. *J Exp. Med.* 1974;**139**:679.
127. Barcinski MA, Rosenthal AS. *J. Exp. Med.* 1977;**145**:726.
128. Kappler JW, Marrack PC. *J. Exp. Med.* 1978;**148**:1510.
129. von Boehmer H, Haas W, Jerne NK. *Proc. Natl. Acad. Sci. USA* 1978;**75**:2439.
130. Matsunaga T, Simpson E. *Proc. Natl. Acad. Sci. USA* 1978;**75**:6207.
131. Hedrick SM, Watson J. *J. Exp. Med.* 1979;**150**:646.
132. Hodes RJ, Hathcock KS, Singer A. *J. Immunol.* 1979;**123**:2823.
133. Erb P, Vogt P, Matsunaga T, Rosenthal A, Feldmann M. *J. Immunol.* 1980;**124**:2656.
134. Urba WJ, Hildemann WH. *Immunogenet* 1978;**6**:433.
135. Vidovic D, Klein J, Nagy ZA. *J. Immunol.* 1985;**134**:3563.
136. Schwartz RH. *Scand. J. Immunol.* 1978;**7**:3.
137. Thomas DW, Shevach EM. *Proc. Natl. Acad. Sci. USA* 1977;**74**:2104.
138. Wilson DB, Fischer-Lindahl K, Wilson DH, Sprent J. *J. Exp. Med.* 1977;**146**:361.
139. Ishii N, Baxevanis CN, Nagy ZA, Klein J. *J. Exp. Med.* 1981:154.
140. Ishii N, Nagy ZA, Klein J. *J. Exp. Med.* 1982;**156**:622.
141. Clark RB, Shevach EM. *J. Exp. Med.* 1982;**155**:635.
142. Vidovic D, Matzinger P. *Nature* 1988;**336**:222.
143. Ishii N, Baxevanis CN, Nagy ZA, Klein J. *Immunogenet.* 1981;**14**:283.
144. Nagy ZA, Baxevanis CN, Ishii N, Klein J. *Immunol. Rev.* 1981;**60**:59.
145. Rock KL, Benacerraf B. *J. Exp. Med.* 1983;**157**:1618.
146. Debré P, Kapp JA, Dorf ME, Benacerraf B. *J. Exp. Med.* 1975;**142**:1447.
147. Rock KL, Benacerraf B. *J. Exp. Med.* 1984;**160**:1864.
148. Babbitt BP, Allen PM, Matsueda G, Haber E, Unanue ER. *Nature* 1985;**317**:359.
149. Schaeffer EB, Sette A, Johnson DL, Bekoff MC, Smith JA, Grey HM, Buus S. *Proc. Natl. Acad. Sci. USA* 1989;**86**:4649.
150. Lemonnier P, Neauport-Sautes C, Kourilsky FM, Démant P. *Immunogenetics* 1975;**2**:517.
151. Murphy DB, Herzenberg LA, Okumura K, Herzenberg LA, McDevitt HO. *J. Exp. Med.* 1976;**144**:699.

152. Tada T, Taniguchi M, David CS. *J. Exp. Med.* 1976;**144**:713.

153. Klein J, Figueroa F, CS David. *Immunogenet.* 1983;**17**:553.

154. Klein J, Juretic A, Baxevanis CN, Nagy ZA. *Nature* 1981;**291**:455.

155. Baxevanis CN, Nagy ZA, Klein J. *Proc. Natl. Acad. Sci. USA* 1981;**78**:3809.

156. McKenzie IFC, Henning M. *Immunogenet.* 1976;**3**:253.

157. Benacerraf B, Germain RN. *Immunol. Rev.* 1978;**38**:70.

158. Okuda K, David CS. *J. Exp. Med.* 1978;**147**:1028.

159. Rich SS, Rich RR. *J. Exp. Med.* 1976;**143**:672.

160. David CS, Cullen SE. *J. Immunol.* 1978;**120**:1659.

161. Juretic A, Protrka N, Walden P, Nagy ZA, Klein J. *Scand. J. Immunol.* 1983;**18**:515.

162. Waltenbaugh C. *J. Exp. Med.* 1981;**154**:1570.

163. Ikezawa Z, Baxevanis CN, Arden B, Tada T, Waltenbaugh CR, Nagy ZA, Klein J. *Proc. Natl. Acad. Sci. USA* 1983;**80**:6637.

164. Steinmetz M, Minard K, Horvath S, McNicholas J, Frelinger J, Wake C, Mach B, Hood L. *Nature* 1982;**300**:35.

165. Ploegh HL, Orr HT, Strominger JL. *Proc. Natl. Acad. Sci. USA* 1980;**77**:6081.

166. Steinmetz M, Frelinger JG, Fisher D, Hunkapiller T, Pereira D, Weissman SM, Uehara H, Nathenson S, Hood L. *Cell* 1981;**24**:125.

167. Carroll MC, Katzman P, Alicot EM, Koller BH, Geraghty DE, Orr HT, Strominger JL, Spies T. *Proc. Natl. Acad. Sci. USA* 1987;**84**:8535.

168. Stephan D, Sun H, Fischer-Lindahl K, Meyer E, Hämmerling G, Hood L, Steinmetz M. *J. Exp. Med.* 1986;**163**:1227.

169. Carle GF, Olson MV. *Nucleic Acids Res.* 1984;**12**:5647.

170. Steinmetz M, Moore KW, Frelinger JG, Sher BT, Boyse EA, Hood L. *Cell* 1981;**25**:683.

171. Strominger JL. *J. Clin. Invest.* 1986;**77**:1411.

172. Ploegh HL, Orr HT, Strominger JL. *Cell* 1981;**24**:287.

173. Hood L, Steinmetz M, Malissen B. *Ann. Rev. Immunol.* 1983;**1**:529.

174. Steinmetz M, Minard K, Horvath S, McNicholas J, Srelinger J, Wake C, Long E, Mach B, Hood L. *Nature* 1982;**300**:35.

175. Spies T, Sorrentino R, Boss JM, Okada K, Strominger JM. *Proc. Natl. Acad. Sci. USA* 1985;**82**:5165.

176. Kelly AP, Monaco JJ, Cho S, Trowsdale J. *Nature* 1991;**353**:571.

177. Deverson EV, Gow IR, Coadwell WJ, Monaco JJ, Butcher GW, Howard JC. *Nature* 1990;**348**:738.

178. Trowsdale J, Hanson I, Mockridge I, Beck S, Townsend A, Kelly A. *Nature* 1990;**348**:741.

179. Spies T, Morton CC, Nedospasov SA, Fiers W, Pious D, Strominger JL. *Proc. Natl. Acad. Sci. USA* 1986;**83**:8699.

180. Müller U, Jongeneel CV, Nedospasov SA, Fischer-Lindahl K, Steinmetz M. *Nature* 1987;**325**:265.

Chapter 7

Antigen Processing and Presentation

Although antigen presentation and partially also antigen processing are functions of the MHC, their discussion deserves a separate chapter, because the goal of the research to be described under this title was to elucidate a particular biological mechanism, in contrast to classical MHC research that aimed at the characterization of a gene system. Thus MHC research, although it touched upon several immunological phenomena, was basically genetics, whereas the study of antigen processing and presentation belongs to the realm of immunology, or in a broader context to cell biology. Nevertheless, this separation remains somewhat artificial, particularly if one considers that none of the previous studies came as close to the understanding of the true biological function of MHC as the ones on antigen processing and presentation.

7.1 THE RULES OF PEPTIDE BINDING TO MHC MOLECULES

7.1.1 T Cell Epitopes

The notion that the antigenic determinants (or epitopes) for T cells are different from the ones seen by B-cell immunoglobulins had been around for a long time before the nature of T-cell epitopes was recognized. The seminal observation came again from Benacerraf's lab: as early as in 1959, Gell and Benacerraf[1] showed that ovalbumin (OVA)-sensitized guinea pigs could mount a delayed type hypersensitivity reaction to both native and denatured OVA equally well, whereas only native OVA could induce anaphylaxis. Their conclusion was that the antigenic requirements for cellular and humoral immune response were different. This translates precisely into physically different T- and B-cell epitopes in contemporary language. The reader should be reminded that T and B cells were not yet known at that time.

> 'The deeper you venture into history, the more you realize how strong Benacerraf's influence was on the entire field', comments Dr. G. 'One gains the impression that he discovered just about everything worth discovering in immunology.'
>
> 'Once I managed to grab the word, I would like to take the opportunity and make a comment on the history of immunological terminology. A good example

A History of Modern Immunology. http://dx.doi.org/10.1016/B978-0-12-416974-6.00007-7

at hand is how antigenic determinants became epitopes. Obviously the original term implies that certain parts of a molecule determine antigenicity. But some immunologists frowned and claimed not to understand this, because in principle any area on the surface of a protein could be recognized by an antibody. It was then Jerne, if I remember correctly, who suggested to use the uncommitted term epitope, being something that is recognized by a paratope. "Oh yes, this we understand" said most immunologists, from which I can only conclude that they were better in Greek than in Latin. Ironically, it has turned out later that T-cell epitopes do determine the immunogenicity of the whole protein, i.e., they are true determinants. Yet it was the term epitope that survived. Why? Probably because this is shorter.'

The study of antigenicity then went to dormancy for more than a decade, but the puzzle posed by the Gell and Benacerraf observation caught the fancy of some immunologists including very imaginative ones, such as Hans Wigzell and Eli Sercarz. In the 1970s a few studies were performed, all confirming that antibodies require the antigen to be intact, whereas T cells are satisfied with denatured antigen or even fragments thereof.[2–4] Subsequently, Sercarz and colleagues[5] identified B- and T-cell epitopes in hen egg-white lysozyme (HEL) by using HEL peptides obtained by cyanogen bromide cleavage. Besides showing that B- and T-cell epitopes localized in different fragments, they also demonstrated by using species variants of HEL that T-cell recognition was sensitive to single amino acid differences.

'Sorry to interrupt you again, but I cannot resist to say at this place a few words about Eli Sercarz, who was one of the most original figures in immunology', cuts in Dr. G. 'This applies to both his appearance and his mind. Eli was big, sloth-like, wore long hair like a hippy, and his social behavior was characterized by a lightly embarrassed absent-mindedness. All this endowed him with an awkward charm so that you could not help but like him. Throughout his professional life, Eli did only one thing: he investigated the immune response to HEL. And by doing this he discovered a series of important general principles in immunology. He demonstrated to all of us that the talented can gain a good understanding of the world by merely looking at it through a pinhole.'

The conclusion from the studies up to this point has been that while immunoglobulins recognize conformational determinants on the surface of proteins, the antigenic information for T cells resides in short linear amino acid sequences. However, this interpretation did not account for the finding that T cells were also able to utilize intact proteins as antigens. To explain the latter, it was proposed that globular proteins first had to be rendered antigenic for T cells by degradation into short fragments: the concept of 'antigen processing' was born.

Subsequent efforts were focussed on a more precise definition of T-cell epitopes. The first epitopes to be identified were the dominant epitope of HEL, corresponding to sequence 46–61 by Unanue and colleagues,[6] and the dominant OVA epitope in sequence 323–339 by Howard Grey and his group.[7] The epitopes were also manufactured as synthetic peptides, and were shown to induce the same T-cell response as the intact proteins. These findings were then extended to class I epitopes by Alain Townsend and colleagues in England: they have shown that the epitopes of influenza nucleoprotein recognized together with class I MHC molecules by cytotoxic T cells correspond to short peptides of the antigen.[8,9] It thus seemed generalizable that T cells recognize antigen in the form of MHC-bound short peptide sequences.

The HEL 46–61 peptide was then used by Unanue and colleagues to demonstrate a selective binding of a T-cell epitope to a particular class II MHC molecule in their groundbreaking study[10] (discussed in Section 6.2.6). Shortly thereafter, Grey and colleagues[11] reported that the OVA 323–339 peptide behaved similarly, i.e., showed selective binding to certain class II molecules.

These studies have led to a view of T-cell epitopes as being peptides, some residues of which bind to the MHC molecule, while others are exposed for recognition by the antigen receptor of the T cell. The hypothesis was also testable experimentally. The approach taken was to test a series of single amino acid substituted analogues of the epitope in two different assays: first, the response of a T cell clone (or T cell hybridoma) to the analogue peptide, and second, the inhibition of presentation of the original epitope by the analogue. An analogue that was not stimulatory for T cells was assumed to have lost either MHC binding or T-cell recognition. If the same analogue was inhibitory in the competition assay, the implication was that it still bound to MHC, and thus the tested residue should be involved in contacting the T-cell receptor. If the analogue failed to compete, it was assumed not to bind to MHC. Thus, this experimental system permitted to classify each amino acid of the peptide epitope as either MHC contact residue or T-cell contact residue. Indeed, this approach, when applied to the two 'star' epitopes, HEL 46–61 and OVA 323–339, resulted in the identification of MHC and T-cell contact residues, and even residues that were contacted by both MHC and T cell, whereas some positions in the peptides turned out to be neutral.[12,13] However, the interpretation of the results remained somewhat uncertain, because the conformation of MHC-bound peptides was unknown. In fact, the data on the HEL epitope were consistent with an α-helical peptide conformation, whereas the OVA data suggested an extended conformation. Thus peptide conformation had remained a hotly debated issue that could only be resolved by X-ray crystallography of peptide–MHC complexes many years later.

At this point, the tenor of epitope studies was clearly taken over by the Grey group. They have demonstrated in an extensive study[14] that peptide binding to a particular MHC molecule always correlates with a T-cell response to the same peptide–MHC complex, and from this they have concluded that the long sought for mechanistic explanation for MHC restriction is indeed a specific interaction between the peptide and the restricting MHC molecule. Furthermore, they have shown that each MHC molecule possesses a single peptide binding site, which can bind many different peptide sequences as long as they have the proper MHC contact residues.

All these pioneering studies launched the so-called 'peptide revolution' yielding an ever-increasing list of characterized T-cell epitopes that has filled a sizable database by now.

'Howard Grey was a quiet man, who had resided for ages in Denver, and whose epithet in immunology circles was "a solid biochemist",' adds Dr. G. 'This was perhaps meant to be a recognition of his qualities, but it was not entirely flattering, because immunologists thought at that time that the public display of eccentric personality was an obligatory attribute of scientific greatness. Howard was definitely not the person to put up at egomaniac shows, but he was a clear thinker. He knew that the puzzle of T-cell recognition could be approached from two sides: from the receptor and the ligand, respectively, and that he could only reasonably contribute to the latter. And this is what he did. I should also mention here at least one more person, who significantly contributed to Howard's studies. This was Alessandro Sette, an Italian postdoc, who shortly before was only famous for his driving of his subcompact Autobianchi like a madman in the chaotic traffic of Rome. But his thinking was just as fast as his driving, and his ambition was enormous. He added a great deal of dynamics to the Grey group, an essential constituent of top performance.'

7.1.2 Peptide-Binding Motifs for Class I MHC Molecules

The epoch-making study of Unanue and colleagues[10] demonstrating that a peptide epitope can bind to a particular MHC molecule but fails to bind to another allotype (allelic form) of the same molecule has clearly indicated a certain degree of specificity in peptide–MHC interactions. But this specificity appeared unusual: on the one hand, the binding of a particular peptide to a given MHC molecule was specific, on the other hand, the same MHC molecule was expected to bind a large number of various peptide sequences to fulfill its antigen-presenting function. For most immunologists, who viewed specificity on the basis of antigen–antibody interactions as a perfect complementarity between two protein surfaces, it was difficult to envisage how these two, virtually contradictory properties of peptide–MHC interaction could be reconciled.

A possible solution to this dilemma was offered by a model emerging from epitope studies. It has proposed that the side chains of specific amino acids at fixed (anchoring) positions of the peptide should interact with the MHC binding site, whereas the remaining peptide positions should not be relevant for MHC binding, and could thus be occupied by any amino acid residue. The side chains of the latter have been assumed to point outwards from the binding site and are thus available for recognition by T cells. The prediction from this model has been that diverse peptides binding to a particular MHC molecule should all have the same or a physical-chemically equivalent residue at the anchor positions, or conversely, shared residues at the same positions of a diverse set of MHC-binding peptides should represent anchor residues. The anchor residues together with their peptide position were proposed to constitute a so-called binding motif. A motif was assumed to be characteristic of a particular MHC molecule, and to be different from that of another MHC molecule, or even from that of another allotype of the same molecule.

The model was put into test first for class I MHC molecules due to a fortunate incident. Namely it has turned out that peptides binding to class I molecules are all uniform in size: they are nine amino acids long for most MHC types, with the exception of only a few MHC types that bind eight amino-acid-long peptides. The pioneering work on class I binding motifs was performed by Rammensee and his colleagues.[15] They isolated the class I molecule to be tested from a cell line by immunoprecipitation with a monoclonal antibody, eluted its peptide content by acid treatment and purified the peptides using reversed-phase high-performance liquid chromatography. The heterogeneous peptide mixture was then subjected to Edman degradation, a method by which amino acids from the N-terminus are cleaved off one by one, and identified. They performed this analysis for three different murine (K^d, K^b, D^b) and one human (HLA.A2.1) class I molecule. The results have clearly demonstrated in each peptide mixture the existence of two anchor positions, at which only a single, or two closely related amino acids could be identified. At the remaining, non-anchor positions a variable number (4–14) of different amino acids were found, indicating that these positions were probably not involved in interactions with the MHC molecule.

A representative sample of class I binding motifs is compiled in Table 7.1. The analysis of this motif information permits a few interesting conclusions even in the absence of knowledge about the structure of the MHC binding site.

Perhaps the most striking aspect of motifs is that the overall peptide binding mode is highly conserved across all class I allotypes, isotypes (H-2K, D, L, and HLA.A, B, C), and even across species. All class I molecules appear to bind peptides via two anchors, one of which is always located at the C-terminus of peptides at position 9 (or position 8 in octamers), and the other one close to the N-terminus, in most cases at position 2. In addition to the obligatory anchors, some motifs possess one or more auxiliary anchors at various peptide positions that may increase binding affinity. The majority of anchor residues have non-polar side chains of different sizes (small: A, P, V; large: L, I, M) or aromatic rings (F, Y). These side chains can be envisaged to extend into hydrophobic cavities of different sizes in the MHC molecule, and engage in hydrophobic interactions. Some anchor positions are occupied by charged amino acids (basic: K, R, H; or acidic: D, E) that may form salt bridges with residues of the opposite charge in the MHC molecule. Altogether, this simple

TABLE 7.1 Peptide Binding Motifs for Class I MHC Molecules

MHC Molecule[a]	Peptide Position									References
	1	2	3	4	5	6	7	8	9	
H-2K^d		Y, F[b]							I, L, V	15,20
H-2K^k		E						I, V	--[c]	20,21
H-2D^b					N				M, I, L	15,20
H-2L^d		P, S							F, L, M	20,22
HLA.A*01		T, S[d]	D, E				L		Y	23,20
HLA.A*0201		L, M				V			V, L	15,20
HLA.A*0206		V							V	20,24
HLA.A*0207		L	D						L	20,25
HLA.A*0217		L	P						L	21,26
HLA.A*2902		E	F						Y	20,26
HLA.A*3001		Y, F							L	20,27
HLA.A*6601	E, D	T, V							R, K	20,28
HLA.B*07		P	R						L, F	20,29
HLA.B*0703		P	R					E	L	20,30
HLA.B*0705		P							L	20,30
HLA.B*08			K		K, R				L	20,31
HLA.B*1801	D	E			L				F, Y	20
HLA.B*2701		R							Y	20,32
HLA.Cw.*0102		A, L							L	20,33
HLA.Cw*0401		Y, P, F				V, I, L			L, F, M	34

a: Murine (H-2) and human (HLA) molecules. b: Single letter code for amino acids. c: no position 9 (octamer peptide). d: auxiliary anchors are underlined.

and rather archaic binding mode may enable the binding of a large number of different peptides with sufficient affinity.

Another interesting conclusion is that, despite the conserved binding mode, the binding motif for each class I molecule is unique. The difference between individual motifs is in some cases substantial (hydrophobic vs. charged anchor, or different anchoring positions), whereas in other instances it is minimal or restricted to auxiliary anchors. Usually, the motifs of closely related MHC subtypes exhibit only subtle differences (as illustrated in Table 7.1 by subtypes of HLA.A*02 and HLA.B*07). But completely identical binding motifs occur very rarely, and even in those cases the sets of preferred residues at non-anchor positions are different. The consequence of this arrangement is that each MHC molecule will bind a distinct set of peptides, and that the sets bound by different MHC molecules will overlap with each other.

It follows from their binding mode that MHC molecules cannot distinguish between self peptides and peptides derived from intracellular pathogens. Indeed the bulk of peptides eluted from class I molecules turned out to match with sequences from abundant self proteins.[16,17]

'The champion of class I motifs, Hans-Georg Rammensee, started his carrier as a PhD student in my laboratory', adds Dr. G. 'This is one of the few facts along my scientific carrier that I can be proud of without reservation. Hans-Georg was a quiet youngster, small, lean, and humble, very different from what many think Germans should be like. Perhaps this had to do with his descent, as his ancestors were Huguenots, who had to flee from France to Germany in the eighteenth century to escape the persecution of Protestants. His thesis was on minor histocompatibility antigens, a set of mysterious entities that causes rejection of MHC-identical grafts, and induces a cytotoxic T-cell response. However, they fail to trigger antibody production, and for this reason it appeared hopeless at that time to identify the molecules responsible for rejection. But Hans-Georg was as firm in belief as his ancestors, and finally he was the one who found out that minor histocompatibility antigens were nothing else but peptides from polymorphic self proteins bound to class I MHC molecules.[18,19] Thereby he solved a 30-year-old puzzle in immunology. After his postdoctoral training he took a position at Jan Klein's Department of Immunogenetics in Tübingen, and with his work on class I–peptide interactions he managed to overshadow his gigantic boss. A modern story of David and Goliath.'

7.1.3 Peptide-Binding Motifs for Class II MHC Molecules

The determination of class I binding motifs, efficient and straightforward as it went, could unfortunately not serve as a template for class II motif studies. The complications with class II became immediately apparent upon the characterization of peptides naturally bound to these molecules.

The first study in this direction was performed by Janeway and coworkers.[35] They isolated and sequenced peptides eluted from two murine class II molecules, I-A^b and I-E^b. The first surprise was that these peptides were 13–17 amino acids long, i.e., much longer than the ones binding to class I molecules, and in addition variable in length. The bulk of eluted peptides represented only a small set of sequences, and a single species of peptide occurred often in various lengths, resulting from differential cleavage of their C-termini. Thus, natural class II ligands were clearly not suitable for pool sequencing, because their different lengths made a proper alignment for Edman degradation practically impossible. Furthermore, a motif information could not be extracted from the data due to the limited heterogeneity of sequences. Apart from these discouraging messages, the study revealed some interesting aspects of class II ligands. First, the majority of sequences derived from self proteins, but in contrast to class I molecules that present cytosolic proteins, the class-II-bound peptides were from cell membrane molecules. Second, sequences from foreign proteins taken up by the cells from the culture medium were also detectable. And finally, the sets of peptides bound to the two different class II molecules were clearly distinct.

'Many immunologists found it surprising that this organic chemistry type of study had come from Charlie Janeway's lab', recalls Dr. G. 'The reason for this was that immunology had become compartmentalized into sub-specialities by that time, and most colleagues considered Charlie to be a cellular immunologist. But this assessment was wrong. For Charlie was an all-rounder, belonging to the remaining few, who preferred to think about the immune system as a whole. And the question of class II ligands appeared to him to be the next one to answer, in order to gain new information about the system.'

'Actually, I must admit that I look upon the phenomenon of sub-specialization with some skepticism. It always occurs of necessity, when a field becomes too complex to be kept in mind. Although it may be helpful in going into more detail, it tempts you at the same time to give up thinking about the actual subject of your discipline. I read a funny definition of it in the 1960s in a periodical entitled *The Journal of Irreproducible Results* that used to deal with humorous aspects of science. Unfortunately the journal was not long-lived, because too many colleagues had lost their humor in the fierce competition for research funds. The definition ran thus: "If you keep telling the same nonsense for at least ten years, you'll be considered a specialist".'

'Returning to Charlie, I should mention that he was a special person in many respects. One of his distinguishing marks was the Jr tag behind his name that he kept well into his fifties, and so he was likely to be the oldest junior you could possibly meet. Another was his stentorian voice that would have sufficed for playing a Greek tragedy in an open-air setting. But most importantly, he was the author of an immunology textbook[36] that not only provided evidence for his all-rounder capabilities, but was also the best of its kind ever written. He was deadly ill already, when he wrote this book, and could survive to see just the beginning of its extraordinary success. Meanwhile a whole generation of immunologists has grown up, whose first encounter with their discipline was through Charlie's "Immunobiology", or "Janeway's" as they call it.'

Several additional studies were then performed to characterize peptides binding to different class II molecules, such as I-A^d (Ref. 37) DR1 (Ref. 38), DR2, DR3, DR4, DR7, DR8 (Ref. 39), and DR11 (Ref. 40). All data were in agreement about the average length of class II binding peptides (13–18 residues). The overwhelming majority of peptides were shown to derive from endogeneously synthesized proteins, mostly from the MHC itself or other cell-membrane-bound molecules, as well as from secreted proteins. A few peptides originated from external proteins probably taken up by endocytosis. Sets of peptides of different length from the same protein were repeatedly identified. They appeared to result from differential cleavage at both N- and C-termini. Some peptides were uniquely found in association with a particular class II molecule, whereas others showed degenerate binding to several different molecules. A sad common denominator of all these otherwise interesting studies was the failure to identify any useful binding motif.

Many colleagues, including those working on T cell epitopes, used a different strategy in the expectation of arriving at binding motifs. They started their analysis with a known T-cell epitope, and a peptide-binding assay. (The latter existed in many different formats, but most of them were competition assays, in which unknown ligands were tested as competitors with a labelled indicator peptide for binding to a class II molecule.) Because the epitope under investigation was usually quite long, the first goal was to define a 'core' binding region by sequential truncation at both ends of the peptide. Once the binding core, i.e., the shortest peptide without significant loss of binding affinity was defined, it was subjected to alanine-scan (sequential replacement of each residue with alanine) to identify side chains important for binding. Where a residue was found to be important for binding it was regarded an anchor candidate, and for its validation, all known peptides binding to the same class II molecule (usually 10 to <100) were searched for the presence of the same residue at the expected position.

The most informative study in this vein was the one reported by Jardetzky et al.[41] These authors investigated the binding of a flu hemagglutinin peptide, HA 306–318, and a number of its substituted variants to HLA-DR1. They found that a single tyrosine residue at peptide position 3 (308 in the hemagglutinin sequence) was essential for binding, whereas substitutions at the remaining positions had no or only minimal effect. This was most dramatically illustrated by a peptide in which all residues were exchanged to alanine except the obligatory tyrosine, and yet, it was able to bind to DR1 with an affinity similar to that of the HA 306–318 peptide. They concluded from these data that peptide binding to DR1 required only a single obligatory side chain anchor, and assumed that the remaining peptide interacted with the binding site, predominantly via the conserved peptide backbone. Additional side chains were considered to increase or decrease binding affinity, or to have no effect. Subsequent binding studies have confirmed the existence of an obligatory hydrophobic anchor close to the N-terminus of peptides binding to different DR allotypes.[42,43] This site, referred to as p1, was rather permissive, although some DR allotypes seemed to prefer aliphatic (L, I, V, M), and others aromatic (F, Y) side chains. Some studies have also suggested that additional, auxiliary anchors may exist at relative positions 4, 6, and 9 of

DR binding peptides.[42–44] The conserved features of peptide binding to DR molecules, i.e., the p1 anchoring site and interactions with the peptide backbone, were attributed to the monomorphic DR α-chain shared by all DR allotypes, and different side chain preferences at other sites were assumed to be due to the polymorphic DR β-chains. By this interpretation, different DR molecules would be able to bind the same set of peptides on the one hand (a phenomenon termed 'promiscuity'), but show some degree of selectivity on the other. Both of these characteristics had been observed before in DR-binding peptide epitopes.

The obligatory p1 anchor served as a good reference point to align DR-binding peptides, and permitted also an attempt by Rammensee and colleagues[45] to define DR binding motifs by pool sequencing of naturally bound peptide mixtures. In fact, their study pushed the pool-sequencing technology to its limits, because a single anchor was usually found in at least three adjacent sequencing cycles instead of a single one, due to the different lengths of peptides in the pool. Nevertheless this study did result in some motif-information, and also confirmed certain data obtained with synthetic peptides.

'Altogether, the experiments discussed so far revealed some characteristics of peptide binding to class II molecules, but the binding motif information extracted from these data remained incomplete and somewhat vague', comments Dr. G. 'The reasons for this were clear for everybody involved. First, as already pointed out, the length differences of class II binding peptides made an objective alignment almost impossible. Second, the sequence diversity of peptides binding to a particular class II molecule was too low. Considering, for example, a nine-amino-acid-long binding core, the total combinatorial diversity of class II binding peptides would be 20^9 , i.e., $\sim 5 \times 10^{11}$, and thus the ~10 to 100 sequences per class II molecule available for these studies represented a minute, statistically insignificant sample. Thus any anchor identified could have been in error resulting from the infinitesimally small sample size. Third, because the binding peptides did not necessarily use all anchoring sites, auxiliary anchors could not be identified with any degree of certainty. Under these conditions it is a small miracle that many pieces of information from these studies have remained valid. This success could, however, be ascribed to the "art of experimentation" rather than the experimental system used.'

The breakthrough in class II motif studies was brought about by a novel technology: the construction of phage display libraries comprising vast numbers of random peptides.[46–48] By this technology, random oligonucleotides are inserted into the pIII gene of filamentous phages (e.g., the M13 bacteriophage of *E. coli*). This gene encodes a minor coat protein, protein III, expressed in five copies on the surface of the phage. The random nucleotide sequences translate into random peptides of defined length at the N-terminus of protein III, known to extend from the phage surface, and thus accessible for binding to antibodies or other receptors. Random peptide libraries constructed this way contain 10^7–10^8 different peptide sequences. Thus this method had the potential to circumvent the two major problems of class II motif studies, namely variable peptide length and too small sample size. Selection of tightly binding phages from the library is achieved by a procedure termed panning, a version of affinity purification. Phages are allowed to bind to a biotinylated receptor, the complexes are immobilized on a streptavidin-coated surface, unbound phages are washed away, and the bound ones eluted. Usually 3–4 rounds of panning result in a very strong enrichment of peptide sequences binding to the receptor with high affinity.

'This technology was adapted to the study of class II motifs by a PhD student, Juergen Hammer, in Francesco Sinigaglia's laboratory', adds Dr. G. 'Juergen belonged to the new generation of molecular biologists, who were no longer just "gene cloners", but preferred to think in terms of large-scale genetic screening procedures. He chose the right laboratory for his studies at Hoffmann La Roche Inc., first, because there was a strong industrial interest in gene libraries, and second, because Francesco belonged to those few colleagues, who succeeded in maintaining high scientific standards in an industrial setting. In addition to being bright, Juergen was also very efficient, and this combination was key to his success. According to Francesco "he was the best student I have ever seen". Later, after I had had the opportunity to "borrow" him as a postdoc for one year, I could only confirm Francesco's statement.'

'Juergen chose to construct a random nonapeptide library displayed on the M13 phage for class II binding studies. The length of nine amino acids was a critical element of design, because this was long enough to encompass all expected anchor positions, but much shorter than the average class II binding peptides. This way the number of conserved main chain interactions was significantly reduced, and the contribution of individual side chains to binding could be assessed much more clearly. The library contained $>2 \times 10^7$ different sequences, i.e., it was large enough to minimize the possibility of sampling error. As a kind of validation, he panned first the library on DR1, for which the most detailed binding motif information was available from previous studies. The results[49] confirmed the previously found anchor sites at positions 1, 6, and 9, and identified another hydrophobic anchor at position 4. Moreover, the motif obtained was extremely clear, because it was based only on the tightest binding sequences. For example, at position 1 only aromatic residues were detected, because the aliphatic residues that also allow binding of longer peptides,[43] provided insufficient affinity to qualify as good binders in the nonapeptide library. At further anchor positions, one or two best-fitting residues were identified, and all non-fitting or suboptimally fitting residues found before,[43,45] were eliminated by the phage library approach. And these results did not reflect the limit of the technology, as we have found out later that additional minor anchors can be identified by increasing the stringency of the washing steps after panning.[50] He then extended his studies to DR4 and DR5, (DR11) and the resulting motifs revealed that the anchors at p1 and p4 were conserved among the tested DR allotypes, whereas the p6 anchor was allotype specific.'[51]

The most conclusive HLA-DR binding motifs are summarized in Table 7.2. The data permit the following conclusions about the rules of peptide binding to DR molecules:

1. At p1, two different patterns occur: either a preference for aromatic side chains (Y, F, W) or for aliphatic residues (I, L, M, V) plus F, but no Y and W.
2. The preference for R at the p2 auxiliary anchor site seems to be conserved.
3. The p4 site is largely conserved, it requires hydrophobic residues with some exceptions (e.g., the acidic residue D in DRB1*0301).
4. The p6 site shows allotype-dependent variations.
5. The presence of p7 and p9 anchor sites varies by allotype: some have either p7 or p9, others have both or neither. Usually hydrophobic side chains are preferred at these two positions (except p9 in DRB1*0405 that requires acidic residues D or E).

Perhaps it is worth mentioning that motif information is only available for a dozen DR allotypes,[54] whereas the majority (additional >100) has not been investigated for peptide binding.

The peptide-binding modes of the additional human class II isotypes (DQ and DP) have remained largely undefined. The few studies undertaken in this direction suggest that the binding mode of DQ (and its murine analogue I-A) may be fundamentally different from that of DR (analogous to I-E in mice), and consequently, the peptide repertoires bound by these two isotypes are complementary with little overlap.[55–58] Thus, whereas different allotypes of the same class II isotype bind peptides with a degree of cross-reactivity, there appears to be a clear inter-isotype selectivity. Interestingly, among class I isotypes this degree of selectivity cannot be observed: they have very similar peptide-binding modes, and are thus more 'interchangeable'. Probably this explains why the so-called 'immune response gene-effect' (i.e., the association of certain immune responses with a single MHC isotype; see in Section 6.2.5) was only observed with class II but not with class I MHC. The peptide-binding mode of DQ molecules was finally elucidated by crystallographic studies, but equivalent information for DP molecules is not available.

'The history of class II binding motifs provides a good example for the incompleteness of scientific quest', points out Dr. G. 'It would be hard to overlook that the class II molecules for which detailed motif information was generated were almost exclusively the ones genetically associated with autoimmune disease. Thus the primary driver of these studies was to find out whether the disease association of these molecules was related to peptide binding specificity or not. The remaining molecules (i.e., the great majority) were deemed to have too low scientific impact to make the investment worthwhile. The causes behind such a decision can be manifold, for example, technical, financial, or personal aspects commonly referred to as the "human factor". Therefore, many areas of scientific investigation

TABLE 7.2 Peptide Binding Motifs for HLA-DR Molecules

HLA-DR Molecule[a]	Peptide Position									Reference
	1	2	3	4	5	6	7	8	9	
DRB1*0101	Y, F, W[b]	R		M, L		A, G, S	L, I, V		L, M, A	49,50,51
DRB1*0401	Y, F, W	R		M, L, A, V		T, S, N	L, I, V, Q, M, N		–	50,51,52,53
DRB1*0404	I, L, M, F, V	R		M, L, I, F		T, S, N, V	L, I, M, N		–	53
DRB1*0405	Y, F, W	R		M, F		T, S, N,	F, Y, L, N		E, D	54
DRB1*1101	Y, F, W	R		M, L, V		R, K	–		–	50,51
DRB1*0301	I, L, M, F, V	n.d.[c]		D		R, K, E, Q, N	–		F, Y, L	44,54

a: allele designations for the polymorphic β chains are shown. b: single letter code for amino acids. c: not detected by the method used.

remain, as a rule, only partially explored, except when a fast, simple, and possibly cheap method is available that enables a complete "harvest".'

7.2 THE MOST REVEALING CRYSTALLOGRAPHIC STUDY IN THE HISTORY OF IMMUNOLOGY: THE THREE-DIMENSIONAL STRUCTURE OF MHC MOLECULES

7.2.1 The Peptide-Binding Site of Class I Molecules

The abundant peptide-binding information generated for MHC molecules would not have permitted, per se, to form an idea about the structure of the peptide-binding site. The most common belief about the latter was that it might be analogous to the antigen-combining site of immunoglobulins. This notion was obviously based on sequence homologies between MHC and immunoglobulin. But a number of colleagues were even skeptical about the existence of a specific MHC-binding site at all. Under these circumstances, the exploration of the three-dimensional structure of MHC molecules was highly desirable.

The first successful crystallographic study was performed with the human class I molecule, HLA-A2, in Don Wiley's laboratory at Harvard University. The protein chemistry part of this work was done at Jack Strominger's Biochemistry Department. The results were presented as two adjacent leading articles in *Nature* by Bjorkman et al.[59,60] in 1987. It is important to note that, at that time, the peptidic nature of both class-I- and class-II-associated T-cell epitopes was already known, but a specific interaction between peptides and MHC was only shown for class II (see Section 7.1.1). Thus the characterization of ligand and binding site proceeded simultaneously, although not in perfect synchrony, obviously for technical reasons.

The first paper[59] described the overall structure of the four extracellular domains of the class I molecule ($\alpha 1$, $\alpha 2$, $\alpha 3$, plus $\beta 2$ microglobulin; $\beta 2m$), and at the same time provided an eye-opener for immunologists. As expected on the basis of sequence homologies, the two membrane proximal domains ($\alpha 3$, $\beta 2m$) had immunoglobulin folds. However, the membrane distal $\alpha 1$ and $\alpha 2$ domains had a structure that immunologists had neither seen nor expected before. These two domains turned out to be structurally similar, each of them consisting of four antiparallel β-strands followed by a long helical region. The two domains are paired by intramolecular dimerization so that the four β-strands from each domain form a single, eight-stranded β-pleated sheet, and this is topped by the two α-helical regions (one from each domain). This structure is located on the top of the molecule with the helices facing away from the cell membrane (Fig. 7.1). A large groove between the α-helices was proposed to provide a binding site for peptides. This was all the more likely, because a region of unresolved electron density was noted in the groove that was not accounted for by the HLA chain itself. This density was interpreted as bound ligands that co-purified and co-crystallized with HLA-A2.

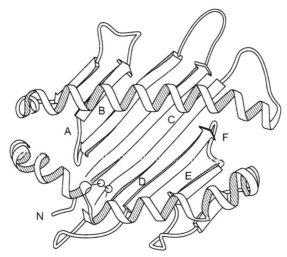

FIGURE 7.1 Schematic representation of the peptide-binding site of the HLA-A2 class I molecule. The binding site is shown as viewed from the top of the molecule, showing the surface contacted by the T-cell antigen receptor. The α1 and α2 domain helices, the amino terminus (N) of the molecule, and the approximate location of specificity pockets A through F, are indicated. From Reference 59, pocket locations according to Reference 61. (Reprinted by permission from Macmillan Publishers Ltd: *Nature* **329**, issue 6139, © 1987.)

'The beauty about this structure was that it was fully self-explanatory', points out Dr. G. 'Even laymen could conceive that here was an unusual-looking binding site resembling the mouth of a catfish, the size and shape of which was appropriate for accommodating a peptide.'

'Shortly after the discovery I met Pam Bjorkman at Lee Hoods laboratory in Pasadena, and she asked me the following question: "What do you think, why was the electron density in the groove unresolved?" "I guess you will tell me" was my answer. "It was unresolved, because each HLA molecule in the crystal bound a *different* peptide." Thus this observation has provided the first direct proof for the hypothesis that MHC molecules are non-specific, or more exactly oligospecific peptide receptors. Admittedly, before Pam's explanation I had found this concept hard to believe.'

The follow-up report[60] dealt with the purported peptide binding site in more detail. A very interesting fact borne out by this study is that 15 of the 17 polymorphic amino acid positions in class I molecules (i.e., positions showing high variability in 22 human class I sequences) are located in the binding site region. Five of them are on the central β-strands, and are thus likely to interact with the peptide directly. Further polymorphic sites are located on the helices, and six or seven of them could participate in peptide binding, whereas three or four of them are facing the solvent. The latter could make direct contacts with the antigen receptor of T cells. Even the remaining two polymorphic residues that are not located on helices or β-strands are close enough to have an indirect influence on the binding site. These data have strongly suggested that the polymorphism of MHC is associated with peptide binding, and that the latter may represent the evolutionary driving force for the former. Furthermore, a number of highly conserved residues were identified in the binding site, but at that time it was unclear whether they were involved in peptide binding or served to maintain the molecular structure.

To obtain more precise information about the interaction of the binding groove with its ligands, the structure of HLA-A2 was refined to 2.6 Å resolution[61] (from 3.5 Å), and the structure of two additional class I molecules, HLA-Aw68 (Ref. 62) and HLA-B27 (Ref. 63), was determined at high resolution. These studies led to a new level of understanding.

The most important news was the identification of six 'pockets' or sub-sites within the binding cleft (denoted A through F). Pockets A and F were located at the extreme ends, whereas B and C at the junction of the β-sheet with the α1 helix, and D and E close to the α2 helix (Fig. 7.1). The pockets were shown to be lined with side chains of MHC residues, and appeared suited to bind individual side chains from peptides. Since information about the bound peptides (see 'motifs' in Section 7.1.2) became available simultaneously with these studies, one could envisage that pocket A would bind the N-terminal peptide residue, p1, pocket B would accommodate p2, pocket C p6, pocket D p3, pocket E p7, and pocket F the C-terminal p9 (in case of nonamer peptides). The surface of some pockets was found to be predominantly hydrophobic, but others, especially those at the ends (A and F) exhibited clusters of polar atoms. Many residues lining the pockets, particularly the central ones, were identified as polymorphic, and could thus account for binding specificity differences between MHC molecules.

Under improved resolution, the previously unresolved 'extra electron density' in the groove also gained a better definition. It could be interpreted as a mixture of nonameric peptides in extended conformation, with clear definition of the main chain and of several side chains. Peptides eluted from class I molecules were reported to be nonamers[15] at almost exactly the same time, and thus the two sets of data confirmed each other nicely.

Despite improved resolution, the final details could not be deciphered by the use of MHC crystals binding a mixture of different peptides, because different side chains at the same peptide position still resulted in a 'blur', and the peptide main chain could also assume different conformations depending on the sequence. Therefore, crystals of MHC molecules complexed with a single peptide were required. This technically difficult task was first accomplished at the Scripps Institute in La Jolla, by crystallographer Ian Wilson together with the bright Swedish MHC biochemist Per Peterson, who had moved there from Uppsala shortly before. They managed to crystallize the murine class I molecule H-2K^b together with two different virus-derived peptides.[64,65] One year later, Wiley and colleagues reported their results on five different crystallized peptide–MHC complexes.[66] Taken together, these two sets of data provided answers, as final as technically possible, to all open questions.

Perhaps the most important observation of these studies was that both ends of the peptide were bound tightly via a network of hydrogen bonds formed between side chains of highly conserved MHC residues and the NH3- and COOH-termini of peptide, as well as backbone atoms of the first and last two peptide residues. This binding mode appeared to be universal, applying to all human and murine class I molecules. Fixing of the ends was the obvious cause for the extended conformation of peptides in the groove. The backbone amide and/or carbonyl groups of additional peptide residues were also shown to form hydrogen bonds with MHC side chains. Indeed, in some peptide–MHC complexes, the backbone of every single peptide residue was hydrogen-bonded to MHC. The fixation of peptide ends was further stabilized by the interaction of pocket B with the p2 side chain, and of pocket F with the p9 side chain. (Pocket A was found to interact only with the peptide NH3-terminus, while the side chain of p1 was solvent exposed.) The selective or specific aspects of peptide binding were shown to result from interactions between polymorphic pockets and peptide side chains. Interestingly, the class I cleft turned out to be 'closed' at both ends by large conserved residues (Y and W) in pockets A and F, with the result of restricting the length of accepted peptides to 9 ± 1 residues. Altogether, the class I binding site was shown to engage in a large number of interactions with the peptide, some of which were peptide sequence-independent (via the peptide backbone and termini), and others specific (via peptide side chains). This ambivalency of the binding site explains how a single class I type can form tight complexes with a large number of peptides with diverse sequences.

An enigmatic finding from these studies has been that 73–83% of the solvent-accessible surface of peptides is buried upon binding to MHC, raising the question of how the T-cell receptor can find sufficient variability of presented antigens. The answer given by crystallography was perfectly satisfactory, although more complex than immunologists would have wished. Namely, it has turned out that while the termini of peptide are fixed and almost completely buried, its central portion (p4–p7) is exposed, and in addition, the peptide backbone in this region undergoes substantial, sequence-dependent conformational adjustments. The conformational variations include both sideward shifts toward the $\alpha 1$ or $\alpha 2$ helix, and a twisting of the main chain along its length. The combined effect of these displacements is to alter the position as well as the orientation of peptide side chains. In other words, every single peptide side chain in this region can be presented to T cells in a number of fundamentally different ways. Thus, the diversity of antigenic surface seen by T cells would probably exceed by at least one order of magnitude the combinatorial variability of amino acids at four positions ($20^4 = 1.6 \times 10^5$).

'There was only one question, in which the two cystallographer groups did not agree completely', adds Dr. G 'and this concerned the effect of peptides on the overall conformation of the binding site. While both groups agreed that the peptide sequence-dependent conformational changes in the α1 and α2 domain main chain were small, Wilson considered these changes significant,[65] but Wiley argued that they were either within the estimated coordinate error, or could be explained by crystal contacts.'[66]

'The idea that ligand conformation should be instrumental for T-cell recognition is deeply rooted in immunology. It dates back to the "altered self" hypothesis,[67,68] according to which T cells recognize, instead of foreign antigens, antigen-induced modifications of self molecules. This hypothesis might be praised as a visionary foresight of peptide–MHC complexes, but as stated, it could not lead anywhere conceptually, indeed, it represented a nice piece of immunological agnosticism. Nevertheless, it had many followers, who would have warmly welcomed some support from crystallography. It was good luck that Wiley managed to nip this in the bud!'

7.2.2 The Peptide-Binding Site of Class II Molecules

The three-dimensional structure of a class II molecule was first reported in 1993, 6 years after that of class I. Although a class I homology-based model of class II molecules was already published in 1988, this model,[69] besides being hypothetical, could not precisely account for the differences in terms of peptide binding between the two classes. Therefore, scientists of the class II arena could not have had a more ardent wish than to see finally the crystal structure of a class II molecule.

The first class II molecule to be crystallized was HLA-DR1, and this was again achieved in Don Wiley's laboratory.[70] Because this work coincided almost perfectly with the discovery of class II binding motifs, the two approaches benefited from each others' results significantly.

As predicted by the model[69] of 1988, the overall structure of DR1 turned out to be similar to that of HLA class I. The two domains of the DR1 α-chain, α1 and α2, superimposed closely on the α1 domain of class I and β2-microglobulin, and the two β-chain domains, β1 and β2, on the α2 and less closely on the α3 domain of class I. The binding site, as that of class I, was shown to be composed of an eight-stranded β-sheet floor, and two antiparallel helical regions at the sides. Half of the site was contributed by the α1 and the other half the β1 domain of the two class II chains.

However, a number of differences between class I and class II were also noted, particularly at the ends of the peptide-binding site. These differences help explain why class I binds short, nonameric peptides, whereas class II prefers longer 15–24-residue peptides. First, two N-terminal turns of the α1 domain helix of class I are replaced by a stretch of extended chain in class II, resulting in a more open 'left' end. Second, the C-terminal end of class II α1 helical region bends more toward the floor than the corresponding class I region, opening up the 'right' end of the site. Third, the β1 helical region of DR1 also ends in an extended chain, instead of the short helix seen in class I, further widening the right end. In addition to these differences in the secondary structure, the large conserved amino acids that bind both termini of the peptide in the class I site are not found in class II sequences. Also absent from class II are a nearly conserved tryptophan and a salt bridge that close the left end of the class I binding site. All these changes enable the class II site to bind peptides of arbitrary length.

The class II binding site also contained 'extra electron density' that appeared straight and thin, consistent with peptides in an extended conformation. Its length corresponded to 15 peptide residues contacting the binding site, and additional residues projecting out of both ends of the site. One prominent peptide side chain was seen at about the third position of a 15-mer that identified a binding pocket located at the extreme left end of the site. This pocket, surrounded predominantly with hydrophobic residues, corresponds to the p1 anchoring site identified by peptide-binding studies. Three clusters of polymorphic residues were also seen in the binding site that were assumed to interact with further peptide side chains. In addition, a number of hydrogen bonds between conserved MHC residues and the peptide backbone were identified as side-chain-independent, 'universal' components of binding.

The fine details of class II–peptide interaction were then analyzed in crystals of HLA-DR1 complexed with a single peptide.[71] The peptide chosen for this study was HA306-318 from influenza virus hemagglutinin, an extensively characterized immunodominant epitope.

'In fact, the HA306-318 peptide was so instrumental to class II studies that everyone in the field knew its amino acid sequence by heart. I can still remember it (PKYVKQNTLKLAT) from a distance of 16 years' adds Dr. G.

The HA peptide was seen to be bound to DR1 as an extended strand with the N- and C-termini projecting out of the ends of the binding site. All peptide residues, except the C-terminal 318T, appeared to contact the protein. A surprising finding was that the peptide assumed a twisted conformation in the binding site, so that the successive side chains projected from the backbone about every 130°. This conformation is characteristic of the type II polyproline helix. As a consequence of the main chain twist, approximately every third side chain projected away from the binding site, whereas the remaining residues projected towards or across the site (Fig. 7.2). As was observed with class-I-bound peptides, the bulk of the HA peptide was buried in the DR1 groove, approximately 35% of it remaining solvent-accessible. The total area potentially available for interaction with the T-cell receptor was about the same (400–500 Å^2) as for class I–peptide complexes.

The 'universal' component of peptide binding was shown to be provided by 15 hydrogen bonds between the DR1 protein and main chain atoms of the HA peptide. They were spaced almost evenly along the peptide, and 12 of them involved conserved amino acid residues of the protein. There were three bidentate hydrogen bonds, formed between conserved asparagins and both carbonyl

(a)

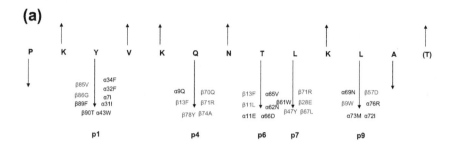

(b)

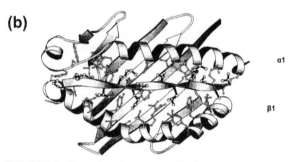

FIGURE 7.2   Interactions between peptide HA306-318 and the HLA-DR1 binding site. (a) Every peptide residue except 318T contacts the binding site. Side chains (arrows) of individual residues point either up toward the solvent, or down toward the binding site. Side chains of five residues extend into sub-sites or pockets in the binding site shown as p1, p4, p6, p7, and p9, according to the relative peptide positions. Protein residues lining each pocket are shown, polymorphic residues in grey. Based on Reference 71. (b) Localization of the HA peptide in the HLA-DR1 binding site. The peptide assumes an extended conformation with a twist, similar to a polyproline type II helix. Helices formed by the α1 and β1 domain of HLA-DR1 are indicated. From Reference 71. (Reprinted by permission from Macmillan Publishers Ltd: *Nature* **368**, issue 6468, © 1994.)

oxygen and amide nitrogen of the respective peptide residues. Disruption of any of the bidentate bonds (e.g., by backbone N-methylation of the respective peptide residue[72]) resulted in a drastic loss of binding affinity, underlining the critical role of these bonds, possibly in maintaining the twisted peptide conformation.

Within the binding site several smaller cavities or 'pockets' were identified, five of which accommodated side chains of the bound HA peptide (Fig. 7.2).

The side chain of peptide residue 308Y was buried in a large prominent hydrophobic pocket at the left end of the site, identified also in the previous study.[70] This pocket corresponding to the position 1 anchoring site (p1) demonstrated in binding studies (see Section 7.1.3) is a major determinant of peptide binding to HLA-DR molecules. Much of this subsite is conserved, explaining why many different DR molecules prefer a hydrophobic side chain at this position. Specificity of this pocket is modulated by a glycine/valine dimorphism at position β86 of the protein: DR molecules with β86G (e.g., DRB1*0101, 0401,

0405) prefer large aromatic side chains (F, Y, W) but can also bind aliphatic side chains (L, I, M) with lower affinity, whereas molecules with β86V (e.g., DRB1*0301, 0404) prefer smaller hydrophobic side chains (I, L, M, V, F) and cannot accommodate Y and W (see Table 7.2).

Four additional HA peptide side chains (311Q, 313T, 314L and 316L) were sequestered in pockets of the DR1 binding site. These pockets were smaller, more shallow and less hydrophobic than p1, and more permissive for different side chains. The side chain of 311Q lay in a large shallow pocket (p4 in Fig. 7.2) that could also bind a variety of aliphatic side chains, but seemed to disfavor positively charged residues (K, R) probably because of electrostatic repulsion with β71R. Polymorphism of this pocket can change its specificity, for example DRB1*0301 accepts a negatively charged residue (D) presumably because of the A to R substitution at position β74. The side chain of 313T was completely buried in a shallow pocket (p6 in Fig. 7.2) with a preference for small residues. The shallow pocket p7 accepted the side chain of 314L that was not completely buried by the interaction. Finally, the side chain of 316L pointed into a small hydrophobic pocket (p9 in Fig. 7.2).

In summary, the almost complete concordance of peptide-binding data involving several different DR molecules with the three-dimensional structure of HA306-318 in HLA-DR1 indicates that DR molecules may bind peptides in essentially the same conformation as DR1 binds the HA peptide. The twisted conformation of the main chain is probably a critical element of binding, because this allows the direction of different peptide side chains towards the appropriate binding pockets. One major pocket (p1) appears to be essential for binding, while the remaining four pockets can remain unused, or when used are rather permissive for a variety of side chains. Because of this permissiveness and the sequence-independent main chain interactions, a large number of peptides with diverse sequences can bind to HLA-DR molecules.

Don Wiley and his group used X-ray crystallography as a tool to address an additional series of biological questions. For example, they studied the interaction of DR molecules with the class-II-associated invariant chain,[73] the binding of class II molecules with 'superantigens' (proteins that crosslink class II molecules with T cell receptor V regions and cause massive T-cell activation),[74,75] and the interaction of autoimmune disease-associated DR molecules with autoantigenic peptides.[76,77]

'Don Wiley was an outstanding figure of structural biology in the twentieth century' points out Dr. G. 'His broad biological interest, ranging from viruses to MHC molecules, always provided the primary motivation for him to find a structural basis for the phenomena of his choice. Indeed, he was more than a crystallographer in the traditional sense: he can be considered as a founder of a new branch of science, nowadays referred to as three-dimensional biology.'

'A brief meeting I had with Wiley on peptide–class II interactions convinced me promptly about his scientific and human qualities. He was extremely lucid and fast in thinking, open in discussions, and his sympathetic, vital personality made him appear at least 15 years younger than his age. It was a great loss and a shock for the community that he left us so early and under so dramatic circumstances. As known, he was reported lost in November 2001 in Memphis, where he attended a meeting, and his body was found weeks later in the Mississippi river. Influenced by the events of that year, some suspected an attack by terrorists. What actually happened has remained a mystery, but Wiley's memory is too valuable for us to permit any further speculation.'

The peptide-binding mode of HLA-DQ and of its murine homologue I-A was far more difficult to determine than that of HLA-DR even by X-ray crystallography. The reasons for this were twofold. First, a clear peptide-binding motif could not be determined for most DQ and I-A molecules. And second, in contrast to DR molecules that are composed of a polymorphic β and a monomorphic α chain, DQ and I-A molecules are made up of two polymorphic chains, and thus display less constant features.

Because previous studies had identified a very different peptide repertoire bound to DQ/I-A compared to HLA-DR (see Section 7.1.3), the expectation was that the peptide-binding mode of these two class II isotypes should differ fundamentally from one another. However, this assumption was not unequivocally supported by crystallographic studies.[78–81] The overall structure of DQ/I-A molecules turned out to be, with minor differences, like that of HLA-DR, including the presence of five pockets, p1, p4, p6, p7 and p9, in the binding site. Peptides were bound in the groove in an extended type II polyproline conformation, as observed in other class II structures. The hydrogen-bonding network between the DQ proteins and the main chain of peptides was also comparable to that seen in DR–peptide complexes.

The most distinctive structural feature of QA/I-A molecules compared to others in class II was the presence of a β bulge on the β-sheet floor, located in the first strand of the α1 domain. The bulge was formed by two residues protruding above the β sheet: a tyrosine replacing glutamine at the α 9 position of HLA-DR, and an inserted glycine next to it. Sequence comparisons suggested that the β bulge should be a conserved feature of all DQ and I-A molecules. This seemingly minor structural change was shown to result in an altered hydrogen-bonding network that pulls the middle portion of the peptide deeper into the groove. The groove itself was found to be narrower than that of HLA-DR mostly due to the acquisition of proline residues in the α-helical walls. Some of these proline residues were found unique to DQ and I-A molecules, and appeared to be essential for maintaining the structure of the groove and its capability to bind peptides.[82]

A surprising feature of peptide binding to DQ and I-A molecules borne out by these studies was that most pockets in the binding groove were only partially filled. Although some pockets exhibited side-chain preferences, for example, p1 of I-A^k for D,[78] p4 of DQ8 for Y,[81] and p9 of DQ8 and I-A^{g7} for E,[80,81] in general, a precise filling of pockets did not seem to be required for high-affinity binding. In fact, even poly-alanines were shown to bind to these molecules with reasonable affinity.[81]

The conclusion from these studies has been that peptide binding to DQ and I-A molecules is characterized by a very loose specificity: apparently none of the five binding pockets in the binding groove needs to be fully occupied for stable association with peptides. Consequently, the selectivity of peptide binding to these molecules is not explained by polymorphic differences in peptide-binding pockets, but is rather due to steric collisions of particular peptide side chains with the binding site. The three-dimensional structure of DQ/I-A molecules does not fully explain their unique peptide-binding mode, although the narrow binding groove and the deep position of bound peptide are likely to contribute to an increased stability of binding.

7.3 ANTIGEN PROCESSING AND LOADING PATHWAYS

7.3.1 Initial Evidence for Antigen Processing

As pointed out already, the concept of antigen processing has emerged from the necessity to explain a set of experimental findings showing that T cells can recognize denatured antigens just as well as native proteins, and small peptide fragments equally well as the whole protein (see Section 7.1.1). These observations suggested that the antigenicity of proteins for T cells would lie in the primary amino acid sequence, in contrast to B-cell epitopes that seemed to depend on the secondary/tertiary structure of proteins. Provided that T cells recognize short amino acid sequences, native proteins could only be recognized equally well, if the immunogenic sequences were located exclusively on the protein surface. This hypothesis would predict that, at least in some instances, when the protein surface lacks T-cell epitopes, the whole native protein should be non-immunogenic for T cells. However, this was not observed in reality. Therefore, an alternative concept was introduced proposing that native proteins would not be recognized by T cells at all, before they became 'processed', i.e., broken down into short peptides. Under this hypothesis processing was considered to be an obligatory step taking place during the time that elapsed between the administration of antigen and the T-cell recognition event.

It may be of interest to point out that the notion of antigen processing had deeper roots too. Michael Sela[83] working with his synthetic amino acid copolymers noted already in the 1960s that the immunogenicity of polymers depended strictly on their metabolizability. This finding that might have appeared enigmatic at that time, became easy to interpret by processing, and thus it can be regarded as an early experimental foundation on which the concept of antigen processing is based.

The first experiments specifically addressing the concept of antigen processing were performed by Ziegler and Unanue.[84,85] These authors studied the uptake and ingestion of *Listeria monocytogenes* by macrophages, and detected the appearance of T-cell relevant antigen on the cell surface by the binding of *Listeria*-specific T cells to macrophages. In this experimental system, *Listeria*-primed T cells exhibited antigen-specific, class II MHC-restricted adhesion to macrophages previously fed with *Listeria*, but failed to bind either to macrophages alone or to the native bacteria. The key observation from these studies was a time-lag of 30–60 minutes between the uptake of bacteria and the presentation of antigen. During this time the bacteria were ingested and partially catabolized. The appearance of T-cell relevant antigen was inhibited by ammonia and cloroquine, agents that are known to increase the pH in lysosomes, and thereby inhibit the activity of lysosomal enzymes. The data have been interpreted to indicate that T-cell epitopes arise by lysosomal degradation of antigens and subsequent appearance of the 'processed' antigenic fragments on the cell surface. However, the evidence obtained from these experiments was circumstantial, and thus did not convince everybody.

An Occam's razor type of approach to the problem of processing was then taken by the Denver immunology unit comprising at that time Howard Grey's group and the Kappler and Marrack couple.[86] To define antigen processing more precisely, they subjected a model antigen, ovalbumin (OVA), to different treatments, such as denaturation with urea, reduction and alkylation, chemical degradation, or protease digestion. The preparations thus obtained were compared with native OVA for antigenicity using a series of OVA-specific T-cell hybridoma as responding cells and a B-cell lymphoma (A20) as antigen-presenting cell (APC). When live A20 cells were used as APC, all antigen preparations were more or less equally active. In contrast, glutaraldehyde-fixed APCs that were unable to catabolize OVA could present chemically or enzymatically fragmented OVA but neither the native nor the denatured antigen. These results have suggested that antigen fragmentation is a necessary and sufficient processing step to produce a T-cell-relevant form of antigen.

'For fairness sake, I should point out that the "cell-free processing" approach taken by the Denver group also provided only indirect evidence' comments Dr. G. 'Yet it was sufficient to convince most immunologists about antigen processing as being biological reality. In retrospect, the almost unanimous acceptance of this mechanism is not easy to rationalize. Certainly, immunological thinking at that time already incorporated the notion that T cells recognize antigen in a special form, and thus antigen processing seemed to make teleological sense. However, the biological necessity behind antigen processing and presentation was not really understood yet, and therefore, the predilection for this concept could have only reflected a kind of collective immunological instinct.'

Years later, the gap between native protein antigen and peptide epitopes was closed by studies demonstrating that the most abundant peptides eluted from class II molecules of APC fed with native hen egg-white lysozyme (HEL) corresponded to the immunodominant epitopes of HEL.[87,88]

Up to this point, antigen processing and presentation were understood as a sequence of events starting with the uptake of antigen, followed by partial degradation of the antigen in lysosomes, loading of the resulting peptides onto class II molecules, and finally, the translocation of peptide-loaded class II molecules to the surface of APC. However, this picture was further complicated by the finding that viral antigens were shown to be presented by class I MHC molecules also in the form of peptides.[89] Moreover, the immunogenic viral proteins were localized in the cytoplasm or nucleus of infected cells and not in lysosomes, indeed they were synthesized in the host cell, and not taken up from outside by endocytosis.[90] Another study showed that an exogenous protein, normally presented only by class II, when targeted artificially to the cytoplasm became presented by class I molecules.[91] These results have led to the concept that the loading of peptides onto class I and class II MHC molecules may occur by two separate pathways: class I molecules are loaded at a thus far unknown location with peptides generated in the cytosol, whereas class II molecules acquire peptides derived from proteolytic fragmentation of endocytosed molecules probably within lysosomes. Of course, this idea sounded familiar for immunologists, who knew very well that T-cell activation via class I and class II MHC molecules, respectively, have entirely different functional consequences. The novel aspect was, however, that the two classes of MHC molecule were proposed to provide antigenic information from two separate intracellular compartments, namely, the cytosol and the endocytic vesicular system.

Subsequent years witnessed a new wave of MHC research aimed at the characterization of the two antigen-processing and -loading pathways. Immunology revealed new facets in the course of these studies. For example, for the first time in its modern history, it abandoned the lymphocyte, and turned its attention to the previously underrated 'accessory cell'. Furthermore, instead of focussing only on the cell surface, it ventured into the cytoplasm. Altogether, this research resembled general cell biology more than immunology. The final result from this novel approach was an impressive collection of data, on which our present knowledge about antigen processing and loading is based.

7.3.2 The Class I Pathway

The first question to be raised about the class I pathway was, how proteins would be processed into peptides in the cytosol. The most likely candidates for cytosolic processing appeared to be the proteasomes, large protease complexes of 20–30 subunits that are present in the cytoplasm in great numbers.[92,93] The assumed role of proteasomes in antigen processing has been substantiated by data demonstrating that two proteasome subunits (termed LMP-2 and LMP-7) are encoded within the MHC,[94–97] and their expression is co-regulated with that of MHC molecules by γ-interferon.[98] There have also been data demonstrating that the LMP subunits are responsible for protein cleavage next to a hydrophobic residue that would fit into the C-terminal F pocket of the class I binding site.[99] However, class I loading with peptides has been shown to occur also in the absence of LMPs,[100,101] and thus the latter do not seem to play an exclusive role in the production of class-I-binding peptides. Nevertheless, the proteasomes have remained the most likely machinery for cytosolic antigen processing.

The proteins available for cytosolic processing are those synthesized endogeneously, including host proteins as well as proteins of pathogen (e.g., virus) origin. Exceptions are secreted and cell membrane proteins that translocate into the endoplasmic reticulum (ER) lumen upon translation, and are therefore not available for processing in the cytosol. Exogenous proteins are, as a rule, not processed in the cytosol for class I presentation, with the exception of a few that can traverse membranes.

Class I MHC molecules are known to assemble in the ER and follow the constitutive secretory pathway through the Golgi complex to the cell surface.[102] It has also been shown that the association of peptides with class I occurs in the ER.[103,104] Thus the question has arisen how the processed peptide fragments can reach from the cytosol to the class I binding sites that are located in a different cellular compartment. This question was answered by the discovery of a new transporter molecule termed TAP (transporter associated with antigen processing). The TAP molecule is a heterodimer belonging to the ABC (ATP-binding cassette) transporter family. It is encoded by two closely linked genes within the class II region of MHC (next to LMP).[105] Cell lines carrying a mutation of either gene are unable to assemble stable class I molecules and fail to present intracellular antigens. TAP is localized to the ER and *cis*-Golgi,[106] and has been shown to be responsible for the transport of short peptides from the cytosol to the ER lumen.[107,108] These peptides are then loaded onto class I molecules.

Thus, class I molecules are 'fully loaded' already at the site of their own assembly in the ER. Indeed, peptide binding itself is part of the assembly process, without which a stable, conformationally correct class I-β2 microglobulin complex cannot form.[109] The binding of peptide to class I resembles the association of protein subunits rather than a classical receptor–ligand interaction, and accordingly, the resulting complexes are very stable. Before moving to the Golgi complex, class I molecules must undergo 'quality control' provided by a chaperone molecule termed calnexin. Calnexin retains class I molecules not properly associated with peptide and β2 microglobulin in the ER.[110]

The pathway described above (Fig. 7.3) appears to be solely responsible for class I presentation of peptides produced by the protein catabolic machinery of the cytosol. But would the opposite also apply? Namely, would all peptides presented by class I be originated from the cytosol? This does not seem to be the case. There is a set of data demonstrating that antigens taken up in the form of particles (e.g., bacteria, cellular debris) by phagocytosis can be presented by class I molecules although the antigens never reach the cytosol.[111–114] In this 'alternative' pathway the class I molecules are most likely loaded within the vacuolar compartment, but the details of the loading process have not been elaborated. The biological significance of this pathway is not quite clear, one

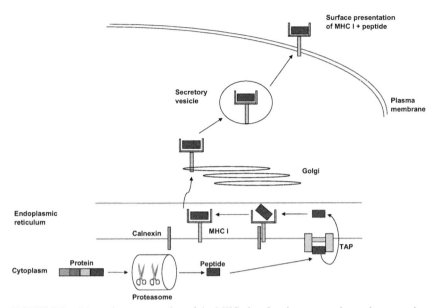

FIGURE 7.3   Schematic representation of the MHC class I antigen processing and presentation pathway. Based on References 99, 102–104, 107, 108, 110.

can only assume that it allows for the induction of cytotoxic T-cell responses to intracellular pathogens that remain in the endocytic vesicle system.

7.3.3 The Class II Pathway

The reader, who is willing to pay a tribute of admiration for the ingenuity of nature would probably find the class II presentation pathway even more instructive and amazing than the class I pathway. For the class II pathway (Fig. 7.4) provides some unusually clear examples of how nature has solved certain defined mechanistic problems.

The major 'operational' problem about this pathway must have been that class II molecules were destined to bind peptides in the endosomal compartment, and thus a mechanism had to evolve to keep their peptide binding site unoccupied, from the point of their assembly in the endoplasmic reticulum (ER) throughout their intracellular transport to the Golgi apparatus and finally to endosomes. This task was assigned by nature to the so-called invariant (Ii) chain.

The Ii chain was discovered in 1979 by Pat Jones in Hugh McDevitt's laboratory, as a constant set of spots in class II immunoprecipitates electrophoresed in two dimensions.[115] Conspicuous was that the constant spots coincided with all different allelic forms of class II molecules, the latter giving rise to greatly variable sets of spots. It was thus reasonable to assume that the invariant moiety might be physically associated with all class II molecules. Genetic studies have

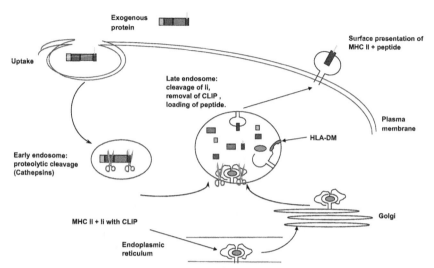

FIGURE 7.4   Schematic representation of the MHC class II antigen processing and presentation pathway. Based on References 115–120,122,126,133.

shown that the Ii protein is encoded outside the MHC, but the *Ii* gene shares promoter/enhancer elements with class II genes suggesting a co-regulation. The Ii molecule itself has turned out to be a type II transmembrane glycoprotein of more than 200 amino acids. Unfortunately, the biochemical characterization of this molecule did not provide any clue to its function, and so the latter remained an enigma for another decade. Finally, cell biology studies in the early 1990s permitted an insight into the function of this mysterious protein. The intracellular path of Ii was shown to start in the ER, where it combines with class II αβ heterodimers, and remains associated with them during their transport through the Golgi complex. Upon reaching the endosomal compartment, the Ii chains are proteolytically cleaved away from class II molecules.

During its coexistence with class II molecules, the Ii chain seems to perform a series of different functions. First, it acts as a chaperone, helping the class II α and β chains to fold into proper heterodimers, promoting the transport of properly folded heterodimers through Golgi, and directing their glycosylation.[116] Second, the cytoplasmic domain of Ii seems to be involved in targeting the class II molecules to acidic endosomes, where the processing of antigens takes place.[117,118] Finally, and most interestingly, the Ii chain, as long as it is associated with class II molecules, effectively shields the binding site of the latter from binding peptides.[119,120] All these functions have been deduced from experiments with mutant cell lines and knockout mice deficient of Ii that exhibit a series of aberrations, including misfolding and deficient transport of class II molecules, lower cell surface expression, and defects in antigen presentation.[121]

The part of Ii that covers the class II binding site corresponds to sequence 81–105, and is referred to as CLIP (class II MHC associated Ii peptide).[122] The mechanism by which CLIP protects class II molecules from binding of peptides is simple: it occupies exactly the same site that is required for the binding of other peptides,[123,124] i.e., it acts as a competitive antagonist. Analysis of the CLIP sequence has revealed that its core binding region (sequence 91–99) forms a 'supermotif' that permits the binding to many, or possibly all, class II molecules.[125] It is thus conceivable that this sequence is the result of a tight and thorough evolutionary selection, in which the selective pressure was on the ability to interact with *all* class II peptide-binding sites (the 'punishment' side must have been that class II molecules unable to bind CLIP became non-functional in the presentation of endosomal antigens).

However, the elegant evolutionary solution for shielding of the class II binding site had its price: namely, after proteolytic cleavage of the Ii chain CLIP remains bound, and therefore, an additional mechanism is required that would facilitate the exchange of CLIP with other peptides present in the endosome. To solve this problem nature reached back to a toolbox that was most obvious for the purpose, namely the MHC itself. The molecule of choice was HLA-DM (H-2M in mice), an $\alpha\beta$ heterodimer highly homologous to class II proteins, and is also encoded by genes in the class II region of MHC.[126] Its three-dimensional structure is similar to that of 'classical' MHC molecules, with the difference that the peptide-binding site is almost completely occluded except for a single large pocket in its center.[127,128] HLA-DM molecules are expressed in the endocytic vesicles to which class II molecules migrate, and become associated with the latter after cleavage of the Ii chain. Details of how they perform their function are unclear, but it is certain that their binding to class II molecules is followed by an accelerated removal of the CLIP peptide, and in addition, of all peptides that lack appropriate anchor residues.[127–129] For this reason HLA-DM is often referred to in the literature as a 'peptide editor'. In addition to its catalytic function, HLA-DM seems to stabilize empty class II molecules, even co-migrates with the latter to lysosomes, until they find a tightly binding peptide.[130,131] Upon binding of a peptide with appropriate anchors, DM molecules detach from class II. The function of DM molecules was also confirmed in vivo, in H-2M-deficient (knockout) mice. These mice were shown to express normal amounts of cell surface class II molecules, but most of them were associated with the CLIP peptide.[132]

However, HLA-DM turned out not to be the ultimate player in class II loading. For completion of the loading process an additional MHC-encoded class II like molecule, HLA-DO (H-2O in mice), was shown to be required as a negative regulator of HLA-DM.[133]

'As promised at the beginning of this section, the class II loading pathway does provide a couple of interesting insights into the working principles of evolution', adds Dr G. 'First, as exemplified by HLA-DM, and DO, evolution always prefers to work on genes with a track record of success, instead of making new ones from scratch. In these instances, copies of class II genes produced by gene duplication seem to have been modified until the proteins they encoded became suitable to perform completely different functions. This is one of the most commonly used strategies of evolution that can be traced back in many different molecular systems. The second, perhaps even more interesting aspect is that the functions of Ii, DM, and DO give us an idea of how interlinked mechanisms could have evolved. The principle here is that evolution strives for functionality, not for perfection. Thus, the Ii chain satisfactorily performs the function of shielding the peptide-binding site of class II molecules, but leaves the CLIP peptide behind. To remove the latter, another mechanism provided by HLA-DM was therefore required. However, the HLA-DM-mediated peptide exchange might have been working "too well", and thus it required negative regulation performed by HLA-DO. The picture arising from this example shows us that evolution tends to correct the shortcomings of one mechanism by a second one, and the weakness of the second one by a third one, and so forth. This procedure – that prompted Susumu Ohno[134] to call evolution a tinkerer – finally leads to the incomprehensible complexity commonly called life.'

Concerning the exact location of the class II peptide loading compartment, a certain degree of uncertainty has remained in the literature. At least three different locations were reported, namely, early endosomes,[135] early lysosomes,[136] and a specialized compartment distinct from these two, referred to as CIIM[137] or CIIV.[138,139] There are two possible ways to reconcile these data: first, peptide loading may occur in all three compartments, or alternatively, it occurs in different compartments in different types of antigen-presenting cells (i.e., dendritic cells, B cells, and macrophages). Another subject of debate was whether peptides would be loaded to newly synthesized class II molecules,[140] or to those recycled from the cell surface.[141] Since these two possibilities are not mutually exclusive, it is reasonable to assume that both could occur in real life.

7.4 THE CASE FOR A SPECIALIZED ANTIGEN-PRESENTING CELL

Around 1970, when in vitro studies of lymphocyte responses became technically feasible, a new surprising finding caused excitement in the immunological community. This was the observation that T and B lymphocytes were not sufficient for the induction of immune responses. At least one, third cell type was shown to be required, which did not participate itself in the immune response but was indispensable for its initiation.[142–145] This ill-defined, non-lymphoid cell type was termed 'accessory cell'.

The identity of the accessory cell was a hotly debated issue in the 1970s. The findings that these cells were in the blood and in spleen cell suspensions, but they were neither lymphocytes nor polymorphonuclear leukocytes suggested that monocytes/macrophages might perform the accessory function. However, cell separation experiments yielded contradictory results. For example, some immune responses seemed to require phagocytic while others non-phagocytic accessory cells,[143] and in certain experimental systems the removal of adherent cells (mostly macrophages) resulted in an improvement of accessory function,[144] instead of its loss. The nature of the accessory function itself was also unclear; most investigators believed that it was equal to antigen presentation, but the finding that antigen-non-specific responses, such as mitogen-induced lymphocyte proliferation also required accessory cells[145] contradicted this. Finally the notion that had developed by the mid-1970s considered the accessory function to be mostly antigen handling, and in addition, the production of 'soluble factors' that might modify the various manifestations of immune response. On mostly intuitive grounds, the accessory cell was considered to be the macrophage, and the observed potent immunostimulatory effect of antigens associated with macrophages[146] supported this view.

Of the two proposed functions of accessory cells, namely, antigen presentation and the production of 'factors', the former was conceptually more appealing and technically more feasible to investigate. Therefore, subsequent years witnessed a burst of studies on antigen presentation. The results brought again a surprise: aside from macrophages, many different cell types turned out to be able to present antigen, including B cells,[147] B-cell lymphoma,[148,149] Langerhans cells of the skin,[150] splenic dendritic cells,[151] vascular endothelial cells,[152] and even astrocytes of the central nervous system.[153] It seemed that any cell type, as long as it expressed class II MHC molecules, was able to activate helper T cells, suggesting that a cell lineage-specific mechanism was not required for antigen presentation. Thus, these findings seemingly argued against the existence of a particular, dedicated antigen-presenting cell (APC). However, all these data had one weakness in common: they utilized in vivo primed T-cell lines and clones as a readout for antigen presentation, and therefore, the only justifiable conclusion they permitted was that the cell types listed above were able to restimulate T cells that had already been activated before. The question of whether any of these cell types could prime naïve, resting T cells remained difficult to answer, because primary T-cell responses to soluble protein antigens were virtually impossible to be induced in vitro. Thus, the search for a specialized APC required a different experimental approach.

One possible way to identify the 'professional' APC appeared to be the separation and characterization of different cell types present in the peripheral lymphoid organs (spleen, lymph nodes). Using this approach, Ralph Steinman and his colleagues at Rockefeller University were able to purify lymphoid dendritic cells, and to show that they represented a separate cell lineage, distinct in terms of morphology and cell surface markers from lymphocytes and monocytes.[154–156] Dendritic cells were shown to express MHC class II constitutively in large copy numbers,[157] and this property rendered them a good candidate for professional APC, even though they were present in small numbers (~1% of total nucleated cells) in the lymphoid organs. But the most convincing argument came from data demonstrating that the T-cell stimulatory capacity of dendritic cells was ~100-fold higher than that of unseparated cells from lymphoid organs,[158] and because they comprise ~1% of the latter, these data suggested that dendritic cells were responsible practically for the entire antigen-presenting capacity.

The detailed physiology of dendritic cells was then worked out in the subsequent decade, and can be briefly summarized as follows (reviewed by Steinman[159]). Dendritic cells are found at various locations in the body, including the blood, afferent lymph, lymphoid organs as well as the interstitium of most non-lymphoid organs (except the brain). They may have different names, e.g., skin dendritic cells are termed Langerhans cells, those in the afferent lymph veiled cells, and in the lymphoid organs they are referred to as interdigitating cells. Organ-resident dendritic cells take up antigens very effectively and synthesize MHC molecules simultaneously. After antigen uptake, they stop MHC synthesis, thereby 'freezing' the antigenic spectrum presented, and migrate via afferent lymph to the T-dependent areas of lymphoid organs. The antigens remain immunogenic on their surface for a long time (at least 1–2 days). The positioning of dendritic cells literally forces recirculating T cells leaving the bloodstream at this location to meet antigen, and thus optimizes the chance of finding T cells specific for the presented antigens. The priming of naïve T cells seems to occur at these locations. In addition to antigen presentation, dendritic cells also have the capacity to form stable clusters with antigen-specific T cells facilitating thereby the priming process. It is also possible that they provide additional thus far unknown 'signals' or 'factors' necessary for priming. Once primed, T cells redistribute again in the body, and exercise their effector function on various types of cells carrying the same antigens.

'The discovery of dendritic cells was very important for immunology, and found application in subsequent vaccination and immunotherapy strategies', adds Dr. G. 'Indeed, it was nominated for a Nobel Prize in 2011, but regrettably Ralph Steinman died 3 hours before the announcement of the Nobel Committee. Although the rules of the Nobel Foundation exclude posthumous awarding, for the first time in history, an exception was made in Ralph Steinman's case.'

'Dendritic cell studies represented a typical example of data-driven research, in which the experimental findings necessitated the development of a concept, and not the other way around. The principle that could be considered here is that the most important processes of life take place in organs, and not in cell suspensions. (Cellular immunologists tend to forget this time and again.) Accordingly, the initiation of immune response seems to occur exclusively in lymphoid organs. Therefore, a cell is required that carries the antigenic information to the lymphoid organs, and this is the dendritic cell. Why immune responses cannot be turned on in situ, e.g., at the site of an infection, is not fully understood. One possible explanation is that a low-frequency-specific T cell would hardly have a chance to meet its antigen, were the latter not positioned "in the doorway" where every T cell has to pass through. Another argument may be that immune responses are potentially dangerous for the host, and thus their initiation must occur under strictly controlled conditions provided only by the specific microenvironment (whatever it means) of lymphoid organs. Clearly, we are still far from fully comprehending the role of lymphoid organs.'

7.5 ANTIGEN PROCESSING AND PRESENTATION: PHENOMENA THAT BEG FOR A CONCEPT

'To trigger... T cells, antigen-presenting cells have to capture antigens, process them and display their fragments in association with MHC molecules'.[160] This sentence or countless variants thereof introduces almost every publication written in the field, indicating that we are dealing here with a kind of axiom in immunology. Indeed, the facts recapitulated in this statement stand firm as a rock. Yet, the sentence, the way it is formulated, leaves a vague feeling of dissatisfaction behind. So what could be the problem with it?

'Nothing, at least from the teleological point of view', answers Dr. G. 'But if you try to place this sentence into an evolutionary context, it seems to suggest that the mode of T-cell recognition must have driven the development of antigen presentation, or in other words, the defense mechanism must have preceded the invader, which does not make much sense. So it must have been the evolutionary biologist in you, who was dissatisfied.'

What could then have been the selective pressure for antigen presentation?

'There is no a priori requirement for antigen processing and presentation. If we want to designate a convincing evolutionary driver for its development we have to approach the question from a different angle. The most likely starting point could have been the need to fight against intracellular pathogens (e.g., viruses). This need must have arisen very early in evolution, perhaps already in protozoa.[161] Therefore, a defense system had to develop that could distinguish between infected and uninfected cells just by looking at the cells from outside, and eliminate the infected ones early enough to prevent further spread of infection. Since intracellular pathogens do not reveal their hiding place voluntarily – this would be to their disadvantage – the defense system had no option other than sampling the intracellular contents in the form of degradation products that can reach the cell surface via physiological waste disposal mechanisms.[162] This could have been the driving force for the recognition of peptides by the defense system, or to put it this way, I cannot think of a better one. Experimental immunologists, who draw their conclusions from observations, perceive this as a requirement for antigen processing and presentation.'

Let us now investigate another highly popular, axioma-like sentence: 'The function of . . . MHC molecules . . . (is) the display of antigenic peptides for recognition by T cells'.[163] Would you agree with this statement?

'The teleological argument behind this statement is the following: MHC molecules present peptides to T cells, consequently, they are antigen-presenting molecules. However, teleology, powerful as it may be, is not sufficient for the analysis of biological phenomena, at least not after Charles Darwin. The question to be asked here is whether antigen presentation could have been the initial evolutionary driving force for the MHC, and the answer is a clear "no". Two different lines of evidence support this conclusion. First, the overwhelming majority

(>99%) of peptides eluted from MHC molecules represents sequences from self proteins instead of foreign antigens. Peptides bound to class I molecules are usually fragments of cytosolic proteins,[15,164,165] whereas those eluted from class II originate from cell membrane-bound or secreted self proteins.[35,37–39] Altogether, MHC-bound peptides represent a comprehensive and balanced sample of the proteomic content of the cell.[166] Second, foreign antigen-derived peptides usually occupy <10% of cell surface MHC molecules, even under conditions where the foreign antigen has been added to the presenting cells at unphysiologically high concentrations.[167,168] The efficiency of foreign antigen presentation is very low: it has been calculated that ~750 foreign protein molecules have to be processed for the presentation of one single immunogenic peptide.[168] Had the selective pressure been antigen presentation on the MHC, it would be expected to perform this job much more efficiently by now. For example, MHC molecules would have evolved into structures with high specificity, such as immunoglobulins.'

'If we take the data above at face value, we can only conclude that the primary function of MHC appears to be the transport of intracellular breakdown products to the cell surface. The intracellular waste comprises mostly peptides remaining after protein catabolism, but it can include other types of macromolecules, for example, lipids and glycolipids that are transported by "non-classical" MHC molecules (e.g., CD1) to the cell surface.[169] Of course, the intracellular debris can also include pathogen-derived material, and this will be transported with the same efficiency. Thus the representation of antigenic peptides on the cell surface will depend on its intracellular concentration relative to other (self) peptides.'

Why are then MHC molecules referred to as antigen presenting molecules in every immunology textbook?

'This question is somewhat difficult to answer. For the data discussed above were generated by immunologists, and everyone in the field was aware of them. Yet there is hardly any publication[170] that would mention peptide transport as a possible function of MHC. Immunologists usually regard the display of peptides on MHC as an identity card of the cell to be controlled for correctness by the immune system. In support of this view are data demonstrating a remarkable stability of peptide–MHC complexes: peptides appear to be an integral part of the MHC structure,[109,171] and their dissociation rate is so slow that some authors[172] consider the interaction with some exaggeration as irreversible (nota bene, the interaction is non-covalent). However, stability is not only a requirement for constant peptide display, but also for the transport itself, as peptides are not supposed to be lost during the intracellular migration of MHC molecules toward the cell membrane. But after all, one cannot blame immunologists for giving their findings an immunological interpretation.'

With the unorthodox answers you have given so far, you have practically obliged yourself to outline a function for the MHC that is justifiable from the evolutionary point of view.

'I can give it a try, even though I'll have to go a very long way back, because the starting point lies in the age of Prokaryotes some 2000 million years ago.'

'It is well known that protein synthesis produces a large amount of waste. According to estimates, an average of one-third of newly synthesized proteins (values vary from 15% to 70%) come off from the ribosomes defective,[173] and additional trash arises by misfolding, erroneous post-translational modifications, and senescent proteins. Therefore protein catabolism and the disposal of non-reusable material (i.e., everything except single amino acids) belong to the most fundamental requirements for cellular health. This housekeeping function is as old as the cell, as evidenced by the finding that *Archaebacteria*, belonging to the most ancient forms of prokaryotic life already possess proteasomes,[174] and the latter are essential for their viability and growth.'[175]

'MHC molecules appear to be the last member in a catabolic waste disposal chain starting with proteolytic degradation, and ending with the transport of the remaining fragments out of the cell. Because the peptide fragments to be transported represent an enormous variety of amino acid sequences, the primary selective pressure on the MHC must have been to bind as many different sequences as possible.[161] Traces of this evolutionary force can be discovered in contemporary MHC, namely, the interaction of *all* MHC-binding sites with peptides exhibits a "non-specific" or "universal" element: hydrogen bonding with the peptide termini and/or backbone.[64-66,71] Of course, the ideal solution would have been a universal binding site that can interact with all peptides. However, the requirement for a tight binding (peptides should not be lost before reaching the cell surface) rendered this solution unfeasible, because for sufficient binding energy hydrophobic and charged interactions were needed in addition to hydrogen bonds. Furthermore, steric collisions of side chains at certain peptide positions with atoms of the binding site would have been unavoidable. Thus the peptide-transporting function set the stage for MHC diversification from the very beginning.'

'Contemporary MHCs encode two or three different molecules per class (e.g., HLA-A, -B, -C for class I, and HLA-DR, -DP, -DQ for class II in human) suggesting that this may be the minimal number of molecules required for effective peptide transport. These molecules, sometimes referred to as isotypes, must have arisen by gene duplication and subsequent diversification, and the selective pressure of binding an ever-increasing portion of the peptide-universe acted on all of them en bloc. This implies that the two or three binding sites must have different binding modes complementing each other, i.e., they bind sets of sequences with as little overlap as possible. There is experimental evidence in support of this notion.[16,17,58] Because of the multicomponent nature of the system, there were different combinatorial solutions to achieve the required broad binding spectrum, and to my opinion, this could have been the origin of MHC polymorphism. The same selective pressure must have kept the successful allele combinations together on the same chromosome, i.e., recombination between them was disfavored. This feature, termed linkage disequilibrium in genetics, is one of the hallmarks of MHC loci.'

'The timepoint at which defense systems "discovered" the primordial MHC as an informer of intracellular infection remains unknown. But this must have been a relatively recent event that probably occurred within the past few hundred million years. Thus the antigen-presenting function can be considered as a secondary use of the peptide transporter system, an evolutionary hitchhiking, so to say. The second function called also an additional selective pressure into existence, namely the struggle of intracellular pathogens to evade the presentation of their peptides.[176] This evolutionary force presumably drove the MHC toward more specificity, i.e., it acted opposite to the pressure on the peptide transporter function.'

'An interesting parallel to the proposed dual function can be observed in MHC polymorphism. It is known that there are major alleles at each MHC locus that differ substantially (in up to 30% of their sequence) from one another, indicating that they should be rather ancient. How old they exactly are is unknown, all we know is that they are certainly older than the species carrying them.[177,178] We used to call the products of these alleles "serologically distinguishable", because they reacted differently with antibodies. More recent sequencing efforts have revealed that each major allele represents, in fact, a family of two to 20 closely related members differing from each other by just a few codons. Thus the closely related members of allele families appear to be recent additions to MHC polymorphism. It is tempting to speculate that the major alleles have evolved in response to the needs of peptide transport, while the minor variants are marks of the fight with intracellular pathogens.[161] The latter selective pressure demands a relatively quick adaptation, faster than the spontaneous mutation rate. Indeed, the minor variants have probably arisen by gene conversion (i.e., by copying of a short sequence from one gene into another). It is worth pointing out that the minor variations are unlikely to affect the overall binding mode of the prototype molecule, they only cause changes in the binding of small peptide subsets. This can be regarded as a way evolution attempted to reconcile the two counteracting selective forces working on MHC.'

The hypothesis above has solely been included here, because it is interesting and seems to make sense from the evolutionary point of view. However, it has to be emphasized that this is Dr. G's private opinion that differs at least in part from what most immunologists believe.

REFERENCES

1. Gell PG, Benacerraf B. *Immunology* 1959;**2**:64.
2. Schirrmacher V, Wigzell H. *J.Exp.Med.* 1972;**136**:1616.
3. Goetzl EJ, Peters JH. *J. Immunol.* 1972;**108**:785.
4. Ishizaka K, Okudaira H, King TP. *J. Immunol.* 1975;**114**:110.
5. Maizels RM, Clarke JA, Harvey MA, Miller A, Sercarz EE. *Eur. J. Immunol* 1980;**10**:509.
6. Allen PM, Strydom DJ, Unanue ER. *Proc. Natl. Acad. Sci. USA* 1984;**81**:2489.
7. Shimonkevitz R, Colon S, Kappler J, Marrack P, Grey HM. *J. Immunol.* 1984;**133**:2067.
8. Townsend ARM, Rothbard J, Gotch FM, Bahadur G, Wraith D, McMichael AJ. *Cell* 1986;**44**:959.
9. Bastin J, Rothbard J, Davey J, Jones I, Townsend A. *J. Exp. Med.* 1987;**165**:1508.
10. Babbitt BP, Allen PM, Matsueda G, Haber E, Unanue ER. *Nature* 1985;**317**:359.
11. Buus S, Colon S, Smith C, Freed JH, Miles C, Grey HM. *Proc. Natl. Acad. Sci. USA* 1986;**83**:3968.
12. Allen PM, Matsueda GR, Evans RJ, Dunbar JB, Marshall GR, Unanue ER. *Nature* 1987;**327**:713.

13. Sette A, Buus S, Colon S, Smith JA, Miles C, Grey HM. *Nature* 1987;**328**:395.
14. Buus S, Sette A, Colon SM, Miles C, Grey HM. *Science* 1987;**235**:1353.
15. Falk K, Rötzschke O, Stevanovic S, Jung G, H-G Rammensee. *Nature* 1991;**351**:290.
16. Jardetzky TS, Lane WS, Robinson RA, Madden DR, Wiley DC. *Nature* 1991;**353**:326.
17. Hunt DF, Henderson RA, Shabanowitz J, Sakauchi K, Michel H, Sevilir N, et al. *Science* 1992;**255**:1261.
18. Wallny HJ, Rammensee HG. *Nature* 1990;**343**:275.
19. Rötzschke O, Falk K, Wallny HJ, Faath S, Rammensee HG. *Science* 1990;**249**:286.
20. MHC ligand database www.syfpeithi.de
21. Norda M, Falk K, Stevanovic S, Jung G, Rammensee HG. *J. Immunother. Emphasis Tumor Immunol.* 1993;**14**:144.
22. Corr M, Boyd LF, Frankel SR, Kozlowski S, Padlan EA, Margulies DH. *J. Exp. Med.* 1992;**176**:1681.
23. Falk K, Rötzschke O, Takiguchi M, Grahovac B, Gnau V, Stevanovic S, et al. *Immunogenet.* 1994;**40**:238.
24. Sudo T, Kamikawaji N, Kimura A, Date Y, Savoie CJ, Nakashima H, et al. *J. Immunol.* 1995;**155**:4749.
25. Savoie CJ, Kamikawaji N, Sasazuki T. *Immunogenet.* 1999;**49**:567.
26. Boisgerault F, Khalil I, Tieng V, Connan F, Tabary T, Cohen JH, et al. *Proc. Natl. Acad. Sci, USA* 1996;**93**:3466.
27. Krausa P, Münz C, Keilholz W, Stevanovic S, Jones EY, Browning M, et al. *Tissue Antigens* 2000;**56**:10.
28. Seeger FH, Schirle M, Gatfield J, Arnold D, Keilholz W, Nikplaus P, et al. *Immunogenet.* 1999;**49**:571.
29. Maier R, Falk K, Rötzschke O, Maier B, Gnau V, Stevanovic S, et al. *Immunogenet.* 1994;**40**:306.
30. Smith KD, Epperson DF, Lutz CT. *Immunogenet.* 1996;**43**:27.
31. Malcherek G, Falk K, Rötzschke O, Rammensee HG, Stevanovic S, Gnau V, et al. *Int. Immunol.* 1993;**5**:1229.
32. Garcia F, Galocha B, Villadangos JA, Lamas JR, Albar JP, Marina A, et al. *Tissue Antigens* 1997;**49**:580.
33. Barber LD, Percival L, Valiante NM, Chen L, Lee C, Gumperz JE, et al. *J. Exp. Med.* 1996;**184**:735.
34. Falk K, Rötzschke O, Grahovac B, Schendel D, Stevanovic S, Gnau V, et al. *Proc. Natl. Acad. Sci. USA* 1993;**90**:12005.
35. Rudensky AY, Preston-Hurlburt P, Hong SC, Barlow A, Janeway Jr CA. *Nature* 1991;**353**:622.
36. Janeway Jr CA, Travers P, Walport M, Shlomchik M. *Immunobiology*. New York: The Immune System in Health and Disease, Garland Science, imprint of Taylor & Francis Books, Inc.; 2001.
37. Hunt DF, Michel H, Dickinson TA, Shabanowitz J, Cox AL, Sakaguchi K, et al. *Science* 1992;**256**:1817.
38. Chicz RM, Urban RG, Lane WS, Gorga JC, Stern LJ, Vignali DAA, et al. *Nature* 1992;**358**:764.
39. Chicz RM, Urban RG, Gorga JC, Vignali DAA, Lane WS, Strominger JL. *J. Exp. Med.* 1993;**178**:27.
40. Newcomb JR, Creswell P. *J. Immunol.* 1993;**150**:499.
41. Jardetzky TS, Gorga JC, Busch R, Rothbard J, Strominger JL, Wiley DC. *EMBO J.* 1990;**9**:1797.
42. Hill CM, Hayball JD, Allison AA, Rothbard JB. *J. Immunol.* 1991;**147**:189.

43. O'Sullivan D, Arrhenius T, Sidney J, del Guercio MF, Albertson M, Wall M, et al. *J. Immunol.* 1991;**147**:2663.

44. Geluk A, van Meijgaarden KE, Janson AAM, Drijfhout JW, Meloen RH, RRP de Vries THM Ottenhof. *J. Immunol.* 1992;**149**:2864.

45. Falk K, Rötzschke O, Stevanovic S, Jung G, Rammensee HG. *Immunogenet.* 1994;**39**:230.

46. Scott JK, Smith GP. *Science* 1990;**249**:386.

47. Devlin JJ, Panganiban LC, Devlin PE. *Science* 1990;**249**:404.

48. Cwirla SE, Peters EA, Barrett RW, Dower WJ. *Proc. Natl. Acad. Sci. USA* 1990;**87**:6378.

49. Hammer J, Takacs B, Sinigaglia F. *J. Exp. Med.* 1992;**176**:1007.

50. Hammer J, Belunis C, Bolin D, Papadopoulos J, Walsky R, Higelin J, et al. *Proc. Natl. Acad. Sci. USA* 1994;**91**:4456.

51. Hammer J, Valsasini P, Tolba K, Bolin D, Higelin J, Takacs B, et al. *Cell* 1993;**74**:197.

52. Hammer J, Bono E, Gallazzi F, Belunis C, Nagy Z, Sinigaglia F. *J. Exp. Med.* 1994;**180**:2353.

53. Hammer J, Gallazzi F, Bono E, Karr RW, Guenot J, Valsasini P, et al. *J. Exp. Med.* 1995;**181**:1847.

54. Rammensee HG, Friede T, Stevanovic S. *Immunogenet.* 1995;**41**:178.

55. Sidney J, Oseroff C, del Guercio MF, Southwood S, Krieger JI, Ishioka GY, et al. *J Immunol.* 1994;**152**:4516.

56. Kwok WW, Nepom GT, Raymond FC. *J. Immunol.* 1995;**155**:2468.

57. Nelson CA, Viner NJ, Young SP, Petzold SJ, Unanue ER. *J. Immunol.* 1996;**157**:755.

58. Raddrizzani L, Sturniolo T, Guenot J, Bono E, Gallazzi F, Nagy ZA, et al. *J. Immunol.* 1997;**159**:703.

59. Bjorkman PJ, Saper MA, Samraoui B, Bennett WS, Strominger JL, Wiley DC. *Nature* 1987;**329**:506.

60. Bjorkman PJ, Saper MA, Samraoui B, Bennett WS, Strominger JL, Wiley DC. *Nature* 1987;**329**:512.

61. Saper MA, Bjorkman PJ, Wiley DC. *J. Mol. Biol.* 1991;**219**:277.

62. Garrett TPJ, Saper MA, Bjorkman PJ, Strominger JL, Wiley DC. *Nature* 1989;**342**:692.

63. Madden DR, Gorga JC, Strominger JL, Wiley DC. *Nature* 1991;**353**:321.

64. Fremont DH, Matsumura M, Stura EA, Peterson PA, Wilson IA. *Science* 1992;**257**:919.

65. Matsumura M, Fremont DH, Peterson PA, Wilson IA. *Science* 1992;**257**:927.

66. Madden DA, Garboczi DN, Wiley DC. *Cell* 1993;**75**:693.

67. Zinkernagel RM, Doherty PC. *Contemp. Topics Immunobiol.* 1977;**7**:179.

68. Matzinger P, Bevan MJ. *Cell. Immunol.* 1977;**29**:1.

69. Brown JH, Jardetzky T, Saper MA, Samraoui B, Bjorkman PJ, Wiley DC. *Nature* 1988;**332**:845.

70. Brown JH, Jardetzky TS, Gorga JC, Stern LJ, Urban RG, Strominger JL, et al. *Nature* 1993;**364**:33.

71. Stern LJ, Brown JH, Jardetzky TS, Gorga JC, Urban RG, Strominger JL, et al. *Nature* 1994;**368**:215.

72. Falcioni F, Ito K, Vidovic D, Belunis C, Campbell R, Berthel SJ, et al. *Nature Biotech.* 1999;**17**:562.

73. Ghosh P, Amaya M, Mellins E, Wiley DC. *Nature* 1995;**378**:457.

74. Jardetzky TS, Brown JH, Gorga JC, Stern LJ, Urban RG, Chi Y, et al. *Nature* 1994;**368**:711.

75. Kim J, Urban RG, Strominger JL, Wiley DC. *Science* 1994;**266**:1870.

76. Dessen A, Lawrence CM, Cupo S, Zaller DM, Wiley DC. *Immunity* 1997;**7**:473.

77. Smith KJ, Pyrdol J, Gauthier L, Wiley DC, Wucherpfennig KW. *J. Exp. Med.* 1998;**188**:1511.

78. Fremont DH, Monnaie D, Nelson CA, Hendrickson WA, Unanue ER. *Immunity* 1998;**8**:305.

79. Scott CA, Peterson PA, Teyton L, Wilson IA. *Immunity* 1998;**8**:319.

80. Corper AL, Stratmann T, Apostolopoulos V, Scott CA, Garcia KC, Kang AS, et al. *Science* 2000;**288**:505.

81. Lee KH, Wucherpfennig KW, Wiley DC. *Nature Immunol.* 2001;**2**:501.

82. Nelson CA, Viner N, Young S, Petzold S, Benoist C, Mathis D, et al. *J. Immunol.* 1996;**156**:176.

83. Sela M. *Adv. Immunol.* 1966;**5**:30.

84. Ziegler K, Unanue ER. *J. Immunol.* 1981;**127**:1869.

85. Ziegler K, Unanue ER. *Proc. Natl. Acad. Sci. USA* 1982;**79**:175.

86. Shimonkevitz R, Kappler J, Marrack P, Grey H. *J. Exp. Med.* 1983;**158**:303.

87. Demotz S, Grey HM, Appella E, Sette A. *Nature* 1989;**342**:682.

88. Nelson CA, Roof RW, McCourt DW, Unanue ER. *Proc. Natl. Acad. Sci. USA* 1992;**89**:7380.

89. Townsend AR, Gotch FM, Davey J. *Cell* 1985;**42**:457.

90. Morrison LA, Lukatcher AE, Braciale VL, Fan DP, Braciale TJ. *J. Exp. Med.* 1986;**163**:903.

91. Moore MW, Carbone FR, Bevan MJ. *Cell* 1988;**54**:777.

92. Kopp F, Steiner R, Dahlmann B, Kuehn L, Reinauer H. *Biochem. Biophys. Acta* 1986;**872**:253.

93. Tanaka K, Ichihara A, Waxman L, Goldberg AL. *J. Biol. Chem.* 1986;**263**:15197.

94. Glynne R, Powis SH, Beck S, Kelly A, Kerr LA, Trowsdale J. *Nature* 1991;**353**:357.

95. Ortiz-Navarrete V, Selig A, Gernold M, Frentzel S, Kloetzel PM, Hämmerling GJ. *Nature* 1991;**353**:662.

96. Martinez CK, Monaco JJ. *Nature* 1991;**353**:664.

97. Kelly A, Powis SH, Glynne R, Radley E, Beck S, Trowsdale J. *Nature* 1991;**353**:667.

98. Garzynska M, Rock KL, Goldberg AL. *Nature* 1993;**365**:264.

99. Driscoll J, Brown MG, Finley D, Monaco JJ. *Nature* 1993;**365**:262.

100. Arnold D, Driscoll J, Androlewicz M, Hughes E, Creswell P, Spies T. *Nature* 1992;**360**:171.

101. Momburg F, Ortiz-Navarrete V, Neefjes J, Goulmy E, van de Wal Y, Spits H, et al. *Nature* 1992;**360**:174.

102. Neefjes JJ, Stollorz V, Peters PJ, Geuze HJ, Ploegh HL. *Cell* 1990;**61**:171.

103. Nuchtern JG, Bonifacino JS, Biddison WE, Klausner RD. *Nature* 1989;**339**:223.

104. Cox JH, Yewdell JW, Eisenlohr LC, Johnson PR, Bennink JR. *Science* 1990;**247**:715.

105. Kelly A, Powis SH, Kerr LA, Mockridge I, Elliott T, Bastin J, et al. *Nature* 1992;**355**:641.

106. Kleijmeer MJ, Kelly A, Geuze HJ, Slot JW, Townsend A, Trowsdale J. *Nature* 1992;**357**:342.

107. Neefjes JJ, Momburg F, Hämmerling GJ. *Science* 1993;**261**:769.

108. Shepherd JC, Schumacher TNM, Aston-Rickardt PG, Imaeda S, Ploegh HL, Janeway Jr CA, et al. *Cell* 1993;**74**:577.

109. Townsend A, Öhlén C, Bastin J, Ljunggren HG, Forster L, Kärre K. *Nature* 1989;**340**:443.

110. Degen E, Cohendoyle MF, Williams DB. *J. Exp. Med.* 1992;**175**:1653.

111. Gooding LR, Edwards CB. *J. Immunol.* 1980;**124**:1258.

112. Carbone FR, Bevan MJ. *J. Exp. Med.* 1990;**171**:377.

113. Debrick JE, Campbell PA, Staerz UD. *J. Immunol.* 1991;**147**:2846.

114. Pfeifer JD, Wick MJ, Roberts RL, Findlay K, Normark SJ, Harding CV. *Nature* 1993;**361**:359.

115. Jones PP, Murphy DB, Hewgill D, McDevitt HO. *Immunochemistry* 1979;**16**:51.

116. Anderson MS, Miller J. *Proc. Natl. Acad. Sci. USA* 1992;**89**:2282.

117. Lamb CA, Yewdell JW, Bennink JR, Cresswell P. *Proc. Natl. Acad. Sci. USA* 1991;**88**:5998.

118. Roche PA, Teletski CL, Karp DR, Pinet V, Bakke O, Long EO. *EMBO J.* 1992;**11**:2841.

119. Roche PA, Cresswell P. *Nature* 1990;**345**:615.

120. Teyton L, O'Sullivan D, Dickson PW, Lotteau V, Sette A, Fink P, et al. *Nature* 1990;**348**:39.

121. Viville S, Neefjes J, Lotteau V, Dierich A, Lemeur M, Ploegh H, et al. *Cell* 1993;**72**:635.

122. Riberdy JM, Newcomb JR, Surman MJ, Barbosa JA, Cresswell P. *Nature* 1992;**360**:474.

123. Bangia N, Watts TH. *Int. Immunol.* 1995;**7**:1585.

124. Kropshofer H, Vogt AB, Hämmerling GJ. *Proc. Natl. Acad. Sci. USA* 1995;**92**:8313.

125. Malcherek G, Gnau V, Jung G, Rammensee HG, Melms A. *J. Exp. Med.* 1995;**181**:527.

126. Kelly AP, Monaco JJ, Cho S, Trowsdale J. *Nature* 1991;**353**:571.

127. Sloan VS, Cameron P, Porter G, Gammon M, Amaya M, Mellins E, et al. *Nature* 1995;**375**:802.

128. Denzin LK, Cresswell P. *Cell* 1995;**82**:155.

129. van Ham M, Grüneberg U, Malcherek G, Bröker I, Melms A, Trowsdale J. *J. Exp. Med* 1996;**184**:2019.

130. Denzin LK, Hammond C, Cresswell P. *J. Exp. Med.* 1996;**184**:2153.

131. Kropshofer H, Arndt SO, Moldenhauer G, Hämmerling GJ, Vogt AB. *Immunity* 1997;**6**:293.

132. Fung-Leung WP, Surh CD, Liljedahl M, Pang J, Leturcq D, Peterson PA, et al. *Science* 1996;**271**:1278.

133. Liljedahl M, Winqvist O, Surh CD, Wong P, Ngo K, Teyton L, et al. *Immunity* 1998;**8**:233.

134. Ohno S. *Evolution by gene duplication.* 1970. Springer, Berlin, Heidelberg, New York.

135. Guagliardi LE, Koppelman B, Blum JS, Marks MS, Creswell P, Brodsky FM. *Nature* 1990;**343**:133.

136. Harding CV, Geuze HJ. *J. Immunol.* 1993;**151**:3988.

137. Rudensky AY, Maric M, Eastman S, Shoemaker L, DeRoos PC, Blum JS. *Immunity* 1994;**1**:585.

138. Amigorena S, Drake JR, Webster P, Mellman I. *Nature* 1994;**369**:113.

139. Amigorena S, Webster P, Drake J, Newcomb J, Creswell P, Mellman I. *J. Exp. Med.* 1995;**181**:1729.

140. Davidson HW, Reid PA, Lanzavecchia A, Watts C. *Cell* 1991;**67**:105.

141. Harding CV, Unanue ER, Slot JW, Schwartz AL, Geuze HL. *Proc. Natl. Acad. Sci. USA* 1990;**87**:5553.

142. Mosier DE. *Science* 1967;**158**:1573.

143. Shortman K, Diener E, Russell P, Armstrong WD. *J. Exp. Med.* 1970;**131**:461.

144. Miller CL, Mishell RI. *J. Immunol.* 1975;**114**:692.

145. Lipsky PE, Ellner JJ, Rosenthal AL. *J. Immunol.* 1976;**116**:868.

146. Unanue ER. *Adv. Immunol.* 1972;**15**:95.

147. Chesnut RW, Grey HM. *J. Immunol.* 1981;**126**:1075.

148. McKean DJ, Infante AJ, Nilson A, Kimoto M, Fathman CG, Walker E, et al. *J. Exp. Med.* 1981;**154**:1419.

149. Glimcher LH, Kim KJ, Green I, Paul W. *J. Exp. Med.* 1982;**155**:445.

150. Stingl G, Katz SI, Clement L, Green I, Shevach EM. *J. Immunol.* 1978;**121**:2005.

151. Sunshine GH, Katz DR, Feldmann M. *J. Exp. Med.* 1980;**152**:1817.

152. Hirschberg H, Braathen LR, Thorsby E. *Immunol. Rev.* 1982;**66**:57.

153. Fontana A, Fierz W, Wekerle H. *Nature* 1984;**307**:273.

154. Steinman RM, Cohn ZA. *J. Exp. Med.* 1973;**137**:1142.

155. Steinman RM, Cohn ZA. *J. Exp. Med.* 1974;**139**:380.

156. Steinman RM, Lustig DS, Cohn ZA. *J. Exp. Med.* 1974;**139**:1431.

157. Nussenzweig MC, Steinman RM, Unkeless JC, Witmer MD, Gutchinov B, Cohn ZA. *J. Exp. Med.* 1981;**154**:168.

158. Van Voortis WC, Valinsky J, Hoffman E, Luban J, Hair LS, Steinman RM. *J. Exp. Med.* 1983;**158**:174.

159. Steinman RM. *Ann. Rev. Immunol.* 1991;**9**:271.

160. Lanzavecchia A, Roosnek E, Gregory T, Berman P, Abrignani S. *Nature* 1988;**334**:530.

161. Nagy ZA. *Scand J. Immunol.* 2008;**67**:313.

162. Cohn M. *Mol. Immunol.* 2005;**42**:1419.

163. Germain RN, Hendrix LR. *Nature* 1991;**353**:134.

164. Jardetzky TS, Lane WS, Robinson RA, Madden DR, Wiley DC. *Nature* 1991;**353**:326.

165. Hunt DF, Henderson RA, Shabanowitz J, Sakauchi K, Michel H, Sevilir N, et al. *Science* 1992;**255**:1261.

166. Hickman HD, Luis AD, Buchli R, Few SR, Sathiamurthy M, VanGundy RS, et al. *J. Immunol.* 2004;**172**:2944.

167. Porgador A, Yewdell JW, Deng Y, Bennink JR, Germain RN. *Immunity* 1997;**6**:715.

168. Dadaglio G, Nelson CA, Deck MB, Petzold SJ, Unanue ER. *Immunity* 1997;**6**:727.

169. Dutronc Y, Porcelli SA. *Tissue Antigens* 2002;**42**:1419.

170. Bartl S, Baltimore D, Weissman IL. *Proc. Natl. Acad. Sci. USA* 1994;**91**:10769.

171. Sadegh-Nasseri S, Germain RN. *Nature* 1991;**353**:167.

172. Lanzavecchia A, Reid PA, Watts C. *Nature* 1992;**357**:249.

173. Saveanu L, Carroll O, Hassainya Y, van Endert P. *Immunol. Rev.* 2005;**207**:42.

174. Dahlmann B, Kopp F, Knehn L, Niedel B, Pfeifer G, Hegerl R, et al. *FEBS Lett.* 1989;**251**:125.

175. Zhou G, Kowalczyk D, Humbard MA, Rohatgi S, Maupin-Furlow JA. *J. Bacteriol.* 2008;**190**:8096.

176. Nagy ZA, Lehmann PV, Falcioni F, Muller S, Adorini L. *Immunol. Today* 1989;**10**:132.

177. Figueroa F, Günther E, Klein J. *Nature* 1988;**335**:265.

178. Lawlor DA, Ward FE, Ennis PD, Jackson AP, Parham P. *Nature* 1988;**335**:268.

Chapter 8

The Intricate Behavior of T Cells

The period from about 1970 until the mid-1980s can be viewed as the age of T cells in immunology research. During these 15 years, T-cell studies dominated the immunological literature, many fascinating aspects of T-cell biology have been discovered, and toward the end, the long and often frustrating attempts to identify the T-cell antigen receptor were also crowned with success. Of course, not all questions found their answer. For example, the nature of the ligand for T cells (i.e., peptides bound to MHC) was recognized as late as 1985, and the precise way T cells recognize their ligand was clarified by crystallographic studies in the second half of the 1990s. Furthermore, several questions of T-cell biology, including for example the role of T cells in immune tolerance and in autoimmune disease were addressed after 1985, and some of them are still the subject of intensive research. Thus, although 'the age of T cells' has been over for a long time, 'the T-cell story' cannot be regarded as complete until today.

8.1 MAJOR HISTOCOMPATIBILITY COMPLEX RESTRICTION OF T-CELL RECOGNITION

It was long before immunologists had any idea about the nature of the T-cell antigen receptor, when the single, most important discovery about T-cell recognition had been made. This was the observation that antigen recognition by T cells involved the MHC in a mysterious way: the phenomenon known as MHC restriction.

8.1.1 Discovery

Everything started with a short and inconspicuous paper in the *Journal of Immunology* by Kindred and Shreffler[1] in 1972. The two authors studied antibody responses in athymic nude mice to so-called T-dependent antigens, the response to which required T-cell help. To provide a source of helper T cells they inoculated the nude mice with thymocytes from different mouse strains. Their key observation was that antibody responses occurred only when the injected thymocytes carried identical MHC with the recipient mice, i.e., they were syngeneic. MHC-disparate (allogeneic) thymus cells were unable to provide help, whereas differences at non-MHC 'background' loci did not seem to matter. The

A History of Modern Immunology. http://dx.doi.org/10.1016/B978-0-12-416974-6.00008-9

conclusion from this study has been that T–B-cell collaboration requires MHC identity of the interacting parties.

'How the famous MHC geneticist Don Shreffler teamed up with the less well known Australian geneticist Berenice Kindred is unknown for me', reflects Dr. G. 'It is also unclear, why and when Berenice switched her scientific interest from the genetics of invariable traits, meant to answer questions such as why we have five fingers on one hand, to the genetics of nude mice, another funny subject. Clearly, Berenice liked to have fun, and her roaring laughter was heard echoing in the corridors of several different scientific institutions, because she also liked change.'

'I may also mention that some colleagues with a preference for down-to-earth physiology criticized the findings of Kindred and Shreffler by saying: "So what, T and B cells in the same individual are always syngeneic, this condition is given anyway." However, they overlooked one important rule, namely, that biological processes hidden under normal physiology can only be discovered if they are interrupted by unnatural experimental conditions. Or as a former, sarcastic mentor of mine used to put it: "Physiology is best studied in decapitated and eviscerated rats".'

The one who immediately grasped the significance of this finding was, of course, Baruj Benacerraf. He launched a project, championed by David Katz, for mapping of the genes that control T–B-cell interaction. In their studies they were able to narrow down the genetic requirement for T–B-cell collaboration to the class II region of MHC.[2–4] The conclusion was narrowed down correspondingly: a successful collaboration between helper T (Th) cells and B cells for antibody production requires identity of the class II region of the two interacting cells. To give a mechanistic interpretation of the data, they proposed that the class II region encodes 'interaction molecules' expressed on T and B cells, respectively. This hypothesis was very much in line with the contemporary interpretation of the MHC class II region, the latter being looked upon as a large collection (almost a flea market) of immune-related genes (see Section 6.3.1). Thus, it seemed that this puzzling finding would not lead anywhere, at least not in the short term, because all one could do was to wait until the relevant class II genes and their products were characterized.

The fortunate turn in history came, when Rolf Zinkernagel, a young Swiss MD with multiple scientific interests went to Australia, as many European scientists did at that time, to broaden his knowledge in microbiology at Gordon Ada's Department at the John Curtin School of Medical Research in Canberra. There he met another young and bright scientist, Peter Doherty, and a collaboration of historical importance began.

Zinkernagel and Doherty studied the cytotoxic (cytolytic) T-cell response of mice to lymphocytic choriomeningitis virus (LCM). They infected mice with the virus and tested the immune spleen cells for a cytotoxic response measured by the release of radioactivity from ^{51}Cr-labeled, virus-infected target cells, in vitro. Their basic finding was that in order for cytolysis to occur, the effector cells had to share MHC with the target cells.[5] Thus the results confirmed the previously demonstrated requirement for MHC identity in Th-cell–B-cell collaboration, and extended it to cytotoxic T lymphocytes (Tc). In the next publication that appeared a few months later,[6] they went one step further, and addressed the possible mechanism behind the phenomenon, by then referring to it as MHC restriction. They considered two possible mechanisms, one being the 'interaction molecule' hypothesis put forward by Katz et al.,[3] and another one, namely that T cells might recognize foreign antigens (in this case LCM virus) together with MHC molecules of the target cell. They termed the latter hypothesis 'altered self'. The experimental approach to distinguish between these two possibilities was the following (Fig. 8.1). They generated Tc in LCM virus-infected MHC-heterozygous F_1 hybrid mice that we designate here schematically (**a x b**) F_1. The F_1 Tc cells were then transferred into LCM-infected recipients of either parental strain (**a** and **b**, respectively). (The recipients were immunosuppressed to prevent a reaction against incompatible MHC molecules of the second parent expressed on the F_1 cells.) By doing this, the (**a x b**) Tc were 'restimulated' with LCM + MHC^a, and LCM + MHC^b, respectively. The Tc cells were then recovered from the recipients, and tested for cytolysis on target cells carrying LCM + MHC^a. Lysis of LCM + MHC^a target cells was only observed when the Tc were restimulated in mice of the **a** parental strain.

What did these results reveal about the mechanism of MHC restriction? Under the interaction molecule hypothesis, such molecules of both **a** and **b** parental type should be expressed on the F_1 T cells, and thus, restimulation should have occurred in both parental strains, i.e., lysis of LCM + MHC^a target cells was expected to occur, no matter whether the Tc cells were previously in **a** or **b** recipients. The finding that this was not the case ruled out the interaction molecule hypothesis (or 'intimacy' hypothesis as Zinkernagel and Doherty

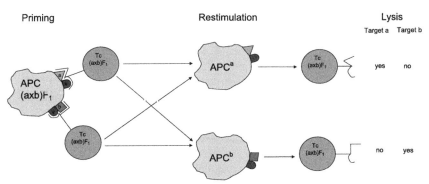

FIGURE 8.1 Principle of the Zinkernagel-Doherty experiment. Immunization of (axb)F_1 mice with LCMV generates two cytotoxic T-cell (Tc) populations each recognizing virus (v) with either parental MHC type, a or b. Transfer of Tc into virus-infected parental strain mice results in restimulation and expansion of the Tc population recognizing virus together with the respective parental MHC type. Based on References 6 and 7.

used to call it). By exclusion, the altered self hypothesis seemed more likely to be valid, even though it was not completely proven. According to the latter model, in the F_1 animals two populations of Tc were generated, one specific for LCM+MHC^a and the other for LCM+MHC^b. The first population was restimulated in **a** recipients and lyzed LCM + MHC^a target cells. The second population might have been restimulated in the **b** parent (Fig. 8.1), but its lytic activity was not tested for lack of appropriate target cells (this missing experimental group was supplied later in a follow-up study[7]).

The altered self concept thus proposed that T cells primed by the simultaneous recognition of foreign antigen plus one particular self MHC molecule reacted to the same antigen–MHC combination upon restimulation as well as in the effector phase. Consequently, the same antigen plus another MHC, or another antigen with the same MHC represented different ligands not recognizable by these T cells. Concerning the nature of antigenic ligand the authors envisaged two possibilities: first, the antigen somehow modifies self MHC molecules and the T-cell receptor (TCR) recognizes modified self MHC as a foreign antigen, and second, the ligand consists of antigen combined with self MHC, and the TCR recognizes both components.

One question left open by the altered self hypothesis was whether MHC identity between T cell and target cell was an absolute requirement, or alternatively, T cells could recognize antigen also in association with a foreign MHC molecule. This question was difficult to address experimentally, because of the strong alloreaction of T cells to foreign MHC. Thus an experimental situation had to be created, in which the T cells were tolerant of the foreign MHC to be tested. The solution to this problem was to use chimeric mice whose T-cell precursors derived from mice of MHC^a were allowed to develop in the body of (**a x b**)F_1 recipients. Indeed T cells from these chimeras were shown to recognize antigen in association with MHC^b (and naturally also MHC^a).[8–11] These data gave further support to the notion that MHC is part of the ligand recognized by T cells.

'Those readers who may not understand at first sight the rationales and reasonings above, should not blame themselves', remarks Dr. G. 'Indeed, at that time the majority of immunologists failed to understand them, and therefore, it took some time before the concept of MHC restriction settled firmly in the community's mind. But once this happened, Zinkernagel and Doherty became the most wanted seminar speakers in the world.'

'The Zinkernagel and Doherty study provided a good example of how powerful the experimental use of F_1-parental strain combinations could be in answering important biological questions. Thus little wonder that the "F_1 experiment" became one of the most popular instruments in subsequent immunological experimentation.'

'Perhaps it is interesting to note that the discovery of MHC restriction thanks its existence to MHC polymorphism. Namely, if different mouse strains expressing allelic variants of the same MHC molecule had not been available, the observation would not have been possible to make. Of course, even if the MHC had been monomorphic, its involvement in T-cell recognition would have been discovered; the question is only: when? But this is just idle speculation, as we know that the MHC must be polymorphic, it follows from its function (see Section 7.5).'

'One benefit Rolf Zinkernagel had of his discovery was that he could count himself amongst those few scientists, who found an appropriate position in their home country. The same applied to Peter Doherty, although later he migrated to the US, the only country at that time that cared for attracting bright people (a policy called "brain-drain" on this side of the Atlantic).'

'Subsequently, Zinkernagel and Doherty clarified many additional questions related to MHC restriction, and 22 years later, when the mechanisms behind this phenomenon became fully understood, they were awarded with the Nobel Prize.'

8.1.2 MHC Restriction of Cytotoxic T-cell Responses

The cytotoxic T lymphocyte (Tc) response represented a favorable experimental model for studies of MHC restriction, in the first place because its readout was a short-term, usually 4 h long, chromium release assay. This duration was too short to allow the development of unwanted reactions against allogeneic cells, and thus it was possible to combine cytotoxic T-cell populations and target cells differing from each other in the entire MHC or parts of it. Because of this technical advantage, the generality of Zinkernagel's and Doherty's finding was proven for Tc responses almost instantaneously.

Indeed, MHC restriction turned out to apply to all murine Tc responses studied, including responses to viruses reported by Blanden and colleagues[12] and Wainberg et al.,[13] to hapten-treated syngeneic cells shown by Shearer and colleagues[14,15] and Forman,[16] and to minor histocompatibility antigens described by Bevan[17,18] and Simpson and colleagues.[19] A couple of years later, MHC restriction of Tc responses was demonstrated also in additional species, namely, in the rat[20] and most importantly in human.[21]

The next obvious task was to determine more precisely, which MHC molecules – or 'restricting elements' as they were called – were involved in Tc responses. This was done by standard mapping strategies of MHC genetics using intra-H-2 recombinant mouse strains as shown in Table 8.1. The mapping studies were performed in two different ways. In the first version, the target cells of standard H-2 types were kept constant, and the Tc were generated in mice carrying different recombinant H-2 types. This strategy was the only option as long as solely tumor cell lines of a few standard H-2 types were considered to be good targets for Tc. In the second version, the Tc were generated in mice of standard H-2 types, and the targets came from different recombinant strains. This was made possible by the observation that mitogen induced T- or B-cell blasts from any mouse strain were comparably susceptible to the lytic activity of Tc[22] and could thus be used as targets. These strategies and variants thereof then became the standard procedure for 'restriction mapping' of Tc responses in the next decade or so.

TABLE 8.1 Mapping Strategies for the Determination of MHC Regions Involved in the Restriction of Cytotoxic T Cell Responses

Cytotoxic T Cell H-2 Type			Target Cell H-2 Type			
K[a]	I	D	K	I	D	Lysis
a[b]	a	a	a	a	a	++
b	b	b	a	a	a	−
a	b	b	a	a	a	+
b	a	a	a	a	a	+
a	a	a	a	a	a	++
a	a	a	b	b	b	−
a	a	a	a	b	b	+
a	a	a	b	b	a	+

[a] MHC (H-2) regions in mouse: K,D class I; I class II
[b] alleles at H-2 regions
Based on References 7, 16, 18 and 23

The results from the mapping studies came out uncommonly clear: in all Tc responses the effector cells and target cells had to share at least one of the class I regions (K or D) in order for lysis to occur.[7,16,18,23] In most instances, two distinct Tc populations were detectable, one that required identity at the K and the other at the D region.[7,16] This could also be demonstrated by competitive inhibition experiments, in which the lysis of ^{51}Cr-labeled target cells was inhibited with unlabeled target cells only, if the latter carried the antigen together with the relevant K or D molecule. (This approach, termed 'cold target inhibition', also became standard in Tc studies.) The interpretation of these data was that in response to antigen x, two different Tc specificities were generated, namely, x+K and x+D.

In contrast to the involvement of MHC class I, the class II region turned out to be irrelevant for the lysis of target cells.

These results thus revealed a remarkably strict coupling of an effector function (cytolysis) to one particular class of MHC molecules. This was not entirely unexpected, because it had been shown a couple of years earlier that Tc generated against allogeneic MHC molecules also preferentially lyzed targets sharing class I molecules with the stimulating allogeneic cells (see Section 6.1.3). Furthermore, the finding made biological sense, because the function of Tc was considered to be the elimination of infected cells, thus the self molecule restricting the recognition of cell-bound pathogen was expected to be present on all somatic cells, and MHC class I satisfied this criterion. However, the mechanism behind the association of the cytolytic function with MHC class I remained unknown, and represented one of the major puzzles of T-cell biology for many years to come.

'Perhaps it is worth pointing out that the studies cited above have formally proven MHC restriction solely at the level of effector–target cell interaction, and thus the statement that the same restriction would also apply upon priming of the Tc precursors was just an extrapolation', adds Dr. G. 'However, this does not diminish the value of the finding, because the extrapolation was based on a fundamental immunologic law, namely, that the very same clonally distributed antigen receptor is expressed on lymphocytes throughout all stages of their development (point mutations being the only permissible changes at late stages of immune response). Had this law turned out to be inapplicable to Tc cells, the entire immunobiology would have had to be revised from 1959 on. Besides, most Tc responses require in vivo priming, a direct observation of which would have been impossible at that time, and is still today a technical challenge.'

8.1.3 MHC Restriction of Helper T-Cell Responses

Providing conclusive evidence for MHC restriction in helper T (Th)-cell responses turned out to be far more difficult experimentally than in the case of cytotoxic T cells. The major problem here was how to get around disturbing allogeneic effects that could arise upon mixing of histoincompatible cells. MHC restriction of Th cells could be studied at two different levels, namely in the Th-cell–antigen-presenting-cell (APC) interaction, and in the Th-cell–B-cell interaction. The assay for the former was antigen-specific T-cell proliferation, and for the latter antibody production in vivo or enumeration of plaque-forming cells (PFC) in vitro. All these assays required the coexistence of interacting cell types for several days, a timeframe more than enough for the development of a mixed lymphocyte reaction (MLR), if the participating cells were allogeneic. Therefore, immunologists had to invest a great deal of ingenuity into complicated experimental protocols in order to eliminate or at least minimize disturbing reactions to allogeneic cells.

'Interestingly, many immunologists did not care too much about positive allogeneic effects, such as a non-specific enhancement of antibody response due to ongoing MLR', points out Dr. G. 'Their major concern was exactly the opposite, namely that in semiallogeneic situations, e.g., $(a \times b)F_1$ T cells in parent a or vice versa, suppressor T (Ts) cells might be generated, which in turn could inhibit the response to antigen plus the MHC of parent b. Thus the observed MHC restriction could have been the result of active suppression, instead of selective recognition of antigen with one parental MHC. The rationale behind this assumption appears somewhat irrational today, in that it is virtually impossible to propose a mechanism by which such Ts cells could arise. However, at that time, shortly after the discovery of Ts cells, immunologists suspected Ts cells to be at work in

every instance, where an expected response did not occur. Therefore, it became
an obligatory routine to rule out the action of Ts cells by appropriate cell-mixing
experiments in every study of MHC restriction.'

Historically, the first study to address MHC restriction in Th-cell–B-cell collaboration was the one performed by Katz and Benacerraf and colleagues,[2–4]
as already mentioned before (Section 8.1.1). The protocol they used (shown
in Fig. 8.2) serves as a good illustration of how complex these experiments
had to be in order to avoid the criticism that the results were inconclusive due
to allogeneic effects. The essence of the set-up was a hapten-carrier system, a
favorite model of Benacerraf. Briefly, carrier-primed Th cells obtained from
strain **a** mice immunized with bovine gamma globulin (BGG) were transferred
to (**a**x**b**)F$_1$ recipients. Note that in this situation the **a** strain T cells could have
been alloreactive to the **b** parental MHC of the F$_1$ recipient, while the recipient
considered the **a** T cells as self. Thus a graft-versus-host reaction could have
developed, and to avoid this, the recipients, together with the transferred T cells,
were irradiated 24 h later, and on the same day injected with hapten-primed B
cells of either **a** or **b** strain. The latter were produced by immunizing with dinitrophenyl (DNP) coupled to another carrier, keyhole limpet hemocyanin (KLH).
Still on the same day, mice were boosted with DNP-BGG, and anti-DNP antibodies were measured 7 days later. The built-in assumption in this protocol
was that irradiation eliminated the reactivity of T cells to both the recipient and
the B cells of strain **b**, while it left the BGG-specific, relatively radioresistant
helper activity of Th cells intact. However, it was suspected that the irradiated
T cells might die sooner or later, and this is why irradiation, B-cell transfer and
boosting all had to happen on the same day. Thus, the protocol was a kind of
tightrope walking.

Nevertheless, the results came out clear-cut: strain **a** Th cells could collabo-
rate with strain **a** but not with strain **b** B cells, and by using intra-H-2 recombinant strains the genetic requirement for collaboration was conclusively mapped

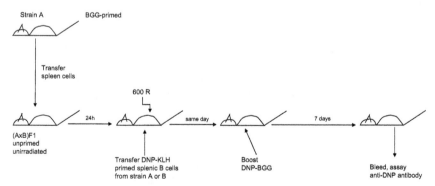

FIGURE 8.2 Protocol of the Katz-Benacerraf experiment. See text for detailed explanation.
Based on Reference 2.

to the class II region. The unfortunate aspect of this study was not in the data, but in their interpretation. Namely, the authors proposed that the genetic restriction affected cell–cell interaction rather than antigen recognition, a hypothesis that was quickly ruled out by Zinkernagel and Doherty.[6] For this reason, many immunologists discredited this work and sought for more conclusive evidence, which in turn led to a proliferation of experiments that were at least as complicated as the Katz and Benacerraf study and yielded sometimes conflicting results.

It is beyond the scope of this book to discuss all subsequent experimental approaches in detail. Suffice it to say that they included both in vitro[24–27] and in vivo[28–30] experiments as well as combinations thereof.[31–33] In some studies, care was taken to remove alloreactive cells from the Th-cell populations before their transfer into allogeneic or semiallogeneic hosts.[30,33] Taken their level of sophistication and complexity, these studies probably represent an insurpassable peak of the art of experimentation in cellular immunology. Nevertheless the results remained somewhat inconclusive: although in the majority of studies MHC class II restriction was shown to apply to both Th-cell–APC and Th-cell–B-cell interactions,[24–26,28–30] in certain studies restriction could only be demonstrated in the Th-cell–APC interaction, whereas no requirement for MHC identity was found in Th–B-cell collaboration.[27,31–33] It has remained unclear, whether this discrepancy was caused by differences in the experimental systems, or alternatively, both restricted and unrestricted Th–B-cell collaboration might have reflected biological reality.

'Immunologists followed these studies with intense interest, because the mode of antigen recognition by Th cells was highly relevant for the mechanism of T–B-cell collaboration', comments Dr. G. 'The requirement for T–B-cell collaboration in the production of IgG antibodies was discovered by Jacques Miller and Graham Mitchell about a decade earlier (see Section 1.3), but the way the two cell types communicated with each other remained largely unexplained. Known was only – based on classical studies by Rajewsky et al.[34] and Mitchison[35] – that the antigenic epitope recognized by the B cell (e.g., a hapten) had to be physically linked to the epitope recognized by the T cell (e.g., a carrier epitope) in order for effective collaboration to occur. Therefore, most immunologists envisaged the communication between the two cells to take place across an "antigen bridge", i.e., one epitope of the antigen bound to the B-cell's surface Ig and the other to the T-cell's antigen receptor (Fig. 8.3). Obviously, if the Th–B-cell collaboration had turned out to be obligatorily MHC restricted, a simple antigen-bridging model could no longer have accounted for the interaction. Because of the discrepancy of experimental findings this question remained open.'

There was also a more limited set of studies, in which MHC restriction of Th cells was investigated exclusively at the level of T-cell–APC interaction. The readout in these experiments was the in vitro secondary proliferative response of in vivo primed Th cells to the priming antigen in the presence of APC. The

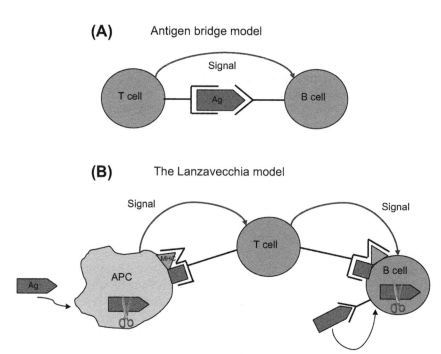

FIGURE 8.3 Models of T–B-cell collaboration. Antigen (Ag) in model B is processed and presented together with MHC class II by APC and B cell in the same way. See text for further explanation. Based on References 34, 35 and 38.

first report along this vein by Rosenthal and Shevach[36] appeared in 1973. In chronological order, this was the third study (after Kindred and Shreffler[1] and Katz et al.[2]), in which a requirement for histocompatibility between interacting cell types was reported. The authors studied the proliferative response of antigen primed T cells from strain 2 and strain 13 guinea pigs to antigen-pulsed APC ('macrophages') of the same strains in a criss-cross manner. They observed antigen-specific proliferation only, when T cells and APC were from the same strain. Although they noted some proliferation of T cells to allogeneic APC in the absence of antigen, i.e., an MLR response, the magnitude of the latter was small, and thus, it did not seriously jeopardize the quality of data and the conclusion drawn from them. Similar experiments were also performed with mice,[37] and the requirement for genetic identity was mapped to the class II region of MHC. In the latter study substantial MLR responses were measured, but these did not seem to be of much concern for the investigators. Altogether, the studies of T-cell–APC interaction were characterized by a more relaxed handling of the problem of allogeneic effect than those of T–B-cell collaboration. Nevertheless, the presence of MLR cast a shadow on the conclusivity of these data.

The final solution for the problem of alloreactivity came in the 1980s, with the invention of T-cell cloning. Although individual T-cell clones could also be alloreactive to defined foreign MHC molecules, this could be determined in advance, and for the purpose of restriction mapping appropriate allogeneic APC could be selected to which the clone did not show any reactivity in the absence of antigen. Thus restriction mapping became a simple routine task, and innumerable reports have provided clear-cut evidence demonstrating that Th cells only recognize antigen together with class II MHC molecules.

These results supplied the second half of the puzzle: whereas the cytotoxic function was found to be coupled to antigen recognition together with class I, the helper function was just as strictly associated with antigen recognition in the context of class II MHC. The latter, again, made sense, because class II molecules were known to be expressed constitutively only on cells involved in the immune response (B cells, APC).

The use of cloned lymphocytes was also instrumental in clarifying the mechanism of T–B-cell collaboration. The experimental system developed for this purpose by Lanzavecchia[38] consisted of tetanus toxoid (TT)-specific human T-cell clones and Epstein-Barr virus (EBV)-transformed, TT-specific cloned human B cells. Such a system could only be built up with human cells, because the cloning of B cells from other species was not feasible. Lanzavecchia was able to show that EBV-transformed TT-specific B cells could present TT very efficiently to T cells. These B cells could also present other antigens, but with 10 000-fold less efficiency. The mechanism accounting for the high efficiency was the specific binding of TT to the surface Ig of the TT-specific B cells followed by Ig-mediated internalization of large amounts of TT. The antigen was then processed and displayed together with class II molecules on the B-cell surface in the same way as in the case of other APC. He also demonstrated MHC restriction of the Th-cell–B-cell interaction, which could then be understood as the recognition by Th cells of the same antigen–MHC complex on both B cells and APC (Fig. 8.3). This study has indicated that in a physiological range of antigen concentrations, it is only the antigen-specific B cell that can present sufficient amounts of antigen to Th cells, and thus, the T–B-cell collaboration is operationally antigen-specific, without the need for a direct antigen bridge between B cell Ig receptor and TCR.

'Antonio Lanzavecchia's paper was a very charismatic one in several respects', points out Dr. G. 'First, it addressed a long-standing open question of immunology. Second, the results with cloned B and T cells were indisputably clear. Third, this was the first study in the history of cellular immunology, in which a human experimental system was used for answering a question of basic immunology. And finally, this was a single author's paper, in the 1980s already very uncommon.'

'Antonio was a young cellular immunologist from Franco Celada's school, and even among Italians, who were for some reason all very good at handling cells, he was probably the best, most careful experimenter. His work literally catapulted him into the "VIP lounge" of immunology, a place where he didn't mind to be anyway.'

8.1.4 Theoretical Implications of MHC Restriction: One Receptor or Two Receptors?

It is not exaggerating to say that the phenomenon of MHC restriction fascinated every immunologist in the world, irrespective of whether he or she worked with T cells or not. The reason for this was the observed dual specificity of T cells. Up to this point in history, immunological specificity – as seen with antibodies – was considered to be directed selectively against foreign substances, while self molecules of the host were not recognized (self–non-self discrimination). Unexpectedly, however, T cells seemed to obey different principles, in that they required the recognition of a foreign antigen and a self MHC molecule simultaneously, and both recognition events appeared to be equally specific. To appreciate the magnitude of surprise this finding caused, it should be remembered that the observation was made in the mid-1970s, when neither the structure of the T cells' antigen receptor (TCR) nor the nature of its ligand were known. Another decade had to pass before the TCR was characterized, and the notion that its ligand was a self MHC-bound foreign peptide started to emerge around the same time. The final answer concerning the way the TCR interacted with its ligand came from X-ray crystallographic studies after the mid-1990s, i.e., another 10–15 years later. Thus the observation of the phenomenon and its explanation were separated from one another by a time span of almost a quarter of a century. During this time immunologists had to develop some concept about T-cell recognition as a guidance to ask meaningful experimental questions. MHC restriction was therefore an ideal 'substrate' for theoreticians to work on, and indeed the most brilliant minds of the field took up the challenge of constructing hypotheses about T-cell recognition.

Finally two different concepts crystallized out for explaining the way T cells recognize antigen: one was termed 'altered self' or 'modified self' or the 'interaction antigen' hypothesis, and the other the 'dual recognition' hypothesis. As ever, the two concepts were formulated such that the validity of one should have cancelled the other, in other words, they were incompatible and competitive, and as a consequence, they divided immunologists into two opposing camps.

Chronologically, the first concept was 'altered self' proposed in 1974 by Zinkernagel and Doherty[6] as an explanation for their results showing killing of virus-infected parental target cells by F_1 cytotoxic T cells (Tc). The model was just a sketch without description in their one-page-long (but Nobel Prize worthy) *Nature* letter. Two different ways for Tc to recognize virus+MHC were envisaged (Figure 8.4):

1. First, the virus would interact somehow with MHC, and the interaction results in a new epitope, a 'neoantigen', that was not present before on either of the two components, and this, in turn, would be recognized by the receptor of Tc.
2. Second, the virus would associate with MHC, and the TCR would recognize both components.

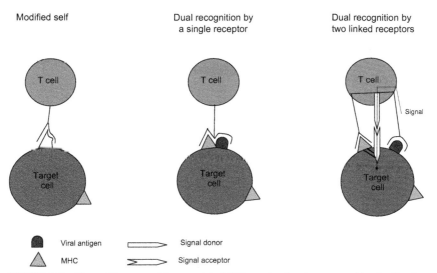

FIGURE 8.4   Three different models to explain MHC-restricted antigen recognition by T cells. See text for further explanation. Based on References 6 and 46.

It is interesting to note that, in a strict sense, only the first version qualifies as 'modified self', whereas the second model is indeed dual recognition by a single receptor site. The latter version was not pursued in subsequent elaborations of the modified self hypothesis because it was 'in between'. And ironically, this has proven to be the case in reality.

In subsequent years, the modified self hypothesis went through several rounds of amendment. At first, two further members of the John Curtin School group, Cunningham and Lafferty,[39] dealt with it in some detail. Their proposal was an opinion rather than a hypothesis, in which they re-emphasized the original finding, namely that T cells primed to an antigenic complex react to the same complex upon a second encounter. Since this could also apply to B cells, they did not see a fundamental difference in antigen recognition between T and B cells. The hypothesis started to take shape in a paper by Matzinger and Bevan,[40] in which the authors interpreted the strong reactivity of T cells to foreign MHC molecules (alloreactivity) as a T-cell response to 'interaction antigens' formed by foreign MHC and non-MHC molecules. Curiously, however, the graphical representation of their model showed MHC and non-MHC antigens as associated but clearly discernible entities recognized by a receptor site of dual specificity. Thus, there seemed to be a gap between their thinking and its visualization, suggesting that the concept of interaction antigen may not have been clearly formulated yet. The final, matured version of the modified self hypothesis was then presented by Matzinger[41] in 1981. Its major assumptions and predictions were the following.

1. T cells recognize neither antigen nor MHC molecules alone, but rather molecular complexes composed of the two.
2. Recognition is mediated by a single TCR binding site for the composite ligand.

3. The initial (germ-line) TCR repertoire may recognize anything, i.e., it is random.

4. MHC restriction is imposed on the TCR repertoire by specialized antigen-presenting cells (APC) that trigger T-cell differentiation only when T cells bind to MHC molecules (or MHC–non-MHC molecular complexes) on the surface of these APC.

5. As pointed out above, alloreactivity was considered to be a crossreaction of self-MHC-restricted T cells to allogeneic MHC+non-MHC molecular complexes.

The dual recognition hypothesis was based on the assumption that MHC restriction could not exist without MHC recognition. Therefore, TCR was thought to have two binding sites, one for foreign antigen and another for self MHC. This model had a number of 'precursors', too, proposed by Zinkernagel and Doherty,[42] Doherty et al.,[43] Janeway et al.,[44] and Blanden and Ada.[45] The first coherent concept based on evolutionary principles was formulated by Cohn and Epstein[47] and Langman,[46] and these were followed by several refinements by Cohn and Langman,[48] Cohn,[49] and Langman and Cohn.[50]

The essence of this concept was that TCR would consist of three physically linked units: a binding site for foreign antigen, another site for the restricting MHC molecule, and a signal donor. On the target cell, the MHC molecule is linked to a signal acceptor. The recognition of MHC by the anti-MHC site would position signal donor onto signal acceptor, and allow the effector signal (activation or killing) to pass through. Signaling itself is initiated exclusively by the anti-antigen site (Fig. 8.4). The assumptions and predictions of this hypothesis were:

1. The ligand of TCR is dual, consisting of foreign antigen and self MHC that may or may not associate with each other.

2. Recognition is mediated by two distinct, physically linked binding sites.

3. The germ-line encodes a TCR repertoire specific for all MHC molecules of the species.

4. Self MHC restriction results from positive somatic selection in the thymus.

5. Alloreactivity is germ-line-encoded, and does not involve the recognition of non-MHC components.

Since the answers to predictions 1 through 5 are now known, we are in the position of scoring the 'hit rate' of the two hypotheses (the 'winner' will be named).

1. Neither
2. Modified self
3. Dual recognition
4. Dual restriction
5. Both only partially.

Thus, both concepts predicted parts of reality almost equally well, although dual recognition was somewhat more explicit in the repertoire questions. On the other hand, the structure of TCR was predicted correctly by the modified self hypothesis. A common weakness of both models was that they did not really deal with the question of how foreign antigens could come to the surface of cells. For this reason, many immunologists, including the discoverers of MHC restriction,[5,6] could not commit themselves to either concept.

In hindsight, one can conclude that this theoretical exercise was surprisingly successful in making predictions about a molecular interaction, neither component of which was known. Of course, the participants were aware of the difficulty of their task, and probably this is why Janeway et al.[44] chose the following Robert Frost citation as a motto for their paper:

'We dance round in a ring and suppose
    But the secret sits in the middle and knows'

8.1.5 Immunology and its Theoreticians

This section belongs entirely to Dr. G.

'First of all let me point out that unlike other branches of science (e.g., physics, biology, genetics, etc.), immunology has hardly any theoreticians. A possible reason for this is that immunology has its roots in medicine, and the latter had developed from empiricism toward science, not the other way around. In addition, a large proportion, if not the majority of immunologists, has a medical background, and these colleagues carry over a pragmatic-empirical view from their education to their science. As a result, a value system has developed in immunology that overestimates experimental data, under-rates concepts, and fails to realize that one cannot exist without the other. A trivial, nonetheless vitally important consequence of this attitude is that granting agencies support almost exclusively experimental studies. As far as I know, at present, the only immunologist who lives on theoretical work is Mel Cohn (and he is well over 80), the remaining few are experimentalists doing theoretical work in their spare time.'

'The situation outlined above explains why most immunologists hesitate to accept or even argue about theories. For them immunological concepts represent a private issue, a duel to be fought out between Mel Cohn and Polly Matzinger. As an interesting contrast, however, there is one single concept that has been accepted, understood and known by everybody: the clonal selection theory of Burnet. And the authors of the two existing selection theories, Jerne and Burnet, enjoyed the status of an oracle: whatever they said was accepted almost unanimously, even if it was wrong (such as the network theory by Jerne). Of course this status was reached only after the clonal selection theory was proven experimentally, i.e., about 20 years later. It seems therefore that the acceptance of theoretical immunologists is similar to that of nineteenth century French painters: namely, the latter, had to die first, before their pictures could be sold.'

'Immunological theory has never been a subject of education, and so all those who contributed to it were originally or have remained experimentalists. Depending on the weight of conceptual work in their activity, they can be considered either theorizing experimentalists or experimenting theoreticians. The first group includes some of the best of us, for example, Av Mitchison, Mike Bevan, Charlie Janeway, and Hans Wigzell. These people were characterized by very sharp thinking, concept-driven experimentation, and a keen interest in the workings of the immune system, but they expected understanding to come from experimental data, and thus were not the ones, who would sit down and work out a theory in detail. It is the second group, experimenting theoreticians, whom I would like to talk about here. But my recollections will not cover all theoreticians in the field, only those whom I know personally.'

'Admittedly, I have always had an inclination for theories and theoreticians, perhaps because in my early career Ben Pernis told me: "If you want to contribute to immunology, you have to know two things: theory and the most recent methods". This was his way of expressing the two most important factors, "know-what" and "know-how", in the proper order. I have found talking with theoreticians always beneficial for at least two reasons: first, I learned a lot, and second, I could be sure that they would speak their mind, free from any political or business interest.'

'One of the most promising theoreticians was Alastair Cunningham, a crystal-clear thinker from the John Curtin School "think tank" in Canberra, Australia. Our "migration routes" crossed twice, at the Basel Institute and in Canada, this is how I got to know him. He started as an experimentalist, but soon devoted himself entirely to theory. At that time he worked at the Ontario Cancer Institute in Toronto, which housed the best Canadian immunology group headed by Rick Miller and Bob Philipps. Alastair could not have even suspected what an influence this place would have on his life! It all started in the mornings, when he went to work, and had to see a crowd of cancer patients waiting in the lobby for their treatment. Being a sensitive man he could read from their faces that the help they needed was not merely medical. So one day he enrolled onto a course of psychology, made a PhD, and specialized in the psychological treatment of cancer patients. This is how immunology lost a leading theoretician in favor of humanity. He also wrote a book *"The Healing Journey"* on his new topic of interest. Of course, the healing power of mind over body is difficult to assess by scientific methods, and is still treated with scepticism by Western medicine. Nevertheless, evidence in support of this concept is accumulating slowly. And apparently it did function in Alastair's own disease, because he recovered from it completely.'

'Perhaps the most colorful personality and most popular recent theoretician in immunology has been Polly Matzinger. Polly had almost too many outstanding qualities to fit into a single person. To start with the simplest, visible one, she was stunningly pretty, like nobody else ever in the field. In addition, she could be very friendly and charming. If she wanted. But if not, you really had bad luck! Since she would have qualified by her looks for show business, she also felt entitled to be sometimes mischievous like a diva. For example, her early claim to fame was a publication in the *Journal of Experimental Medicine*, in which she put her dog as a co-author.[51] After this escapade she could not publish in the *JEM* anymore, and this would have meant the end of her career for many, but not for Polly. For her the only difference it made was that later on she published mostly in *Nature* (and without her dog). Polly was also an excellent businesswoman, who always knew where, when and how to present her data or thoughts to obtain maximal attention. Her publications were written in a crisp and clear style, with a playful ease, so that everyone could understand and enjoy them. But her most important quality was her first-class thinking capability. She was a thinking talent probably by birth, a true biological thinker, who made the impression of thinking not only with the brain but with the whole body. She contributed, in addition to the modified self hypothesis, with many original ideas to the field, all of which were a joy to read. It is not surprising that Polly's ideas quickly became popular in the immunological community. And this was not everything: Polly has remained an experimenter all through her career, and her data were just as original as her theories. Polly's theoretical achievements were often contrasted to those of Mel Cohn, and the organizers of immunology meetings liked to arrange public debates between them. Here, the "show effect" was not so much the content of their debate as the polite but clearly sensible hostility between the two. It is difficult not to talk more about Polly. I only hope she will write up her memoires some day!'

'There were only two permanent, full-time theoreticians in immunology (who, of course, also started as experimenters): Mel Cohn and Rod Langman. Mention has already been made of Mel's activity at the Basel Institute for Immunology. Best known of his theoretical contributions was the two-signal model of lymphocyte activation[52] that was widely accepted and cited. Mel was running the Developmental Biology Laboratory at the Salk Institute, an interesting place to visit. Indeed, I have never missed the opportunity to drop in every time I had something to do at the West Coast. The place had a particularly beneficial effect on me, mostly because people in this group were thoughtful, open, communicative, and in addition, all looked happy. Compared to the fiercely competitive world of immunology, this place was an oasis of freedom and humanity. Although I have always had a high opinion of Mel, based on his behavior "on stage" where he was usually provocative, mocking and ironical, I would never have expected that he could create such an ideal working atmosphere. This shows once again that the hidden qualities of a person are best recognized through reflections by the surrounding people.'

'On one of my visits, I was picked up at San Diego airport by a tall, skinny and lively looking young guy, who introduced himself as Rod Langman. Our very first discussion took place in the car, and although it was not scientific in nature, I would like to reproduce it here, because nothing could serve as a better example to characterize Rod. This happened back in the time of the Cold War, when the US president in charge made a public statement that he could "envisage the possibility of a European war", with the justification that "we also have to sacrifice something". Being on the victims' side I was appalled by this statement and asked Rod what he thought about it. "Sure we have to sacrifice something" was the answer. "But this argument comes from religion, it has nothing to do with politics" I said. He got the point in milliseconds. "You're right, this is boloney", and a few seconds later "one should actually interlink them so tightly that they cannot make a war anymore". So this is what Rod was like: always open to a better idea, and ready to further develop it in a creative manner. From this point on, we had been close friends until his untimely death.'

'Rod established himself in the field by his clear, creative and elegant formulation of the dual recognition hypothesis.[46] Shortly before, he was a post doc in Mel's lab, but his student visa expired, and he left for Canada to wait for his US residence permit. While waiting he wrote up the hypothesis, and Mel did the same,[47] unbeknownst to each other. Only when they, by chance, exchanged manuscripts did it turn out that the concept had two versions, and so they published both. Polly Matzinger and Mike Bevan were also in Mel's lab, when they invented "modified self", the opposing concept.[40] Thus this place was as much central for immunological theories, as Jerusalem for religions. Rolf Zinkernagel was also there, but he, as a real Swiss, remained neutral amidst the theoretical debates.'

'In the subsequent 24 years Mel and Rod worked closely together. Their collaboration covered the entire field of conceptual immunology, and resulted in a number of new theories about antibody response,[53] T-cell recognition,[54] self–nonself discrimination,[55] and computerized models of the immune system.[56] Their theories were sometimes difficult to understand, and were not so easily accepted as Polly's, which by no means indicates that they were less valid. Mel and Rod had an enormous influence on my own thinking: among others I owe them for my evolutionary view of the immune system. I cannot be grateful enough for their friendship and intellectual input!'

8.2 CHASE FOR THE ANTIGEN RECEPTOR OF T CELLS

For a long time, the antigen receptor of T cells used to be merely an abstraction, because its existence was only assumed on the basis of the antigen specificity of T-cell responses. Yet, it was so central to immunology that everyone referred to it as 'the' T-cell receptor (TCR), tacitly implying that this was the only cell surface molecule on T cells that deserved the attention of immunologists. However, the way leading to the isolation and molecular characterization of TCR proved to be long and rough, paved with flaws and disappointments. After several years had passed and the TCR still kept refusing to reveal its identity, immunologists started to call it 'elusive' to conceal their embarrassment. This epithet was introduced by Simonsen and colleagues[57] as early as 1972, and its use became more and more frequent (and justified) with time, until the discovery of TCR in 1984. So it did not surprise anybody, when *Nature* commented the discovery in News and Views[58] under the following title: 'The T-lymphocyte antigen receptor – elusive no more'. Finally it has also turned out that there are two distinct TCR molecules, and thus, even the more precise term 'the' T-cell antigen receptor (or the TCAR) would have been factually incorrect.

8.2.1 Early Attempts at Identifying TCR: 'Ig or not Ig, this is the Question'

According to Burnet's clonal selection theory,[59] antibody specificities are clonally distributed, i.e., one cell produces only one specific antibody. This antibody is expressed on the surface of the respective B-cell clone, and serves as antigen receptor of the latter. Subsequently, this prediction was also confirmed experimentally.[60]

By analogy, most immunologists believed initially that the antigen receptor of T cells (TCR) should also be a clonally distributed immunoglobulin

(Ig). A popular argument in support of this assumption was that the development of a second, extremely diverse molecular species, in addition to Ig, would have been an unreasonably high evolutionary investment. (Although this argument sounded reasonable at that time, meanwhile we have learned that evolution tends to re-use successful exons, genes, and gene systems for different purposes, and that this strategy represents indeed the most economic investment.)

However, attempts to demonstrate Ig on the surface of T cells yielded disappointing results. First of all, by using immunofluorescence techniques most T cells appeared to be surface Ig negative, in contrast to B cells. When more sensitive techniques were used, such as lactoperoxidase-catalyzed surface radioiodination capable of detecting as few as 250 Ig molecules per cell, some authors[61] could demonstrate IgM on T cells whereas others could not.[62]

A subsequent series of experiments then shed serious doubts on the concept of Ig being TCR. One of the new approaches taken by Hudson et al.[63] was to use radioiodinated antibodies against chicken Ig light chain for the detection of surface Ig on chicken T cells by autoradiography. They found that after 7 days of exposure only B cells were Ig-positive. Upon increasing the sensitivity of this technique by long-term exposure, T cells also became positive, suggesting that they did carry surface Ig, but in smaller amounts than B cells. Surprisingly, however, in bursectomized chickens no surface Ig was found on T cells, indicating that the T-cell Ig was not synthesized endogenously but was acquired indirectly from B cells. In another set of experiments, different authors were able to show that T cells activated against allogeneic MHC molecules in vivo[64,65] or in vitro[66,67] carried sufficient Ig on their surface to be detected by immunofluorescence. These findings raised the possibility that T cells would express surface Ig only after specific activation with antigen.[66] The problem with this interpretation was that T cells, in order to become activated by antigen, should have expressed the antigen receptor also in the resting state. Thus, assuming that Ig was the antigen receptor, it should have been present on resting as well as activated cells. But these speculations soon came to a stop, after the demonstration that the surface Ig on in vivo alloactivated T cells was also originated from B cells.[68,69] It seemed therefore that the T-cell Ig almost certainly did not serve as antigen receptor.

Of course, the next question was how the activated T cells acquired Ig molecules, and what the latter had to do there after all. The simplest explanation for Ig acquisition, namely that it occurred via Fc receptors, was ruled out by the demonstration that these alloactivated T cells were Fc-receptor-negative.[70] The puzzle was finally solved by a research project at the Basel Institute for Immunology, in which Dr. G was heavily involved, and so it is his turn again.

'The first question was what experimental model to choose for these studies. The in vivo model consisted of parental thymus cells injected into irradiated F_1 (i.e., MHC heterozygous) recipients. T cells activated against incompatible MHC molecules of the second parent carried Ig on their surface, and could be recovered from the thoracic duct. This model was at hand in Basel, it was brought in by Jonathan Sprent.'

'Jonathan was a young export of the "Australian School", a quiet, serious, critically thinking and hard-working scientist, and a polite person, diagonally opposite to most of the overexcited Basel youth. The latter often criticized him quite vehemently at seminars, not really for scientific reasons, but probably for his being different. In contrast, Harald von Boehmer, who was an aristocrat and as such valued proper behavior, liked and appreciated him very much. Nowadays every immunologist must know the name of Jonathan Sprent, because he has become one of the "living classics" for his numerous significant contributions.'

'His in vivo model had, however, some disadvantages. First, it required thoracic duct cannulation of mice, an operation that probably Jonathan could only perform. This was per se not a serious problem, because he was there, and a whole bunch of cannulated mice were running on a big wheel in Harald's lab. More problematic was the fact that the in vivo model was not as readily amenable to experimental manipulations as an in vitro system.'

'The team therefore decided to use the mixed lymphocyte reaction (MLR) as a model, in which Ig-positive T cells were also demonstrable.[66,67] Thus we started to investigate MLR-activated T cells by two-color fluorescence for Ig and a T-cell marker, respectively, that represented the state of the art technology at that time. Indeed we could see many Ig-positive T cells, but the staining was patchy and weak, sometimes only a few green spots per cell, nothing to compare with the strong, ring-type fluorescence seen on B cells. Fortunately, Ben Pernis, an old immunofluorescence expert, looked at the cells and confirmed that the fluorescence was real, otherwise we could have easily taken it for an artefact. We then used purified T cells as MLR responders, obtained by another brand-new technology: nylon wool column separation.[71] This method, as new techniques in general, was somewhat tricky, but luckily its discoverer Michael Julius was also at the Institute, and with his help we managed to obtain T-cell populations with <1% B-cell contamination. Interestingly, T-cell blasts from B-cell-depleted responder populations were surface Ig negative, indicating that the Ig came from B cells present in the same culture. This result raised the possibility that in MLR cultures, beside T cells, B cells can also become activated by allogeneic MHC molecules to produce antibodies against the stimulating alloantigens. Indeed we were able to show that Ig-negative T blasts from B-cell-depleted responder cells, when treated with specific anti-stimulator MHC antibodies, showed again a patchy-type fluorescence with anti-Ig reagents.[72] The implication was that stimulator alloantigens must have been bound to T cells, and that the bound antigen also had free epitopes available for anti-stimulator antibodies. Thus what we had on the activated responder T cells was a kind of piggy-back, the first layer of which was stimulator antigen, and the second layer on top was anti-stimulator antibody. A nice little "natural artefact" to mislead poor immunologists. Later we could also show that the stimulator antigens were bound to the responder T cells specifically, most likely via the unknown TCR.[73] Hence this experimental system appeared promising for "fishing out" TCR via the bound alloantigens and antibodies. Unfortunately, all attempts in this direction failed. Thus, the TCR finally remained "elusive", but we still achieved one thing: nobody considered surface Ig as a candidate for TCR anymore.'

'These results appeared interesting enough to be presented at a "high-end" immunology meeting, where everybody who counted was present. I immediately picked out from the crowd Av Mitchison, who was sitting in the front row and sleeping. But as soon as I finished talking, he jumped up and asked a question. This surprised me so much that I could hardly give an answer. Years later I realized that this was his favorite show to embarrass speakers.'

'But Mitchison used the "sleeping trick" also for other purposes. For example, once he visited a university somewhere at the edge of British Commonwealth, and the local clinic boss, an immunology aficionado himself, threw a big party in his honor in his lake-side villa (with private yacht harbor, of course). Mitchison arrived at the party in his usual outfit consisting of a pair of trousers that hadn't seen an iron for years, and an old, stretched-out pullover. He greeted the guests nicely, smiled at everybody, but did not talk much, instead he found a comfortable armchair, strategically located in the middle of the living room, sat down and fell asleep. Clearly, Av Mitchison was an active non-conformist and anti-snob. Of course, he could also communicate normally, but only with those selected ones, whom he considered acceptable human beings.'

'After my conference talk, Janos Gergely, Chairman of the Hungarian Immunology Society, a man with a good sense of humor, came to me "Congratulations on your talk" he said "Even God Mitchison seemed to be interested." "True, he is a god, but not in a monotheistic sense" was my answer. So we soon set up an immunological Holy Trinity, in which the Father was Burnet, who stood above and beyond everything and everybody, the Son was Av Mitchison, who attended every meeting and talked to the people, and the Holy Spirit was Niels Jerne, who floated above us invisibly, in his roof-top office at the Basel Institute. However, this was just an oversimplification. For, in reality, immunology had more gods than the late Roman Empire.'

8.2.2 Serological Approaches to the Isolation of TCR

By the mid-1970s it became clear that TCR was structurally unrelated to immunoglobulin, in that it was not recognized by anti-Ig antibodies (although claims of the opposite were also made). In other words, there was no easy way for its molecular characterization. In one respect, however, TCR remained similar to Ig, namely, antigen specificity. Therefore it was reasonable to assume that TCRs, similarly to Ig, must have variable (V) regions that form a large number of different antigen-combining sites. Implicit in this statement is that different V regions of TCR must carry distinct idiotypes recognizable by anti-idiotypic antibodies like in the case of Ig.[74,75] The approach then would have been to generate antigen-specific T cells and use them as immunogen to raise anti-idiotypic antibodies specific for their receptor. Unfortunately, the technical preconditions were not yet in place for such an enterprise: in vitro culture of T cells was still in its infancy, cloning of antigen-specific T cells was achieved only about 5 years later, and monoclonal antibodies were just discovered, but not yet widely used. Under these circumstances only a good idea could get the project starting.

The leading idea in this early phase of TCR hunting came from transplantation immunology, and was referred to as 'the Ramseier principle', named after the Swiss immunologist who proposed it.[76] It originated from the observation that MHC type **a** T cells injected into (**a** x **b**)F₁ animals, although induced a graft-versus-host disease, the hosts after a while learned to get the disease under control. The finding was interpreted as follows: the F₁ hosts must have eliminated **a** anti-**b** T cells by self tolerance, and therefore the **a** anti-**b** TCR expressed on the grafted **a** cells activated against the **b** parental MHC represents a foreign antigen for the host. The latter is then capable of producing anti-idiotypic antibodies against this TCR, and such antibodies in turn suppress the disease. This model was then turned into immunization protocols, for example, **a** T cells activated against **b** in mixed lymphocyte reaction, in vitro, were injected repeatedly into F₁ hosts to raise anti-idiotypic antibodies. Using this or similar systems, some laboratories reported on antisera with the expected anti-idiotypic specificity.[77–79] Unfortunately, these antisera were of limited usefulness for two reasons: first, because activation across whole MHC induced a huge polyclonal response and a correspondingly high number of diverse idiotypes, and second, because the antibodies were raised in mice (or rats) and were thus available in too small amounts for protein chemical studies.

Another popular idea was the 'shared idiotype' hypothesis, according to which antibodies and TCR specific for the same antigen should have idiotypes in common.[77,80,81] Consequently, immunization with anti-MHC antibodies, for example, **a** anti-**b**, should result in anti-idiotypic antibodies that crossreact with **a** T cells activated against MHC type **b** in a mixed lymphocyte reaction. This approach suffered from the same problem as the one above. Namely, the antibody used as immunogen was polyclonal representing a whole array of different idiotypes, and the anti-idiotypic antibody raised against it was probably even more heterogeneous displaying very complicated reactivity patterns. Altogether these early attempts were deemed to remain unsuccessful, because they lacked analytical precision.

At this stage it was clear that the success of the serological approach critically depended on a source of homogeneous antigenic material (e.g., TCR on cloned T cells) to be used as immunogen. The technological breakthrough making this possible was the cloning and in vitro expansion of antigen-specific T cells in culture media supplemented with T-cell growth factor (later interleukin-2; IL-2) that was achieved around 1980 simultaneously, in a number of laboratories.[82–85] Another approach was to 'immortalize' antigen-specific T cells by fusion with T cell tumor lines. The resulting hybridoma could be cloned and grew infinitely in standard tissue culture media. The T-cell hybridoma technology was successfully applied first by Kappler, and Marrack and colleagues,[86] who were able to produce antigen-specific MHC-restricted hybrids that grew in culture without stimulation, and their specificity could be 'recalled', i.e., they produced IL-2 when challenged with antigen presented by spleen cells of the appropriate MHC type.

'John Kappler and Philippa (or Pepa, as she likes to be called) Marrack have probably been the most successful married couple in immunology', remarks Dr. G. 'While both are equally good scientists, they have very different personalities, John being friendly and gentle, and Pepa tough and authoritative. Obviously their harmony is based on complementarity. They provide a good example for a well-known phenomenon, namely that science is often performed in duets. The duets may be of the same or of different sex, but they are always formed between complementary personalities. There have been many duets in immunology, e.g., Mel Cohn and Rod Langman, Eli Sercarz and Alex Miller in the US, Hermann Wagner and Martin Röllinghof in Germany, and Diane Mathis and Christoph Benoist in France, just to mention a few. The benefit from this collaboration modus is that the output of the duet is usually much more than just the sum of productivities of the two.'

Since all leading T-cell laboratories of the world used the anti-idiotype strategy for generating anti-TCR antibody, and they were at a comparable technological stage, it was predictable that more than one of them would also succeed. The year when this happened was 1983. Based on the date of publication the first monoclonal antibodies (mAbs) to TCR were reported by the group of Ellis Reinherz and Stuart Schlossman[87] at the Harvard-affiliated Dana-Farber Cancer Institute in Boston, in February. They produced two mAbs against a human alloreactive cytotoxic T-cell clone. The mAbs bound exclusively to the immunizing clone, specifically inhibited its cytolytic function, and immunoprecipitated two molecules of 49 000 and 43 000 molecular weight (mw) under reducing conditions from the clone. The authors assumed that these two 'clonotypic' molecules make up the antigen receptor of T cells. The clonotypic structures were associated in the membrane with the 20 000 mw T3 (now CD3) molecule[88] expressed in all T cells, and assumed to be involved in the signaling of T cells. The first mAb to a class II-restricted antigen-specific TCR was reported by the Kappler-Marrack team[89] in Denver, in April. This mAb was raised against an ovalbumin (OVA)-specific, I-A^d (murine MHC-II) restricted T-cell hybridoma, and appeared also clonotypic reacting only against the immunizing hybridoma, and not to other OVA-specific T cells tested. It precipitated an 80 000 mw dimer that upon reduction dissociated into 40-44 000 mw monomers. The very thorough and detailed characterization of the mAb left no doubt that the disulfide-bonded dimeric molecule it detected was indeed the antigen-specific class II restricted TCR, or at least part of it. In the very same year four additional clonotypic mAbs with similar characteristics (but raised against different T-cell clones) were reported by Frank Fitch and colleagues in Chicago,[90] Charlie Janeway's group[91] at Yale University, the Reinherz-Schlossman team,[92] and Ron Schwartz[93] at the NIH, followed by a fifth one in early 1984 produced by Mike Bevan's team[94] at Scripps Clinic. The collective observation from these studies was that all clonotypic mAbs reacted with virtually the same ~80 000 mw disulfide-bonded dimer. This molecule was therefore likely to be used for antigen recognition by all T cells.

'The anti-idiotype approach appeared at that time to be (and was indeed) the only feasible strategy for generating TCR-specific serological reagents, and everybody was aware of this', points out Dr. G. 'So it was not surprising that so many labs succeeded almost the same time. This did not really represent true competition, because many labs were in fact not aware of the ongoing work in other groups. The almost inflationary success of the approach resulted solely from the collective knowledge of strategy. Actually any lab that possessed T-cell clones and hybrid-oma technology could have made such mAbs, and indeed many more were produced later, in addition to the "pioneers" listed above. I must admit, I was also about making one, the immunized mice with the expected serum antibodies were there, ready for hybridomas. But the head of the department I used to work at didn't like the project, and while I was out for a week vacation, he ordered the mice be killed.'

'It came as a surprise that a human immunology group won the race, before all the mouse immunology "favorites". Only those colleagues were less surprised who worked with both mouse and human T cells, and therefore knew how much easier the latter are to handle. Indeed, the "robustness" and "willingness" of human T cells might have been a factor in the rapid success of the Reinherz-Schlossman group. It is also interesting that not all T-cell cloner groups pursued the anti-clonotype approach. For example, Harald von Boehmer, a pioneer of T-cell cloning did not use his advantage for making anti-TCR mAbs. Also Garry Fathman, another pioneer of long-term T-cell culturing, although the first to pub-lish a clonotypic antiserum,[95] did not produce mAbs. Not that he didn't want to, but the project probably overlapped with his relocation from Basel to Stanford, and he might have been too busy with setting up his new lab.'

The clonotypic mAbs, although the door-opener for TCR studies, had the disad-vantage of reacting only with an undetectably small fraction of normal T cells. However, they permitted the isolation of purified receptor material, which in turn was used for immunization to obtain mAbs that reacted with measurable portions of normal T cells. Some of these mAbs behaved as anti-allotypic,[96] others apparently recognized all TCR.[97]

Protein chemistry performed with the aid of anti-TCR mAbs revealed that the two TCR chains of similar mw were distinct, separable on the basis of charge: the more acidic chain was termed α and the more basic one β chain.[89,93] Both chains were shown to contain variable and constant regions.[87,98]

With the discovery of the TCR gene complex (to be discussed next), the anti-TCR mAb approach experienced a renaissance. This was because the TCR V-gene usage of T-cell clones could be determined, and these clones could then be used to assign the specificity of mAbs to defined V gene products. Indeed, some of the earlier anti-clonotypes also turned out to recognize particular TCR V regions. Furthermore, a large deletion of TCR $V\beta$ genes was discovered in certain mouse strains,[99] which permitted the immunization of the deficient strain with normal T cells from non-deleting strains.[100] Finally, a series of addi-tional innovative approaches enabled the production of a whole battery of mAbs specific for defined regions of TCR. These antibodies are now commercially available, and represent important tools in research and diagnostics.

8.2.3 The Winner is Again Molecular Biology: The TCR Gene Complex

In 1984 the reading public of the world was relieved, because George Orwell's nightmare vision was proven wrong or at least grossly pre-dated, and immunologists were particularly relieved, as the puzzle of TCR was finally cracked. The solution came from studies of T-cell-specific gene expression. Immunologists, who had been exposed to molecular biology since the discovery of immunoglobulin genes by Tonegawa, now had to learn the meaning of additional, novel approaches, for example, 'subtraction library'. They also had to learn at least two new actors in the field, namely, Mark Davis, a young fellow at the NIH (later at Stanford University) and Tak Mak at the Ontario Cancer Institute in Toronto, who identified the first TCR genes in mouse and human, respectively.

The molecular biological strategy was based on the following assumptions about TCR genes:

1. First, they should be expressed in T cells but not in B cells or other cell types
2. Second, like Ig genes, TCR genes should rearrange somatically
3. Third, as Ig molecules, TCR should have constant and variable regions encoded in separate genes.

The experimental procedure developed on the basis of these assumptions by Mark Davis and colleagues[101] started with the production of labeled cDNA from mRNA of antigen-specific mouse T-cell hybridomas. They used only mRNA from membrane-bound polysomes (~3% of total mRNA), where the TCR transcript was expected to be. The cDNA was then hybridized to mRNA from B cells to 'subtract' all genes expressed in both cell types in common (~98%). The remaining cDNA representing about 0.5% of the input was used as a probe to screen a library of cloned cDNAs. Ten T-cell-specific cDNA clones were identified, one of which hybridized to a region of genome that rearranged in several different T-cell lines. This clone was sequenced and compared with crossreacting clones from a thymocyte library.[102] The results showed the presence of variable (V), constant (C) and joining (J) regions in the gene that were similar in size and sequence to the corresponding regions of Ig genes. The authors concluded that this gene encoded one chain of TCR (the β chain, as it later turned out).

The approach taken by Tak Mak and colleagues,[103] although relying on the same assumptions, was somewhat different. These authors produced cDNA clones from mRNA of a human leukemic T-cell line that was known to express TCR protein. The clones were then grouped on the basis of their relative expression in the same T-cell line versus a human B-cell line. Four virtually T-cell-specific clones were identified, all of which hybridized selectively to T-cell mRNA from different sources, but not to RNA from other hematopoietic or non-hematopoietic cell types. One of these clones was sequenced and found to be homologous to the V, J and C regions of mammalian Ig. This clone was also shown later to hybridize to a region of DNA rearranging in human T cells.

Thus the clone seemed to code for a chain of the human TCR (it happened to be again the β chain).

These two ground-breaking studies were quickly followed by an almost campaign-like series of investigations with the participation of all major molecular biology laboratories including Lee Hood's lab at the California Institute of Technology, Jack Strominger's group at Harvard, and also the lab of 'grand master' Tonegawa (who moved meanwhile from Basel to the Massachusetts Institute of Technology). This concerted effort resulted in a nearly complete information on TCR genes within a few years. The gene encoding the TCR α chain was cloned in both mice[104,105] and human[106] still in 1984, followed the next year by the unexpected finding of a third gene coding for a distinct TCR chain termed γ.[107–109] The γ gene posed a new puzzle, first of all because the γ transcript was found in cells that already expressed both the α and the β genes. This finding taken together with the observation that almost all T cells (about 97%) express the αβ TCR, seemed to suggest that T cells might have two different receptors formed by three different chains. However, in a later study focussing on the remaining 3% αβ-negative T cells, it has been shown that the γ chain is associated with a fourth polypeptide termed δ, thus, this small subpopulation of T cells expresses a second, distinct TCR heterodimer.[110]

But this was not quite the end of finding unexpected TCR chains. In ontogeny, the TCR β gene was found to be expressed first, followed later by the α gene. In the time interval in between the β chain does not remain 'partnerless', it is expressed on the cell surface together with yet another polypeptide chain that was named by its discoverer, Harald von Boehmer, pre-Tα.[111] This novel chain also belongs to the Ig superfamily, and seems to be indispensable during T-cell ontogeny.[112] Its apparent role is to rescue cells containing a productively rearranged β gene from programmed cell death. After rearrangement of the α gene, the pre-Tα polypeptide becomes replaced by a 'proper' α chain. Thus pre-Tα appears to 'prioritize' the lineage commitment of T cells in favor of αβ TCR expression. In this context, it is interesting to note that pre-antigen receptors seem to be a must during lymphocyte development, as B cells also possess a pre-B chain that associates with the μ heavy chain of Ig early in ontogeny.[113]

To identify possible evolutionary relationships between TCR and other proteins, the amino acid sequences of TCR chains (deduced from cDNA) were compared to other known protein sequences. As already mentioned above, the closest similarity found was with Ig, whereas other members of the Ig superfamily, e.g., MHC, appeared more distantly related. The homology between TCR and Ig is highest at sequence positions that are important for maintaining protein structure, for example, the positions of cysteins involved in intra- and interchain disulfide bonds, as well as in sequences flanking the conserved cysteins. Interestingly, however, it could not be unequivocally established whether TCR chains are more similar to heavy or light chains of Ig, and mouse TCR sequences were found equally homologous to mouse Ig and human Ig. These observations suggest that TCR genes and Ig genes have evolved from a common ancestor, but the two gene systems must have diverged before the separation of heavy and light chain genes of Ig, and the time at which this happened was so long ago that the evolutionary distance between mouse and human appears in comparison as a rather short interval.

Molecular biologists worked also with a white-hot fury on the genomic organization of TCR genes and gene segments. These studies that ran parallel in mouse[114–118] and human[118–123] will not be discussed in detail, suffice it to say that they represented another tour de force of molecular biology, in the course of which new 'world records' were established, for example, the longest ever stretch of contiguous DNA was sequenced. The final results, the organization of the TCR gene complex, are summarized in Fig. 8.5.

It is obvious at first sight that the organization of TCR loci is homologous to that of Ig loci (see in Fig. 5.1). In both instances, the protein is encoded in separate V, J, C, or V, D, J, C segments. The functional gene encoding the V region is produced in both cases by somatic rearrangement of V-J and V-D-J segments, respectively. The initial diversity of proteins results from the almost random choice of V, D and J gene segments out of many. Differences between the two gene families exist in the way they generate further diversity. Whereas Ig loci have many more V segments than TCR loci, the opposite is true for J segments. Thus junctional diversity is much higher in the case of TCR genes, and this is further increased by imprecise V-J joining, the use of D segments in

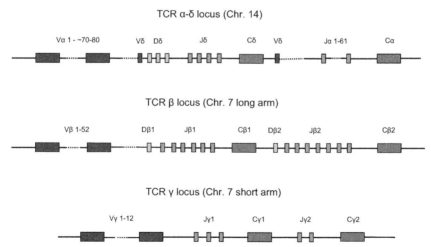

FIGURE 8.5   Genomic organization (and chromosomal location) of human TCR loci. In addition to the two Vδ segment shown, six further Vδ genes are interspersed among Vα. Multi-segment organization of C genes is not shown. Murine TCR loci are homologous to human. Differences exist only in the number of V genes, and in the γ locus, which contains one more functional VJC cluster. Based on References 118–123.

all three reading frames, and frequent N-additions of nucleotides at V-D and D-J junctions. In contrast, somatic hypermutation of V genes that is a major mechanism of Ig diversification does not seem to occur in TCR genes. It seems therefore that while Igs diversify along the entire V region (in all complementarity determining regions, CDR1, 2, 3), the somatic variability of TCR is limited to the junctional (CDR3) region.

Interesting is the organization of the TCR α locus that also contains the δ locus embedded. This arrangement that is conserved between mice and human may be an incidental result of gene duplication. But it has a functional consequence, namely that in case of a productive α rearrangement the entire δ locus will be deleted. Thus, the arrangement of the α-δ locus in contemporary immune systems provides a mechanism for keeping the two T cell lineages, $\alpha\beta$ and $\gamma\delta$, separate. Another interesting feature of TCR loci is that α and β are much more diverse than γ and δ. This again makes functional sense, since $\alpha\beta$ T cells are mostly or perhaps entirely responsible for the recognition of peptides bound to class I and class II MHC molecules. In contrast, $\gamma\delta$ TCRs are often expressed on natural killer-like T cells, and seem to recognize non-peptidic microbial products presented by 'non-classical' MHC molecules (e.g., CD1, Qa-1).[124–127] This T-cell subset localizing in the skin and intestinal epithelia is involved in the immediate local defense against microbes, and thus represents a link between the adaptive and innate immune systems.

'Although the discovery and characterization of TCR genes was one of the most exciting piece of work ever done in immunology, the results did not fully meet the expectations of immunobiologists', adds Dr. G. – 'What immunobiologists anticipated was that this research would shed light on the mechanism of MHC restriction, and this was not the case. TCRs turned out to be homologous to Ig, both at the gene level and in their predicted protein structure, and this finding gave no clue as to why the former are MHC restricted and the latter not. Furthermore, no clear differences were found in TCR V-gene usage in mouse strains of different MHC types[128] (except in a few instances[129]), and often the same V genes were used in T cells recognizing antigen presented by class I and class II MHC, respectively. Thus MHC restriction could not be simply explained by the selective use of different Vα and/or Vβ gene products for the recognition of different MHC molecules. This rather sobering conclusion left immunobiologists with the only hope that perhaps the resolution of the 3-dimensional structure of TCR will help solving the puzzle.'

8.2.4 How T Cells Recognize Antigen: Crystallography of TCR–peptide–MHC Complexes

The crystallization of TCR, in principle a straightforward task, turned out in reality to be much harder than anticipated. Namely, 'native' TCR proteins did not form crystals adequate for X-ray diffraction analysis, and thus a whole series of different protein engineering and expression methods had to be tried before the problem finally yielded to technology. The operation took altogether 11 years, from the publication of the first TCR sequences in 1984 until the first reported TCR structure in 1995.

In the meantime immunologists attempted to gain insight into T-cell recognition by applying indirect methods. For example, TCR was modeled on the basis of its homology to Ig Fab fragments, and this model was fitted over the α helices flanking the peptide-binding site of MHC.[117] Another approach involved the immunization of mice transgenic to a single TCR chain (α or β) with peptides that vary at residues affecting T cell response (but not MHC binding). By sequencing the complementing TCR chain involved in the responses, TCR residues contacting the peptide could be identified.[130] The model that has emerged from these studies proposed the TCR to 'dock' on the α1 helix of MHC with the CDR1 and CDR2 loops of the TCR β chain, and with CDR1 and CDR2 of TCR α on the α2 MHC helix (or β1 in MHC-II), which would position the CDR3 loops of both chains over the bound peptide. Thus this model assigned MHC recognition to the germ-line-encoded part of the V region, and peptide recognition to the somatically varied part. In addition to the proposed parallel alignment of the TCR-binding site with MHC helices, the authors[117] also envisaged the possibility of TCR docking perpendicular to MHC helices, but found this version less appealing and less consistent with data available at that time.

The three-dimensional structure of TCR α and β chain[131,132] confirmed in many respects the predictions based on Ig homology. Indeed, the typical β-sheet sandwich structures termed 'Ig fold' could be identified in both V and with some variations in the C region of TCR chains, the interface between chains was also similar to that between the H and L chains, and the variable CDR loops were located on the top of the molecule. Altogether the TCR structure resembled a membrane-anchored Fab fragment. Again, these results failed to explain why TCR were MHC restricted, and thus the mechanism of MHC restriction slowly began to appear at least as elusive as TCR itself used to be some 20 years earlier. Fortunately, at this point the so far obstinate technology started to show its obedient side, as it turned out that complexes of TCR with peptide and MHC (pMHC) crystallize much more readily than TCR alone. And the analysis of TCR–pMHC complexes finally allowed a glimpse into the structural basis of MHC restriction.

The present knowledge about the way T cells recognize antigen is based largely on the crystallographic analysis of half a dozen TCR–pMHC complexes, four with class I[133–137] and two with class II MHC molecules.[138,139] From the biological point of view most important was the finding that the docking orientation of TCR on MHC was comparable in all complexes. If one considers the MHC α1 helix as North (the upper helix in most graphic representations) and the α2 or (in class II) β1 helix as South, then all TCRs were found to dock diagonally, so that TCRα was at SW and TCRβ at NE

(Fig. 8.6). This alignment positions αCDR1 over the N-terminal part of the peptide and the neighboring MHC surface (mostly the α2/β1 and partially the α1 helix), αCDR2 exclusively over the α2/β1 helix, and βCDR1 over the peptide C-terminus plus parts of the helices, and βCDR2 entirely over the α1 helix (Fig. 8.6). The MHC surface buried by TCR is highly homologous in class I and class II, which permits the use of the same V gene pool in the recognition of both classes. The CDR3 loops of both chains are located side by side, covering the middle portion of the bound peptide, but they contact also the helical walls. This orientation appears to be universal, differences exist only in the angle of TCR contact surface relative to the MHC-bound peptide, which can vary from 45° to 80°. Another highly relevant finding was that about two-thirds of the surface buried by TCR was contributed by the MHC and one-third by the peptide. The number of atomic contacts with MHC also exceeded that with the peptide. Thus TCR has turned out to be a receptor that 'sees' both MHC and peptide together, i.e., neither 'modified self' nor two separate entities as hypothesized earlier.

'These studies have been cardinal for our understanding of T-cell recognition, but their interpretation should be enjoyed with caution', warns Dr. G. 'This is because crystallographers were fascinated by different aspects of the data than immunologists, and thus often shifted the emphasis away from immunological relevance. For example, the poor complementarity of TCR–MHC contact surface

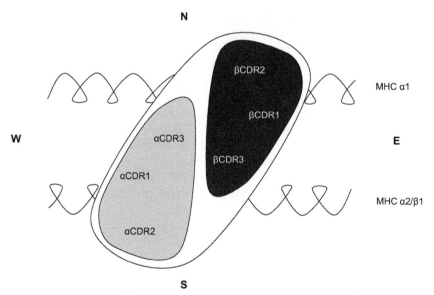

FIGURE 8.6 Schematic representation of the docking orientation of TCR on MHC. Docking of TCR on MHC helices occurs in a diagonal orientation of various angles. Approximate positions of CDR loops of the α chain and β chain, and principal cartographic directions are indicated. Based on References 133–139.

was often overemphasized and taken as a sign of poor specificity, although it translates into low affinity, and the latter does not imply a decay of specificity; if anything the opposite. Also the fact that the different docking angles resulted from different atomic contacts was interpreted as low specificity or preferentially termed "flexibility" or "plasticity", which mean the same. Clearly, the described kind of TCR–MHC interaction, whatever we want to call it, is a fact, and as such probably has functional significance, i.e., it has been selected for. I will expand on this thought later.'

'The structural explanation for the diagonal docking mode was to avoid the two high points of MHC helices located at NW and SE. This way the TCR can contact a large and more or less flat surface. This certainly makes sense, but does not explain why TCRs never dock in a 180° rotated orientation, although this would be stereochemically comparable, with the difference that the α chain would be NE and the β SW. Thus the common docking topology may have a deeper biological meaning, for example, that the recognition of SW by Vα and NE by Vβ are the result of evolutionary selection.'

Particularly informative was the part of crystallographic studies that dealt with the interaction of CDR3 loops with the MHC-bound peptide. As already mentioned, the CDR3 loops are positioned over the middle portion of the peptide, the α-chain loop being closer to the N-terminus and CDR3 β to the C-terminus of peptide. The interface of the two loops forms a pocket in most (but not all) complexes, the size of which is sufficient to accommodate a large amino acid side chain. The occupancy of this pocket has turned out to be important in determining the antigenicity of peptide. For example, the lack of interaction at this single site can turn an antigenic peptide into a partial agonist. In general, antigenic peptides all engaged in strong hydrophobic or electrostatic interactions with TCR. In contrast, a self peptide that was not antigenic made only precarious contacts, and its interface with TCR exhibited poor shape complementarity with large empty spaces in between. These data have established that the number and strength of interactions between the peptide and TCR, in particular the CDR3 loops of the latter, are decisive factors in signaling antigenicity of the peptide to the T cell.

8.3   T-CELL RECOGNITION: FROM FACTS TOWARD UNDERSTANDING

Although most details of T-cell recognition have been uncovered experimentally from the biology down to the level of atomic interactions, the findings have not been quite as revealing as expected. In particular, difficulties tend to arise if one attempts to explain the biology with the available structural data.

For example, MHC restriction at the biological level usually appears MHC-allele-specific, but the TCR V regions responsible for the docking of receptor on MHC molecules do not exhibit obvious allele specificity. The usage of TCR V regions shows no clear correlation with the MHC alleles expressed in the same individual,[128] although quantitative MHC-dependent differences can be demonstrated.[140,141] Thus, with some exceptions.[129,142] it is not possible to assign a particular V region to the recognition of a given MHC molecule. Even more confusing is the finding that the very same V region is capable of docking on both class I and class II MHC molecules,[133,138] but on the contrary, certain V regions can clearly distinguish between the two MHC classes.[143]

Another conceptual problem is posed by the unpredicted diagonal docking orientation of TCR on pMHC. This results in the positioning of CDR2 loops of both chains over the MHC only, but the CDR1 and 3 loops of both chains can contact peptide as well as MHC. Thus, there seems to be no straightforward way for the TCR to distinguish between peptide and MHC, and consequently, between docking and response.

And last but not least, the affinities of TCRs for pMHC range from 10^{-4} to 10^{-6} M, i.e., from barely detectable to low,[144,145] whereas the affinities of antibodies for antigen are between 10^{-8} and 10^{-10} M. Taken that the two structures are highly homologous, why do they work in so widely different affinity ranges?

These few examples illustrate well the complexity of the topic, but are by no means the only open questions. Thus one feels at a loss, when trying to assemble the facts into a coherent picture, and wonders if it is possible at all.

'This sounds like a "Mayday" signal to me', says Dr. G. 'But I must disappoint you, because even to date, as of 2011, there is no completely clear understanding of T-cell recognition. In such complicated cases full of virtual contradictions, the only thing one can do is to try to re-think the function of T cells from square one on, and to assign an evolutionary driving force to each property that turns up on the way. If this is possible, the identified feature could be real, if not, it is likely to be false. I could try such an exercise here, but cannot guarantee that the end will be a revelation.'

8.3.1 T-Cell Function in a Nutshell

'The evolutionary selection pressure for the development of T-cell-mediated immunity has been to provide defense against intracellular infection (mostly by viruses). Because T cells cannot look into the cell, nor can they pull the virus out of the cell, they had to develop means by which they recognize virus-derived material on the cell surface, and destroy the cells displaying such material, before the pathogen could replicate out of control.'

And what about helper T cells?

'Helper T cells use the very same recognition mechanism for a different function (immunoregulation), and thus probably represent a more recent descent of the protective T-cell system. Besides they are also protective on their own right. In this context helper T cells are just one of the countless examples to demonstrate that evolution prefers to re-use successful genes and mechanisms for different purposes instead of making new ones from scratch.'

'Concerning the source of information about intracellular pathogens it is important to realize that the defense system had no choice other than the MHC. The ancestral MHC as part of a house-keeping mechanism to remove intracellular waste must have been there evolutionary ages earlier than the defense system.[146] Thus the latter had to evolve to be able to find the MHC and investigate its contents for the presence of pathogen-derived breakdown products. T cells were therefore destined to a function that is like rummaging in the garbage can. From this reasoning it should be clear that MHC restriction is not just a fancy of TCR; it was dictated by what had been made available by evolution.'

How did the defense system stumble on MHC? Was it just trial and error or could it have been a directed process?

'At present nobody could answer this question, because there are no data that would give us a clue. My preference would be a directed process, but all I can offer in support is a halfway educated guess. The starting point could have been the property of MHC to respond to cellular stress by increased cell surface expression.[147] Cells of the ancient defense system might have sensed the increased density of MHC via low-affinity crossreaction of a cell surface receptor. The resulting cell–cell interaction could have led to elimination of the stressed cell, and provided that the cause of stress was infection, the host enjoyed some survival advantage. Thus the molecular interaction between MHC and the unknown receptor of defensive cells was placed under the control of natural selection. Because cellular stress can also arise from a variety of non-infectious stimuli (heat, radiation, starvation, reactive oxygen species, etc.), the elimination of stressed cells did not always provide a selective advantage, in other words, there was room for improvement by natural selection. It is easy to envisage that subsequent mutations of the receptor leading to the recognition of a pathogen-derived product in addition to MHC could have provided substantially more advantage. At this stage the defensive cell might have been equipped with an invariant receptor similar to the TCR expressed by natural killer-like T cells.[126,127] Somatic variability came into play later, probably following the insertion of a transposon into the receptor gene, as proposed by Lee Hood and colleagues.[148] And here we arrived at the common ancestor of TCR and immunoglobulins.'

'What we have learned so far is that the function of T cells involves two different steps: first, docking on MHC and second, recognizing and responding to pathogen-derived material associated with the MHC. These two steps have very different biology and logistics, so I will have to deal with them separately.'

8.3.2 Specificity Requirements for Docking of TCR on MHC

'Effective TCR–MHC interactions have to meet two specificity requirements: first, TCR should not dock on structures other than MHC, and second, a precise orientation of TCR is to be ensured so that the peptide in the MHC groove can be contacted. The selection pressure for these two features must have been that non-compliance with either incapacitated the anti-viral defense. These specificity elements are proposed therefore to be germ-line-encoded properties of TCR.'

'In real life, TCRs have never been observed to dock anywhere else but on MHC. Furthermore, all TCR–pMHC complexes studied so far, have revealed comparable diagonal orientations of TCR over the MHC helices, with TCR α at SW and β at NE (see in Fig. 8.6). These data indicate (provided that a completely different orientation will not be found in future) that the two TCR chains have been selected separately to recognize two different areas on the MHC contact surface, i.e., *all* α chains SW, and *all* β chains NE. A feasible way to achieve this would be, if conserved amino acid residues on the SW and NE surface of MHC interacted with conserved residues in V regions of the respective TCR chain, as also indicated by recent data.[149,150] Such interactions would permit a proper docking even if only one TCR chain made sufficient contacts with the appropriate MHC area, which has been observed to happen.'[134]

'It is not entirely clear why TCRs assume the observed diagonal docking orientation. Crystallographers argue[134] that this is to avoid the two 'high points' of MHC helices, and allow thereby a flat contact surface, the latter mandatory for reaching peptides that lay deep in the MHC groove. This could indeed provide selective pressure for the evolution of this particular docking orientation.'

'We can thus conclude that the discussed two specificity features have been selected by evolution, and are thus likely to be encoded in the genes for contemporary TCR. It is important to realize that, a priori, there is no additional specificity requirement for correct docking. It was the docking surface that dictated specificity, and because this is relatively conserved among MHC molecules, some TCR V regions appear to distinguish poorly between allelic MHC forms or between class I and class II MHC.'

Why are then MHC-restricted T-cell responses allele-specific?

'When MHC restriction was discovered, it was unknown that the ligand for TCR is a peptide bound to MHC, and that the peptide–MHC interaction exhibits allele-dependent specificity. Virus-infected cells of MHC type **a** and **b** will thus bind and present different viral peptides. A T-cell sensitized to MHC **a**+peptide 1 will not respond to MHC **b** because the latter presents peptide 2 and not peptide 1. This explanation probably applies to the majority of early studies, in which allele-specific response to a complex antigen was shown. But even if the two MHC types were to bind the very same peptide, the orientation of peptide side chains and/or the conformation of peptide backbone may be different, and thus the TCR would sense them as two different antigens. It is therefore extremely difficult to demonstrate a peptide-independent allele-specific recognition of MHC by TCR.'

'Up to this point the specificity requirements for docking should have been reasonably clear, and it is only unfortunate that I must introduce here a third specificity element. This is caused by the polymorphism of MHC and confounds the issue almost hopelessly. It is known that MHC loci are highly polymorphic, and that polymorphism is a requirement for MHC to function as peptide transporter and presenter. The impact of polymorphism on docking is that the docking surface, although relatively conserved, is not invariant: it has a number of polymorphic residues that differ among individual MHC molecules. Because these residues could interfere with the physiology of docking, the evolution of T-cell recognition had to take this unwanted variability also into consideration. The solution was to produce a similar degree of variability in TCR *V* genes. This in turn led to another complication, namely, the docking function had to be subjected to a somatic learning process, during which all TCRs must be tested for their capability to dock on MHC molecules present in the same individual (discussed in Section 8.4.3).'

8.3.3 The Biology of Docking

'The docking function enables TCR to search through the MHC molecules of antigen-presenting cells (APC) for the presence of antigenic peptides.'

'This is a tremendous screening task, if we consider that >99% of MHC molecules are filled with non-informative self peptides. Exactly how tedious this job could be is best illustrated by the use of real numbers. An APC expresses ~250 000 MHC molecules of a particular type, and a T cell ~25 000 copies of TCR. The number of antigenic pMHC complexes necessary for activation of a T cell is ~100–300, i.e., ~1 of 1000 MHC molecules must contain the same antigenic peptide.[151,152] The T cell, by sampling 10% of MHC molecules upon a single docking, can thus safely establish whether the APC has informative ligands or not. If the APC was found negative, the T cell detaches and proceeds to the next APC, or continues circulating. In case 10–30 ligands were found, the T cell must remain attached to the APC, and screen every single MHC molecule to collect 100–300 activating interactions, and this needs on average ten sequential dockings and detachments per receptor on the same APC. Finding the proper ligand is, however, a rare event, if we also consider that only ~1 of 100 000 T cells has a TCR fitting to a particular pMHC complex. We can thus appreciate that the screening process preceding the initiation of a specific T-cell response is like finding a needle in a haystack.'

'One important insight from this numerology is that the screening must proceed very fast. In fact, finding a ligand should not take longer than a couple of hours, because the subsequent expansion of activated T-cell clones to a large protective pool[153] requires several days, and the virus meanwhile replicates. We can conclude therefore that one thing a docking TCR cannot afford is a slow off-rate. In other words, the affinity of TCR for MHC plus a self peptide, i.e., the docking affinity[145] *must be low* for functional reasons. The usual argument that the affinity of TCR is low because "TCRs were not selected for high affinity like antibodies" misses the point, namely that it was selected to be low. As mentioned before, low affinity does not imply poor specificity, rather the opposite, because a crossreactivity of even lower affinity would be equal to no binding.'

'In a simplified world, e.g., if the MHC were a single monomorphic molecule, and TCR had a single pair of V region, the affinity of TCR for MHC would be a parameter selectable by evolution. However, because of the multiplicity of MHC alleles and TCR *V* genes, low affinity can only be selected somatically.'

8.3.4 Peptide Recognition by TCR

'It may not be quite superfluous to point out that the TCR cannot tell what is MHC and what is peptide. All it can see is a familiar-looking surface to dock on. However, it can readily distinguish between invariant and variable components of the contact surface. Invariant is what the receptor was trained to interact with during its somatic selection process, and with respect to a single TCR, this should correspond to the docking surface of one and the same MHC molecule. Variable is by definition everything else, and this should be directly or indirectly peptide-dependent. The TCR also knows *where* to look for variability. This is due to its capability imprinted by evolution to orient itself relative to the MHC surface. As already discussed, the rule here is that the α chain goes SW and the β chain NE, and consequently the somatically varied CDR3 loops of both chains are placed above the middle of the peptide-binding groove (Fig. 8.6). In addition, the CDR1 loops are positioned such that they could contact some N- and C-terminal residues of the peptide. Although the CDR1 loops are not varied somatically, they have different sequences for each V region, and can thus contribute effectively to the detection of peptide-dependent variability of the pMHC surface. We can therefore conclude that the solution chosen by evolution, although somewhat messy for the conceptualizing mind, can subserve the purpose of peptide recognition.'

How does the T cell decide which of the countless variants to respond to?

'All we know about this is based on crystallographic data comparing a non-antigenic self peptide with a few antigenic ones. As discussed before (Section 8.2.4), the self peptide makes only few hydrogen bonds with the CDRs 1α, 1β and 3α, and practically none with 3β of the TCR, and the shape complementarity of interface is poor.[135] In contrast, antigenic peptides usually contact all four CDR1 and CDR3 loops, and engage in interactions with them.[134,139] Contacts with the CDR3 loops appear to be particularly important for sensing the peptide as an activating ligand. Provided that these findings are generalizable, it appears that antigenicity depends on a sufficient number and strength of interactions between TCR and the variant surface of pMHC. If these criteria are not met, the TCR disregards that particular variant and detaches from the MHC.'

There is another troublesome aspect of T-cell recognition. As we have learned, the TCR sees a large invariant surface and a smaller one with some variations. The latter are sometimes so subtle that a single amino acid exchange can turn the antigenic peptide into an inert one. The affinity increment between antigenic and non-antigenic peptides can be as little as three-fold.[154] Thus the TCR must sense minute differences at an extremely poor signal-to-noise ratio. Under these conditions how does it manage to distinguish between docking and peptide recognition?

'Yes, to render T-cell recognition functional must have been an enormous challenge for evolution. The answer was a sophisticated signaling system. The working principle of the latter is not to accept noise, but to treat noise as a qualitatively different signal. Accordingly, T cells can distinguish between at least three different, sequential signals. The first one occurs upon docking: this is a survival signal[155] that tells the T cell "You are doing your job". This signal was set into action during the somatic learning of docking,[156] at which stage its message was "You will be able to do your job". The second type of signal occurs upon incomplete recognition of a peptide, a so-called partial agonist.[157] Such peptides usually have contacts with the CDR1 loops, but insufficient interactions with the CDR3 regions. This signal is telling the T cell "Be alert, there may be something interesting here!" The last one is the activating signal that occurs when the peptide makes sufficient interactions, in particular with the CDR3 loops. It tells the T cell "Respond!" In addition, there is a fourth signal in response to so-called antagonist peptides; this shuts down the T cell.[158] However, the structural basis and biological significance of this TCR antagonism is unknown.'

'We know that all these signals exist in real life, and that they are reflected in different phosphorylation patterns of CD3 chains,[158–160] the signal transduction system of TCR. But how these signals are generated and transmitted to CD3 remains largely unknown. As always, here too, there are two competing views—first, signaling should be initiated by a conformational change of the receptor upon ligand binding, and second, aggregation of ligand-binding TCRs should provide the signal. Considering that TCRs have to fish out a sufficient number of ligands (100–300) from an ocean of non-informative pMHC complexes, and that this fishing expedition may require several successive dockings, it seems almost impossible that an aggregate of signaling size could form at once. Thus the biology would be better served with conformational signaling through each individual liganded TCR, and there is recent evidence[161] to support this notion.'

8.4 THYMUS AND THE T-CELL REPERTOIRE

Having dealt with the intricacies of T-cell recognition in sufficient detail, it is time to pay attention to the events taking place during T-cell ontogeny, prior to the appearance of the mature T-cell repertoire. These developmental steps occur in the thymus, the organ where bone marrow stem cells commit themselves to the T-cell lineage. Because the thymus, ever since the discovery of its immunological role by Jacques Miller,[162] has been the focus of immunologists' interest, there is now detailed knowledge about the ontogenic steps T cells must go through before reaching maturity.

8.4.1 Early Events of Thymocyte Development

The ontogeny of thymocytes is best followed by means of T-cell markers, such as the α and β chain of the T-cell antigen receptor (TCR), CD3, the signaling system of the latter, and the two coreceptors CD4 and CD8 that couple the effector function of T cells to the recognition of MHC class (CD4 specifies helper function and class II recognition, CD8 cytotoxic function and class I recognition; discussed in Section 8.6.2).

The earliest thymocyte progenitors fail to express any of these markers. They are the descendants of multipotent hematopoietic stem cells in the bone marrow, and it is unclear to what extent they are committed to the lymphoid lineage or the T lineage upon arrival at the thymus. However, a final commitment to the latter certainly occurs within the thymus.[163] The first T-cell-specific event in the lives of committed precursors is the rearrangement of the TCR β locus. Successful rearrangement is marked by the cell surface expression of the β chain associated with a surrogate α chain, pre-Tα (see Section 8.2.3), and CD3. Further rearrangements are then put on hold (by switching off the RAG recombinase enzymes), and the thymocytes are signaled to divide, and to proceed to the CD4$^+$CD8$^+$ (double positive [DP]) stage of development.[164] At the DP stage, the recombinases are activated again, and rearrangement of the TCR α locus follows. (T cells expressing γδ TCR are somewhat peripheral to this topic, their ontogeny[165] will therefore not be covered.) Up to this point, thymocyte ontogeny proceeds according to a pre-determined program that does not require antigen recognition.[166] The pre-Tα will then be replaced by a proper α chain, and the resulting DP, TCRα$^+$β$^+$ thymocytes are now ready to undergo different somatic selection processes.

8.4.2 The Germline Repertoire

As pointed out earlier (Section 8.3.2), the capability of TCR to dock on MHC must have been selected for in evolution, and thus MHC-specificity should be encoded in TCR *V* genes.

This idea is not new, it was first proposed by Jerne[167] in 1971. At that time, Jerne was puzzled by the unexpectedly high frequency of T cells responding to foreign MHC molecules,[168,169] and the solution he offered was that the germline *V*-gene repertoire of TCR (then thought to be Ig) should encode specificities for all allelic variants of histocompatibility antigens present in the species. Although he came to this conclusion for a reason different from the one stated here, this does not affect his priority. His explanation for the necessity of such a *V* gene repertoire was that because MHC alleles and *V* genes segregate independently, the latter cannot 'know' which MHC alleles they would meet in a given individual.

'Jerne's explanation is correct, but it is just a hint, and as such, it has remained ever since obscure in many immunologists' minds', points out Dr. G. 'Therefore it may be useful to discuss in some detail the genetic mechanism implied in this hint.'

'Consider a "square one" scenario of two isolated homozygous populations, one with MHC$^{a/a}$ recognized by *V*α$^{a/a}$-*V*β$^{a/a}$, and the other with MHC$^{b/b}$ recognized by *V*α$^{b/b}$-*V*β$^{b/b}$ (superscripts represent allele designation). When the two populations start to interbreed, the F$_1$ hybrids will enjoy some advantage over homozygotes (due to increased defense capacity). However, disaster is pre-programmed for the next interbreeding generations from F$_2$ onwards. This is because the three gene systems (MHC, *V*α, *V*β) segregate independently (are on different chromosomes), and thus a defined proportion of progeny will inherit *V* gene pairs whose products cannot interact with their MHC. For example, MHC$^{a/a}$ homozygous segregants cannot use *V*α^b-*V*β^b, *V*α^a-*V*β^b, and *V*α^b-*V*β^a, and MHC$^{a/b}$ heterozygotes cannot use *V*α^a-*V*β^a, and *V*α^b-*V*β^b.'

'How can evolution respond to this crisis? The most feasible solution is to bring the allelic *V* genes onto the same chromosome by unequal crossing over. *V*α^a+ *V*α^b will then be inherited in a single block, and the same applies to *V*β^a+ *V*β^b.

This simple example illustrates how MHC polymorphism can select for *V*-gene polygeneism, and *against* *V*-gene polymorphism. The final result of this process will be a series of tandem *V*-genes that covers all allelic MHC variants of the species.'

'The crisis due to independent segregation could be significantly ameliorated, if docking were one-sided, i.e., only one of the TCR chains would interact specifically with MHC, as proposed recently by Mel Cohn,[170] and observed also by crystallography.[134] But even in this case, homozygous segregants carrying MHC$^{a/a}$ could not interact with $V\alpha^b$-$V\beta^b$, and the same applies to MHC$^{b/b}$ and $V\alpha^a$-$V\beta^a$. This could still provide sufficient selective pressure for the polygeneism of *V*-segments.'

'It is important to realize that MHC polymorphism in this context does not mean total sequence diversity. Only polymorphism of the docking surface of MHC is relevant for this process. And the presently available ~50 $V\alpha$ and ~50 $V\beta$ genes are probably more than enough for the recognition of all variability occurring on the docking surface of MHC molecules expressed in a species.'

The thesis that TCR *V* genes encode specificities for MHC molecules of the species was not only dictated by theoretical considerations: it was also demonstrated experimentally. In knockout mice that lack the MHC molecules required for repertoire selection, some T cells mature spontaneously,[171] or can be manipulated to mature artificially.[172] These T cells representing the unselected germline repertoire have been shown to respond to any allogeneic MHC molecule with high frequency. Thus the germ-line TCR repertoire appears to be inherently MHC-specific.

8.4.3 Selection of the T-Cell Repertoire in the Thymus

Despite a vast amount of experimental data, this remains the most controversial and mysterious chapter of T-cell biology.

The first hint of a somatic selection process in the thymus came from experiments with bone marrow chimeras. This experimental system was turned loose on immunologists by Harald von Boehmer and colleagues,[173] who demonstrated that a careful removal of mature T cells from bone marrow cell suspensions permits bone marrow stem cells to grow and differentiate in irradiated semi-allogeneic hosts. For example, stem cells of MHC-different strains **a** and **b** could be inoculated into (**a** x **b**)Γ_1 hosts, and the lymphocytes grown out of them functioned normally, and were tolerant of the host and of each other. The major attractivity of this system was that it enabled the study of interactions between histoincompatible cells, for example between MHC-disparate T and B cells,[8] that could not have been done otherwise. Since the mechanism of MHC restriction was the hottest topic of immunology at that time, chimeras immediately became extremely popular, and stayed so for the next decade. But as the amount of data from chimera experiments increased, a mass of contradictory results accumulated in parallel, revealing the internal complexities and limitations of this – originally thought to be straight-forward – experimental system.

Nevertheless, there was one particular experimental setting that repeatedly yielded consistent results. In this type of experiment, adult (**a** x **b**)F$_1$ mice were thymectomized, irradiated, inoculated with F$_1$ bone marrow, and grafted with an irradiated parental type (**a** or **b**) thymus. Mice recovered from these treatments were then immunized, and shown that they generated a cytotoxic T lymphocyte (Tc) response restricted selectively to the MHC type of the thymus (Table 8.2). This experiment was first performed by Zinkernagel et al.[174] using anti-viral Tc as a readout, and Fink and Bevan[175] using minor histocompatibility antigen-specific Tc readout. It was then repeated in many different laboratories using different T-cell responses, with essentially the same results. Quantitative differences existed only in the extent to which the restriction was 'skewed' toward the thymic MHC type. Because the body and the lymphoid compartment of these chimeras were of F$_1$ genotype, the results indicated that radio-resistant cells in the thymus graft determined MHC restriction by some somatic process.

Concerning the mechanism of selective restriction imposed by the thymic MHC type, two competing hypotheses were put forward. Proponents of suppressor T cells thought that the absence of MHC restriction by the second parental MHC type in F$_1$ mice was the result of active suppression. But this possibility was ruled out experimentally.[175] The alternative concept was that T cells 'learn' MHC restriction in the thymus. The learning process was envisaged to be a matching of TCRs with MHC molecules on radioresistant thymic epithelial cells. Thymocytes whose receptors were capable of interacting with thymic MHC would be allowed to develop into mature T cells. This process was often referred to as 'positive selection', as opposed to the deletion of autoreactive T cells in the thymus that was named 'negative selection' (a mechanism of self tolerance).

The terms 'positive and negative selection' established themselves very quickly in the vocabulary of immunologists, but they had remained somewhat

TABLE 8.2 Determination of MHC Restriction by the Thymus

Mouse	Body	MHC Type of Bone Marrow Stem Cells	Thymus	MHC-Restriction of T Cells	
Normal	a x b	a x b	a x b	a	b
Chimera[a]	a x b	a x b	a	a	–
Chimera[a]	a x b	a x b	b	–	b

[a] Adult thymectomized, irradiated, bone marrow reconstituted mice grafted with irradiated neonatal thymus. Based on References 174 and 175

speculative for another decade, until the actual mechanisms could be addressed experimentally. The technological advance that enabled an experimental approach to thymic selection was the development of transgenic and gene-knockout mice. For example, in mice lacking MHC expression, the development of thymocytes was shown to halt at the CD4$^+$8$^+$ (double positive [DP]) TCR$\alpha\beta^+$ stage.[176,177] Similarly, in mice with a disrupted TCR α gene,[178] thymocytes remain at the DP stage. Successful interaction of DP thymocytes with MHC was shown to provide the cells with a survival signal,[156] whereas those T cells whose receptor could not dock on MHC would 'die by neglect'. Furthermore, a TCR specific for a certain antigen–MHC combination was used as a transgene to demonstrate that recipient mice expressing the same antigen–MHC combination deleted the transgene in the thymus.[179] In contrast, in mice expressing the relevant MHC but not the antigen, the very same transgene was positively selected and the thymocytes were allowed to develop into single positive (SP; in this case CD4$^-$8$^+$), mature T cells.[180] The conclusion from these experiments has been that recognition of MHC plus a self antigen results in clonal deletion (negative selection), while recognition of MHC alone results in positive selection.

Had the investigations stopped at this point, everything would have remained clear. However, a new quest was launched for a possible role, if any, of MHC-bound self peptides in positive selection, and this provided for a source of further complications. Basically two contradictory sets of data resulted from these experiments. First, it was shown that mice whose MHC molecules were occupied by a single peptide were still capable of generating a functional TCR repertoire,[181,182] indicating that self peptides were only required for maintaining the structure of MHC, but not for positive selection. Other experiments,[183–186] however, suggested that a diverse set of self peptides would represent a stringent requirement for the positive selection of a normal TCR repertoire. Thus these studies ended up with a paradox that has remained with us ever since. The question arises whether this paradox can be disentangled mentally, after it has proven to be inextricable (and indeed was created) experimentally.

'This particular problem had caused me quite a few sleepless nights', admits Dr. G. 'until I realized that the relevant question to ask is what the consequence of a peptide-directed positive selection would be for the docking-screening function of TCR. The answer is relatively simple: if positive selection occurred for a given MHC molecule plus one particular self peptide, the selected TCR would preferentially or in worst case exclusively dock on the subset of MHC molecules occupied by the selecting self peptide. For example, taking previously used estimates (Section 8.3.3), if ~250 000 copies of a certain MHC molecule are expressed per APC, and they bind ~1000 different self peptides (published numbers[187] are 650–2000), at average each peptide would occupy 250 MHC sites. If a certain T cell were only able to dock on 250 sites, 1000 T cells with different receptors would be required for the full screen of one particular MHC molecule expressed on a single APC. It is important to realize that this exercise only serves docking, i.e., a contact of TCRs with appropriate MHC+peptides surfaces, but it does not imply that any of the docking TCRs would find an activating ligand. Thus several rounds of this docking procedure may be necessary with the participation of different TCRs before an activating ligand would be identified. And even after a complete screen, foreign peptides that do not resemble any of the selecting self peptides would be missed. The situation may be less severe in reality, because some self peptides occupy many more MHC sites. However, the problems remain: first, a peptide-directed positive selection would set up an awkward screening schedule with possible "traffic jams", second, it would be slow, and third, some antigenic peptides would inevitably escape detection. Therefore, any mechanism that prevents a TCR to dock on *all* copies of a given MHC molecule appears to be a threat, and should be selected against.'

But how about those data showing the importance of self peptides in positive selection? They were also generated in respectable laboratories, and their validity seems to be beyond doubt.

'It is important to note that the peptides used in those experiments were partial agonists or the like, i.e., similar to the peptides to which the response was measured. It is known that the affinity border between positive and negative selection (discussed below) permits positive selection of some TCRs recognizing MHC plus partial agonists. The important difference is that whereas docking per se is interpreted by the T cell as a survival (first level) signal, partial agonists provide in addition an alertness (second level) signal (see Section 8.3.4). If one uses partial agonists for positive selection in fetal thymus organ cultures,[184–186] the repertoire thus generated will be skewed toward the agonist, and will comprise many T cells at the second signaling level, which are easier to activate (i.e., to bring to the third signaling level"respond"). It is therefore little wonder that a preferential response was obtained to the agonist. No doubt, normal repertoires could also contain T cells selected on partial agonist self peptides. But these cells could not have bypassed the first-level survival signal either, and thus, by definition, they should be able to dock on the selecting MHC molecule also *without* the partial agonist. My predilection is that the existence of such T cells is a borderline phenomenon, and these cells should therefore represent only a minority in the repertoire.'

Early ideas, influenced by Jerne's hypothesis,[167] envisaged positive selection to be a process whereby products of the germ-line-encoded *V* genes, i.e., ~50 Vα x ~50 Vβ, altogether ~2500 Vαβ pairs would be tested for interaction with the MHC molecules expressed in the same individual. This expectation was further nurtured by the assumption that the *V*-gene encoded, somatically invariable CDR1 and CDR2 loops would be responsible for MHC recognition, and the highly variable CDR3 loops for peptide recognition.[117] One can therefore understand the disappointment immunologists felt when the actual data failed to demonstrate a clear correlation between MHC expression and *V*-gene usage.[128]

Crystallography has, however, demonstrated that all three CDR loops of both chains can interact with MHC (Section 8.2.4), and thus the potential number of different TCRs to be tested for MHC interaction is in the order of 10^{12} (considering also variable D and J segment usage and N region diversity). Because this number exceeds by far the total number of T cells a mouse can have, it is reasonable to assume that in the initial repertoire every single T cell has a different receptor. One consequence of this situation is that the specificity of TCR–MHC interaction can be tuned much more finely than expected on the basis of only CDR1+2 interaction with MHC. Indeed it has been demonstrated that a single residue difference in the CDR3 region can radically change the docking specificity of a TCR.[188] It is therefore highly unlikely that a TCR selected to interact with a particular MHC molecule would also be able to dock on another MHC molecule of the same individual. Of course, T cells whose receptor cannot interact with self MHC will die of neglect (for lack of the survival signal), and they may in fact represent the majority of the initial repertoire.

'For fairness' sake I should mention that positive selection has never been a fully proven mechanism, and thus not everybody believes in its existence', adds Dr. G. 'A prominent opponent was Polly Matzinger, who has proposed that the only positive selection step required is the recognition of a foreign antigen by a T cell in the periphery.[189] This would automatically ensure that the appropriate T cell capable of recognizing the antigen presented by a given MHC molecule will be selected out of a random repertoire. All the T cell would need is an interaction of its coreceptor, CD4 or CD8, with the appropriate class of MHC molecule, and if the TCR fits to the peptide-binding groove of the same MHC molecule, the T cell will be activated. Thus MHC restriction would be established in the periphery instead of the thymus. Polly's view is a logical consequence of her "modified self" hypothesis,[41] according to which TCRs recognize neither peptide nor MHC, but a neoantigen formed by the two (see Section 8.1.4). Thus the TCR repertoire could/should be random under this model. I am not sure whether or not her view has remained unchanged after the crystallographic studies of TCR–peptide–MHC complexes. But one point is now clear: the overall shape of peptide–MHC complexes is very similar, and not random. Therefore, the overall shape of TCR-binding site cannot be random either; it should be sufficiently complementary to be able to dock on peptide–MHC. This must be a property selected by evolution, because the MHC is the only site that can inform the T cell about intracellular infection. And if we accept this, we may as well accept thymic-positive selection as an ontogenic step that enables a better use of the T-cell repertoire.'

Positive selection can only take care of one single aspect of T-cell recognition, namely that all selected TCR should be able to interact with self MHC. However, many of the selected clones will in addition recognize self peptides, and these cells must be purged from the final repertoire in order to avoid autoimmunity. The process in charge of this is what we understand as negative selection. The mechanism by which it is achieved is rather unique. Apparently there is a constant affinity threshold set at ~6 μM for the combined affinities of TCR–MHC plus coreceptor–MHC interaction[190] (~70 μM for the TCR–MHC interaction alone). T cells interacting at higher affinity will be deleted, and those with lower affinity positively selected. As already discussed, T cells recognizing a partial agonist self peptide are in the gray zone: some are deleted, others are positively selected. As a result, all cells in the postselection repertoire will be able to dock on self MHC and receive a survival signal, some cells will also receive an alertness signal, but none will be activated (receive a respond signal) by self pMHC complexes.

But one question remains: why is the affinity threshold set so low? After all, antibodies with 100 000-fold higher affinity are also subject to self–non-self discrimination.

'This is a very valid point', confirms Dr. G 'Self–non-self discrimination is indeed a matter of specificity rather than affinity. But I take Ed Palmer's data at face value, and consider the affinity-dependent mechanism real. Although I could imagine a different way, for example that signaling via CDR3, which is a clear indication of reactivity to a self peptide, would lead to death. The affinity-driven mechanism, in contrast, eliminates not only T cells specific for self peptides, but also those binding strongly to self MHC alone, which may also signal T cells for a response. Thus this mechanism seems to prioritize affinity over specificity, which must have a good reason. I think the answer should be sought again in the biology of docking. As I argued before (Section 8.3.3) the speed of docking and detachment can become a question of life or death, and so the repertoire cannot afford to contain T cells with high affinity (and as a rule a slow off-rate) for self MHC. The primary purpose of negative selection thus seems to be to ensure a fast screening function of TCR, but setting of the upper affinity limit for cell survival settles at a stroke also self–non-self discrimination.'

There is one more rather mysterious aspect of T-cell ontogeny left: the transition of thymocytes from the DP to the SP stage. This occurs during repertoire selection so that the mature repertoire only contains SP cells, and in addition, in the correct combination: class I-restricted cytotoxic T cells are always CD4$^-$8$^+$, and class II-restricted helper cells CD4$^+$8$^-$. The coreceptors CD4 and CD8 are known to distinguish between MHC classes (discussed in Section 8.6.2): they bind to areas of MHC molecules that are conserved within the class and distinct from the other class. As a result CD8 binds to all class I and CD4 to all class II molecules. The SP state marks the commitment of thymocytes to an effector class, i.e., CD8 cells will be cytotoxic and CD4 cells helper. Obviously, the cytotoxic function must be linked to class I MHC recognition, because this class presents peptides derived from intracellular pathogens, which mark the infected cell for destruction. Conversely, peptides from extracellular pathogens are presented by class II MHC, and must be recognized by helper T cells that trigger B cells for antibody production against these pathogens. Linking of the effector function of T cells with MHC class recognition is therefore a sine qua non of immune defense. However, such a linkage is not simple to achieve. The specific problem here is that the TCR repertoire is not inherently class I or class II specific (with some exceptions[143]), and thus TCRs have no way to identify the class of the MHC molecule to which they bind. This situation demands that the receptor of every single T cell be expressed together with the appropriate coreceptor at the SP stage. Thus, a T cell whose receptor learned to dock on a class I molecule during positive selection must express CD8, and the same applies to class II docking and CD4 expression. But how the correct coupling of TCR and coreceptor specificity is achieved mechanistically has remained a mystery.

'The solution of this problem would need more data and less speculation', comments Dr. G. 'Yet, in the absence of the former, one is tempted to make conjectures. Perhaps a good starting point would be the proposition that T cells can read the combined affinities of TCR and coreceptor for MHC, and use this information to decide between positive and negative selection.[190] The best physical arrangement would be for obtaining an integrated affinity signal from the two receptors, if the latter were associated in the cell membrane, and they both bound to a single MHC molecule.[191] Because the combined affinity is ~10–15-fold higher than the affinity of a single member of the receptor dyad, it is easy to envisage that the signal generated upon cooperative binding of the coreceptor to MHC would also be different from the one generated by binding of the coreceptor alone. Such a signal could cause continued expression of the coreceptor, and by default, the lack of it could shut down the other coreceptor. It is also possible that the cooperative binding of TCR and coreceptor would signal the MHC of thymic epithelial cells, and the latter cells would then regulate coreceptor expression on T cells, for example, via cytokines as proposed recently.[192] But as I emphasized above, the final solution of this puzzle requires more data.'

8.4.4 The Mature T-Cell Repertoire

Because the mature T-cell repertoire is still under experimental analysis, this theme is not yet ready for a historical account. Nonetheless a few interesting aspects have already emerged, which can be covered meaningfully in this section.

The first question that has been raised and also investigated experimentally is what the T-cell repertoire looks like after the slaughters of thymic selection. According to estimates,[193] only 1–2% of thymocytes are allowed to survive and develop into mature T cells. Thus the question can also be phrased this way: what distinguishes the few survivors from the majority that fell on the battlefield? One obvious answer following from the nature of positive selection is that, in contrast to the preselection repertoire, every single TCR of the mature repertoire will be able to interact with one particular self MHC molecule. The process of positive selection appears to be contingent on a minimum energy of TCR–MHC interaction,[194] which should be understood as an energy range rather than a sharp threshold. TCR that fall within this range are essentially MHC unrestricted, and as such irrelevant for the mature repertoire. They indeed die for lack of a survival signal ('by neglect').

The remaining T cells will have receptors with a wide variety of affinities (except very low!) for self peptide–MHC (pMHC) complexes, and they are subject to negative selection. As pointed out before (Section 8.4.3), negative selection functions by setting a sharp upper affinity limit for T-cell survival, and thus only those T cells will escape whose receptors have affinities between the thresholds for positive and negative selection. The crux, however, is that every TCR is tested on thousands of self peptides bound to a given MHC molecule, and thus chances are high that its affinity for a particular pMHC complex will exceed the cut-off value, and the T cell will be deleted. Negative selection therefore imposes extremely strong constraints on the specificity of TCR. One consequence of this will be that TCRs cross-reacting with several different peptides are likely to be eliminated, i.e., the mature repertoire will have improved peptide specificity compared to the preselection repertoire.[195] In specific terms, affinity-based negative selection over thousands of self peptides exerts its effect on TCR positions that contact the ligand: amino acid residues interacting weakly with other amino acids (AGSTNQ) are favored and strongly interacting ones (ILVYWRE) disfavored at these positions, as shown in a revealing computer simulation study.[196] Thus in the mature repertoire, TCR with weakly interacting contact residues will be enriched. Upon recognition of antigenic peptides, the weak TCR residues bind to strongly interacting amino acids of the peptides, resulting in multiple interactions of moderate strength, which add up to the total binding energy required for T-cell activation. Since each of these moderately strong interactions contributes significantly to the total binding energy, interruption of any of them can result in abrogation of recognition. Antigen recognition will thus be sensitive to single amino acid exchanges in the peptide, i.e., highly specific. By the same token, strongly interacting residues will also be selected against at TCR interaction points with the MHC, improving thereby the specificity of MHC restriction.

In contrast, repertoire selection on a single pMHC complex allowing only minimal negative selection enriches for TCR that engage in strong interactions at fewer points with their ligand. Antigen recognition by such TCRs is less sensitive to amino acid exchanges at many positions of the ligand, except for the few points of strong interaction. These receptors will therefore be more crossreactive.[149,197]

'The way negative selection shapes the TCR repertoire should be understood as a statistical trend rather than a rigid rule', points out Dr. G. 'In reality not all strongly interacting amino acids of TCR contact points are selected against.[150,198] Furthermore, alternative strategies to escape negative selection seem also to exist. For example some TCRs achieve the required low affinity by interacting with only one of the two MHC helices. Such TCRs are more frequent in the preselection repertoire,[149] but can be found also in the mature repertoire.[134] They may have proper peptide specificity, but are predicted to be more prone to alloreactivity.'[199]

'I should mention at this point that we owe most of these new insights into the nature of T-cell repertoire to the Kappler-Marrack group. Without their steadfast, untiring analytical work we would still be feeling around in the dark.'

Another highly interesting question borne out by crystallographic studies is that the number of peptide residues available for TCR contact usually does not exceed 5. The implication is that the antigenic universe recognizable by T cells is limited to the combinatorial of 20 amino acids at 5 positions, i.e., $20^5 = 3.2$ million different peptide sequences. On the one hand, this may be an underestimate, because MHC anchoring residues could also influence T-cell recognition indirectly,[200] on the other hand, conservative amino acid exchanges may not alter the shape of the epitope. Thus this number appears realistic enough to be used as a cap of the epitope universe for T cells. However, 3.2 million is a very modest number in comparison to the potential sequence variability of TCRs that may be a million-fold higher. Thus, unexpectedly, it is the antigens and not the receptors, which appear to set the limit of T-cell recognition. The question then arises how large the universe of foreign peptides would be after the subtraction of self peptides to which the repertoire is tolerant. This question could now be answered precisely by computational studies utilizing the available genome sequences of several mammalian species and microorganisms, and the peptide-binding motifs for MHC molecules. Unfortunately, a simple illustrative study on this topic that would suit the level of this discussion is not available, despite sufficient theoretical coverage of thymic selection.[196,199,201–204]

'The problem with simple illustrative examples is that they can be proven wrong too easily', warns Dr. G. 'Therefore it is not worth working out any, unless it remains at a very general level, at which quantitation plays the role of only providing a "feel". As a possible starting point lends itself the number of genes in the mammalian genome, i.e., ~30 000, translating into a similar number of protein sequences. The question may then be asked: how many MHC-binding peptide sequences can be identified in a single self protein? To obtain a reasonable estimate, we could utilize the startling observation of T-cell epitope studies (Section 7.1.1), namely that antigen processing yields as a rule a single dominant epitope per protein per MHC molecule, and 1–3 minor or "subdominant" epitopes. Allowing four epitopes per MHC, a heterozygous mouse with six class I and four class II molecules would present 24 class I and 16 class II epitopes per protein. To estimate the total number of class I and class II binding self epitopes, the proteome has to be divided into two pools of intracellular and membrane+secreted proteins, respectively. For simplicity we can consider these pools equal (15 000 each) and thus obtain 360 000 class I and 240 000 class II epitopes, altogether 600 000 self peptide sequences. This number is within the range reported in a quantitative study of T-cell repertoire selection.[204] In reality the number may be smaller, because first, not every protein would produce four epitopes for each class I and class II molecule, respectively, second, there are substantial overlaps between the peptide spectra bound by different MHC molecules, and third, several self proteins are completely shielded from the immune system. The conclusion is then that self tolerance would reduce the diversity of antigenic peptides from 3.2 to ~2.6 million, i.e., by ~20%.'

'I should mention here that other estimates based on the number of experimentally identified MHC-bound peptides come out much lower. For example, if we consider the number of peptides found on a single MHC type (~200–2000 peptides[187,205,206]), then at most 20 000 self peptides would induce tolerance. This is most likely an underestimate, as the methods used for peptide identification are orders of magnitude less sensitive than a T-cell response.[207] Furthermore, different APC subpopulations may present different sets of self peptides.'

'Another question that we may ask is whether the peptide universe reduced by self tolerance (i.e., 2.6 million) would still be sufficient to cover all sequences derived from pathogenic microorganisms. The rule of thumb calculation I can offer here is the following. Consider that a virus infection produces ~3 epitopes per class I molecule,[208] i.e., 18 epitopes in a mouse heterozygous at all three class I loci. If we, again for simplicity, allocate half of the possible sequences (1.3 million) to the class I presentation pathway, we can obtain independent epitope sets for ~72 000 different viral species. The number may even be larger, because the defense against related species may occur via shared/crossreactive epitopes.[209] Applying the same rules to the class II pathway, we obtain 12 epitopes per pathogen for two heterozygous class II loci, and an epitope coverage for ~108 000 different microbial species.'

'We can thus conclude that the theoretical limit of antigen diversity set by the combinatorial of 20 amino acids at five peptide positions (3.2 million) may not cause in reality any limitation to T-cell recognition. This number easily accommodates sequences under self tolerance, and can encompass epitope sets for a huge potential number of microbial species, the latter likely to exceed the number of existing species capable of infecting vertebrates.'

This conclusion is, of course, very reassuring, but is it really a surprise?

'Not at all! For the size of the antigen-combining site of TCR and antibodies is selected by self–non-self discrimination.[210] If the combining site could only encompass tetrapeptides and thus distinguish 160 000 sequences, self–non-self discrimination would not be possible. A size for hexapepetides allowing the distinction of 64 million peptides would be an exaggeration. Thus the pentapeptide size is the optimum.'

Antigenic diversity represents but one side of the coin, the other side being the mature T-cell repertoire itself. The question then arises whether the size of the mature repertoire would match the peptide universe curtailed by self tolerance (~2.6 million).

'As determined by most recent massive parallel sequencing efforts the human mature T-cell repertoire comprises at least 1 million distinct clonotypes.[211] There is no compelling reason to believe that the size of murine repertoire would be different, except that physical limitations would not allow to exceed this number too much in mice (mice have ~50–100 million T cells and thus the average clone size would be 50–100 cells, i.e., at the low end to be protective). The answer is therefore that the mature repertoire cannot cover the potential antigenic diversity on a one-to-one basis. If we also consider that a pathogen-derived peptide should be recognized by more than one T-cell clone in order to minimize mutational escape[212,213] of the pathogen, we would prefer an excess of T-cell clones over antigenic peptides, and not the other way around.'

'What is the way out of this seemingly paradoxical situation? The only possibility to cover a larger antigenic diversity by a smaller T-cell repertoire would be, if a single TCR were allowed to recognize several different peptide sequences, and this appears indeed to be the case.[214] This property of TCR is not really cross-reactivity, because the latter is characterized by few strong interactions between receptor and ligand, and is manifested in responses to several related sequences, as discussed above. In contrast, any single TCR seems to recognize a number of distinguishable sequences with equal specificity, i.e., behaves as polyspecific. This can be envisaged to arise by the receptor's capability to establish a sufficient number of moderate energy interactions with certain points of one ligand, and a similar number of moderately strong interactions at different points of another ligand. Thus both recognition events would be sensitive to single amino acid substitutions in the relevant peptide, in other words specific.'

'It is somewhat difficult to assign a number to the degree of polyspecificity. Perhaps we could use the precursor frequency of naïve T cells[209] for guidance, which is in the order of 10^{-5} for a given antigen. This could indeed correspond to the "resolving power" of the T-cell repertoire, i.e., any TCR would recognize one of every 100 000 random peptides, and thus the repertoire of 1 million clonotypes would be 10-fold polyspecific, allowing for the recognition of 10 million peptides, corresponding to ~4-fold of the total antigenic diversity (2.6 million). Other estimates[204] consider the resolving power of the repertoire to be 10^{-4}, which may be too low to be adequately specific, because it would require 100-fold polyspecificity to cover the epitope universe.'

'One more point to emphasize is that polyspecificity would not compromise self–non-self discrimination, as self-reactive clones, whether mono- or polyspecific, would be deleted by negative selection. The only difference it could make is that a single self peptide may eliminate a number of different TCRs. But considering the vast diversity of TCRs in the preselection repertoire, this may be affordable.'

8.5 ALLOREACTIVITY: THE CONTINUING PUZZLE

Alloreactivity, as manifested in the rejection of tissue grafts between individuals of the same species, has been known for about 200 years, and is thus one of the oldest known immune reactions. It has been a puzzle from the very beginning, because there has been no way to assign an evolutionary driving force to the development of a mechanism whose apparent purpose is to preserve individuality within the species. In 1944, allograft rejection was shown by Peter Medawar[215] to be an immune reaction, and subsequently, Mitchison[216] and Billingham and colleagues[217] discovered that it belonged to the category of cell-mediated immunity. However, the puzzle remained as inscrutable as before, because an immune reaction between individuals of the same species appeared inconceivable, except as a nuisance to transplantation surgeons. Indeed, the only natural situation in which mammals could be envisaged to encounter an allograft was pregnancy, and yet, fetuses were as a rule not rejected due to their paternal MHC type by the mother. (Meanwhile it has turned out that extra mechanisms exist to protect the fetus from maternal T-cell response[218]). The general consensus that developed on the basis of insufficient understanding was that alloreactivity per se was at best useless if not harmful, and it was thus likely to represent merely a 'side-effect' of an unknown, biologically relevant mechanism.

Interestingly, alloreactivity, irrelevant as it appeared biologically, proved to be extremely useful from the scientific point of view. Its experimental use resulted in a series of important discoveries, including, for example, the discovery of the MHC (see Section 6.1.1), the T cells (see Section 1.2), the graft-versus-host reaction,[219] the mixed lymphocyte reaction,[220] and cytotoxic T lymphocytes.[221] The latter two had been for a long time the only T-cell responses that could be elicited in vitro, and have thus provided invaluable tools in the analysis and dissection of cellular immune responses.

8.5.1 Relationship Between Alloreactive and Self-MHC Restricted T Cells

In the late 1960s, alloreactivity gained an unexpected new dimension, when Morten Simonsen[222] and Darcy Wilson[169] found that the frequency of T cells responding to an allogeneic MHC haplotype was ≥1%. Even when considering that a haplotype encompasses more than one MHC molecule, this frequency is 2–3 orders of magnitude higher than expected for any foreign non-MHC antigen. Yet, the response appeared to be allele-specific, in that T cells activated against a particular MHC haplotype did not react to a third-party haplotype. Thus, alloreactivity, in addition to being useless, turned out to be much more vigorous than any other immune response, which made the mystery complete.

The finding of aberrantly high frequencies of alloreactive cells caused a real upheaval in immunology, because there was no concept to account for such a phenomenon. Attempts to explain it by assuming that MHC molecules have 100–1000-fold more epitopes than other antigens, or that alloreactivity does not obey the rules of clonal selection were obviously unsatisfactory. The first theoretical treatment of the problem was presented by Jerne[167] in his 1971 hypothesis to which we keep returning. As already discussed (Sections 5.1 and 8.4.2), Jerne has postulated that TCR *V* genes encode specificities for all allelic MHC variants present in the species. He assumed that in the thymus, TCR specific for self MHC of the host would mutate extensively in order to escape deletion by self tolerance. These mutants would give rise to the repertoire for foreign antigens. In contrast, TCR specific for allogeneic MHC molecules (absent from the host) would remain unmutated, and they would be responsible for the high level of alloreactivity. This hypothesis provided a straight-forward explanation for alloreactivity: as the number of *V* genes should roughly match the number of allelic MHC variants in the species (in the order of 100), the 1% frequency of responsive cells to any foreign MHC molecule appeared self evident. The unattractive side of this concept was that it divided the T-cell repertoire into a useful fraction responding to foreign antigens, and a useless one that was merely alloreactive. Nevertheless, the immunology community accepted Jerne's hypothesis for lack of a better alternative.

The discovery of MHC restriction in 1974 (Section 8.1.1) gave, for the first time, a clue to the true biological function of the MHC in T-cell recognition, and simultaneously placed the phenomenon of alloreactivity into a different light. It became possible to envisage that the very same T cells recognizing a foreign antigen in association with self MHC could also react with allogeneic MHC molecules. There were two alternative views as to the way this could happen.

According to the modified self hypothesis,[40] a large number of non-MHC self molecules can associate with self MHC to form a series of 'neoantigens'. Because the neoantigens formed between MHC^a plus self molecules and MHC^b plus the same self molecules would be different, strain **a** mice would not be tolerant of the neoantigens of strain **b**. Consequently, the two strains would mount a polyclonal response against the multitude of each other's neoantigens. Translated into contemporary language, MHC^a and MHC^b present different peptides of the same self molecules, and this is the cause for the lack of tolerance to allogeneic peptide–MHC complexes, and the high frequency of alloresponse. In essence, the modified self hypothesis considered both self-MHC restricted response to foreign antigens and alloreactivity to be mechanistically the same (both directed against peptide–MHC complexes).

The dual recognition concept[46,47] considered high-frequency alloreactivity to be a germ-line-encoded property of TCR, as proposed before by Jerne, with the difference that under the dual recognition model self MHC restricted and alloreactive responses were mediated by the same receptor in two different orientations. In contrast to the modified self model, alloreactivity was postulated not to involve the recognition of non-MHC moieties (i.e., peptides).

However, as pointed out earlier (Section 8.1.4), these early models of T-cell recognition were constructed in the absence of molecular information, and thus some of their assumptions were in error. For example, it is now clear that the ligand of TCR is not a neoantigen, but a composite surface of peptide and MHC, and that the TCR has a single binding site and not two linked sites. It is therefore not surprising that the predictions of these models for alloreactivity could grasp reality only partially.

Experimental results reported simultaneously gave support to both concepts in only one respect. Namely, it has been demonstrated by Bevan[223] and the Benacerraf group[224] that T cells activated against a foreign antigen plus self MHC crossreact with allogeneic MHC molecules in the absence of the foreign antigen, or vice versa.[225] These data suggested that the very same T cells recognize foreign antigen plus self MHC and allogeneic MHC. Later this finding was confirmed at the clonal level, first by von Boehmer and colleagues,[226] and subsequently in a number of reports.[227–231] Thus alloreactivity has been proven to be an inherent property of the self-MHC restricted T-cell repertoire, instead of being mediated by a useless subset of T cells.

8.5.2 Further Peculiarities of Alloresponses

Based on the early studies, alloresponses appeared to be more or less equivalent to self-MHC restricted responses, except for the great difference in responding cell frequencies. However, subsequent analysis has revealed additional differences between the two types of response.

First of all, a difference was demonstrated in the degree of specificity. Whereas self-MHC restricted responses were found to be exquisitely specific, the responses to allogeneic MHC haplotypes showed crossreactivities with multiple MHC haplotypes to which the T cells were not primed. This was observed in both cytotoxic T lymphocyte (Tc) responses to allogeneic MHC,[232,233] as well as in secondary proliferative responses of T cells activated in the mixed lymphocyte reaction (MLR).[234] The degree of crossreactivity was high, 15–50%, depending on the haplotype tested. The possibility of a non-specific response could be ruled out by mapping studies demonstrating that the crossreactive responses were indeed directed against third-party MHC molecules. The MHC-specific crossreactivity was interpreted to be due to the high clonal heterogeneity of alloresponses, which can include clones reacting to shared epitopes present on several different MHC molecules. However, the point could not be proven in this pre-cloning era of T-cell research. Therefore the possibility has remained open that perhaps the recognition of allogeneic MHC molecules may altogether be less specific than that of foreign antigen–self MHC complexes.

'Studying alloreactivity was at that time considered in immunology circles to be a rather esoteric occupation', recalls Dr. G. 'Indeed only transplantation biologists were interested in it, and a handful of theoretical immunologists for whom the explanation of alloreactivity was an obligatory exercise in every concept of T-cell recognition. The opinion held in main-stream immunology was perhaps best formulated by Lis Simpson[233] in the conclusion of her paper "... anti-H-2 responses ... can hardly have any evolutionary or survival value, because it is unlikely that they have been elicited before the twentieth century... Thus anti-H-2 responses may be an accident, their magnitude a mere reflection of underlying and important anti-altered self responses, and therefore the question of their specificity is not important, nor are they very specific." Curiously, immunologists, despite their crushing opinion of alloreactivity, kept using alloresponses cheerfully, as convenient experimental models in their studies.'

Another perplexing finding has been that alloresponses often make mistakes in the coupling of effector response to MHC class. As known, in self restricted responses, Tc cells always recognize antigen together with class I, and T helper (Th) cells with class II MHC. This rule applies only by and large to alloreactive cells. Here it is possible, by using appropriate responder/stimulator combinations, to identify class II-specific Tc,[235,236] as well as class I-specific Th cells.[237] At that time, the full impact of this observation was not realized, because the coreceptors, CD4 and CD8, involved in MHC class discrimination were not yet known. In retrospect, however, it is interesting to note that class II MHC-specific Tc cells were shown to express the Ly2 (CD8) marker,[238,239] now known to be involved in class I recognition. It is thus conceivable that these cells might have served as class I MHC restricted Tc in the self restricted repertoire. Yet they must have bound so strongly to allogeneic class II molecules that they were able to bypass the requirement for the coreceptor, and even disregard it altogether. This example suggests that the 'mistaken' reactivity of TCR to allogeneic MHC may have higher affinity than its physiological interaction with self MHC plus antigen.

One more odd feature of alloreactivity was born out by studies of MHC mutant mice. In the 1970s, several H-2 mutants, all derived from H-2^b mice, were already known. The mutations were shown to affect the gene encoding the H-2K^b class I molecule, and to manifest in 1–4 amino acid substitutions in this molecule.[240] Surprisingly, alloresponses obtained in wild-type versus mutant strain combinations were very vigorous[241–243] despite the minimal genetic disparity. Indeed, the precursor frequency of anti-mutant Tc proved to be as high as the frequency of Tc responding to a whole MHC haplotype difference[244] (the latter including three fully allogeneic class I molecules). Thus, on a per molecule basis, the minimally different mutant molecules induced more Tc than fully allogeneic molecules with extensive sequence difference. Taken together with the earlier observation that xenoreactivity (e.g., mouse anti-human) was weaker than alloreactivity,[169] the findings with mutant mice suggested that the strength of response to foreign MHC molecules was inversely proportional to the genetic distance, i.e., exactly the opposite of what one would expect from an immune response.

We can thus conclude that the research into alloreactivity until the early 1980s added several fascinating pieces to the puzzle, but a solution was not yet on the horizon.

8.5.3 Alloreactivity: A Pot-Pourri of Different Responses

In the second half of the 1980s, two important discoveries – notably the recognition that MHC molecules bind peptides, and the determination of the three-dimensional structure of MHC – gave new impulse to the analysis of alloreactivity.

The first novel insight came from a retrospective evaluation of wild-type anti-mutant responses. With the new knowledge of the MHC crystal structure it became possible to determine the exact location and orientation of the substituted amino acid residues in the mutant molecules. The surprising result was that in about half of all known H-2K^b mutants, the amino acid exchanges occurred either in the bottom of the peptide-binding site, or in the alpha helices with the side chains of residues pointing into the site.[245] Thus these mutations have turned out to be 'invisible' for the TCR, but could significantly alter the peptide-binding specificity of the affected molecules. These structural considerations have suggested that the alloreactivity of wild-type T cells to 'invisible' MHC mutants is equivalent to a self-MHC restricted response against a series of antigenic peptides. The latter can comprise self peptides not presented by the wild-type molecule, and also identical self peptides bound to both wild-type and mutant MHC in different conformations.[246] The explanation for the high-frequency alloreactivity to 'invisibly' mutant MHC molecules is therefore twofold: first, the response is directed against a multitude of peptides, and second, because the docking surface for TCR is identical on the wild-type and mutant molecule, *all* H-2K^b-restricted T cells should be able to dock on the mutant molecule. Obviously, other types of alloreactivity, in which the TCR docking surface of the stimulating MHC molecule differs at a number of amino acids from self MHC, must be mechanistically distinct from the anti-mutant response. The case of anti-mutant response has raised the possibility, for the first time, that alloreactivity may not be a single phenomenon from the mechanistic point of view, and this is where the scientific impact of this finding lies.

A number of studies were then undertaken to investigate the role of peptides in allorecognition. But the results appeared to be contradictory—whereas the involvement of peptides was demonstrated in certain studies,[247–250] peptide-independent alloreactivity was shown in others.[251,252] These data had stirred up the old theoretical argument about the peptide dependence versus independence of alloreactivity for a while, until the Rammensee group came up with a more comprehensive approach.[253] In their experiments peptides eluted from different MHC molecules were used to reconstruct antigenicity for a series of alloreactive T-cell clones. The results demonstrated a great variety of T-cell specificities ranging from peptide-specific, though peptide-dependent, to peptide-independent clones within a cell population activated against a single class I MHC disparity. In a follow-up study,[254] they showed that peptide-specific alloreactive (i.e., allorestricted) T cells were preferentially activated by small genetic disparities between responder and stimulator, whereas larger differences induced more peptide-dependent and peptide-independent clones. These results have left no doubt about the existence of a variety of different T-cell clones within a single alloreactive cell population.

'Further studies have added more mechanistic details as to how certain T-cell clones achieve alloreactivity. For example, many self-restricted antigen-specific clones, once alloreactive, were shown to react to multiple allogeneic MHC molecules.[255–258] Thus extensive crossreactivity, also at the clonal level, seems to be a rule rather than exception in alloreactivity. Crystallographic studies shed light on the molecular details of allorecognition by a few selected TCR. In one instance, the crystal structures of the same TCR bound to syngeneic MHC plus peptide and allogeneic MHC, respectively, were compared.[259] The β chain of this TCR was shown to make more contacts with the allogeneic than with the syngeneic ligand, hence the allogeneic interaction had higher affinity.[145] It has been repeatedly found that, in syngeneic TCR–MHC/peptide complexes, one of the TCR chains makes only spare contacts with the MHC,[134,259] and thus it seems feasible that this chain might be more involved in alloreactivity, as proposed by Cohn.[260] The crystal structure of another TCR–alloMHC complex revealed a different type of interaction. Here the α chain CDR3 loop was shown to fold away from the peptide-binding site and to contact the MHC instead of the peptide.[261] It is predictable that the more TCR–MHC structures will be investigated the more different kinds of interactions will be found.'

In conclusion, alloreactivity seems to encompass an amazingly wide variety of different types of T-cell–MHC interactions, and therefore it appears futile to look for a unified interpretation of this phenomenon.

'I cannot completely agree with your conclusion', argues Dr. G. 'Admittedly, the phenomenon is very complex, but this does not necessarily mean that it is not interpretable. In any attempt to interpret this complexity one should first deal with its source, which is twofold: the TCR repertoire on the one hand, and the ligand on the other.'

'The repertoire aspect is easiest to conceive by considering that all alloreactive TCRs can dock, besides self MHC, also on allogeneic MHC molecules. Thus, in principle, alloreactive TCRs could have been positively selected also in the respective allogeneic hosts. However, they missed negative selection on the allogeneic MHC molecule and its peptide content. The alloreactive T-cell repertoire is therefore expected to be similar to (although not identical with) a positively selected self-restricted repertoire prior to negative selection.'

Negative selection is known to operate at a defined affinity limit (combined affinity of TCR plus coreceptor ~ 6 μM[262]), i.e., T cells whose receptor interacts with any self peptide–MHC (pMHC) complex with an affinity above this limit will be deleted. The affinity-based mechanism of T-cell tolerance imposes constraints on the post-selection TCR repertoire in at least two ways. First, the mature repertoire will be unlikely to contain TCRs with affinities for foreign peptide+self-MHC that are too much higher than the cut-off for negative selection. Second, negative selection against thousands of self pMHCs will remove TCRs that crossreact with many different peptides, and thus the mature repertoire will be more specific. Implicit in these statements is that the repertoire before negative selection should have TCRs with high affinity and extensive crossreactivity, and indeed this has been shown to be the case in a repertoire that underwent limited negative selection.[150] Similarly, in alloreactivity, TCRs can be identified with affinities that are higher than the affinity for foreign peptide plus self-MHC,[145,263,264] and extensive crossreactivity with multiple allelic variants of MHC molecules is commonly found.[255–258]

'The complexity of ligands is the consequence of MHC polymorphism. The effect of polymorphism can be direct, when the polymorphic residues are located on the TCR contact surface, or indirect when they are located in the peptide-binding groove and thus change the peptide spectrum bound by the respective MHC molecule. Obviously, polymorphic residues located outside these two areas are not relevant for alloreactivity.'

'Depending on the properties of alloreactive TCRs and on the docking conditions they have to face, alloreactivity can be reduced to four mechanistically distinct prototypes of response[265] (Fig. 8.7).'

Type 1: Self-Restricted Peptide-Specific

'This is one end of the spectrum, represented by the response of the wild-type strain to 'invisible' MHC mutants, or vice versa (see above). The docking surface of the mutant molecule is identical with that of the wild-type, i.e., it is self. The response is directed exclusively against the divergent peptide content of the mutant molecule. Hence this group is in every respect equivalent to self-restricted, peptide-specific responses.'

Type 2: Allorestricted Peptide-Specific

The docking surface of MHC has a few amino acid differences compared to self, but these can be accommodated by the TCR without causing much change in docking affinity. This type of response can occur only across MHC allotypes, which have a small number and possibly conservative amino acid differences in the docking surface. Therefore it is preferentially detected in alloresponses to minimal genetic disparity,[254] e.g., in wild-type response against mutants with one or two mutated residues directly accessible for the TCR. Allorestriction can also be demonstrated among normal, self-restricted antigen-specific clones.[256]

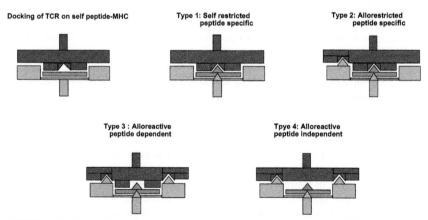

FIGURE 8.7 Schematic representation of four distinct prototypes of alloreactivity. Docking of TCR on self peptide-MHC, a non-signaling interaction, is shown for comparison. Contact(s) of TCR with triangles indicates a signaling interaction. TCR: dark; MHC: light grey; peptide: medium grey. See text for further explanation. From Reference 265.

Observations of type 1 and type 2 responses led earlier to the conclusion that alloreactivity was inversely proportional to the genetic distance (see Section 8.5.2).

Type 3: Alloreactive Peptide-Dependent

This type predominates the response to whole MHC haplotype difference, and is thus the most commonly observed form of alloreactivity. Here, peptides play a subordinate role, serving in most instances only to maintain the conformation of MHC. In this group most of the binding energy required for activation is contributed by interactions between TCR and MHC. These interactions can sum up to an affinity that is one–two orders of magnitude higher than the affinity for peptide plus self-MHC.[145,263,264] Consequently, such interactions cannot occur in the syngeneic context, because the respective T cells would be deleted by negative selection. The interactions with allo-MHC should be preferentially made through polymorphic residues, because TCRs interacting strongly with invariant residues are likely to be deleted by self tolerance. High crossreactivity is expected in this group with respect to peptides, and also with other MHC molecules that share some of the TCR contact residues. Most clones exhibiting multiple alloreactivities[255–258] should belong to this group.

A subgroup of type 3 is represented by alloreactive TCR that mix up class I with class II MHC (see Section 8.5.2). Likely candidates for this subgroup are TCRs that use only one chain for interaction with the docking surface of self MHC (see above). In other words, only one chain of such TCR is positively selected, whereas the other chain is merely entrained.[260] Hence the unselected (entrained) chain could interact strongly with allogeneic MHC be it class I or class II.

I also have to point out here that the existence of type 3 alloreactivity requires that TCR *V* genes encode specificities for polymorphic MHC variants.[260] Were this not the case, this group would be a rarity, and the affinity of TCR–MHC interaction would be low.

Type 4: Alloreactive Peptide-Independent

The existence of this type is dictated by logic but not proven, because the experiments demonstrating such cells[251,252] failed to rigorously exclude the presence of peptides. A formal proof would be furnished by the crystal structure of a TCR–MHC/peptide complex, in which the TCR does not make any contact with the peptide. This structure would also answer the question whether peptide-independent alloreactivity requires a different signaling conformation of TCR[260] or not. But so far such a structure has not been reported. Another often raised question is whether type 4 TCR can recognize empty (peptide-free) MHC molecules. However, this question has limited biological relevance, because empty MHC molecules are unstable, and thus very short-lived.

One final question remains: is it possible that some T cells are not alloreactive at all?

'The answer is "yes" on theoretical grounds,[199] but the question has never been properly addressed experimentally. In most studies, self-restricted antigen-specific T-cell clones were tested for alloreactivity on a panel of eight standard H-2 haplotypes. In the case where no alloreactivity was found, it was tacitly assumed that this was due to the small size of the panel. There was a single study[266] in which a dozen class-II-restricted clones and hybridoma from different sources were tested on Jan Klein's extended panel representing 26 I-A and 20 I-E class II alleles. Interestingly, two-thirds of the cell lines showed no alloreactivity at all, while the remaining ones exhibited multiple alloreactivities. However, the results could not conclusively establish the existence of non-alloreactive T cells, because the estimated number of class II alleles in the mouse population may be at least two-fold higher. Since Klein's panel was the largest in the world, these experiments could not be pushed any further.'

'Perhaps a more promising approach would be to use human T cells and take advantage of the world-wide organization of blood banks for obtaining a huge variety of stimulator cells. But the investment might be more than the answer is worth.'

As a summary of this topic, one can state that the puzzle of alloreactivity had been assembled with a great deal of patience and ingenuity, to reach almost completion by the end of the twentieth century. To provide the two–three missing pieces would, however, require a relatively large effort. The future can only tell whether these pieces will ever be supplied.

8.6 FUNCTIONAL SUBCLASSES OF T CELLS

8.6.1 Ly1 and Ly2,3: Markers to Distinguish Between Helper and Cytotoxic T Cells

By the mid-1970s it had become clear that T cells can perform at least two distinct and assayable functions: they can provide help to B cells in antibody production, and can mediate cytotoxicity against target cells carrying different antigens. The discovery of MHC restriction coupled this functional dichotomy of T cells to the recognition of different MHC classes: cytotoxic T lymphocytes (Tc) were shown to require class I (Section 8.1.2), and T helper (Th) cells class II MHC (Section 8.1.3) for their sensitization as well as effector function against foreign antigens. Responses to allogeneic MHC molecules appeared to follow the same rules, albeit less strictly: Tcs were generated preferentially across class I (Section 6.1.3), and proliferative Th-type responses to class II (Section 6.2.2) MHC disparity. It was therefore reasonable to assume that these two functions were mediated by separate T-cell subclasses, but experimental evidence to prove this point was not available. It was also unclear whether the functional commitment occurred after sensitization to antigen, or else the T cells had been predetermined to express a particular function before they encountered antigen. To be able to address these questions experimentally, techniques were required that allow the identification and separation of the T-cell subpopulations performing different functions.

The answer to this technical demand came from studies of polymorphic differentiation antigens, a long-standing interest of Lloyd Old and Edward Boyse at the Memorial Sloan-Kettering Cancer Center in New York. Three of these antigens, termed Ly1, Ly2 and Ly3, were of particular interest, because they were expressed exclusively on the surface of murine T cells. The Ly1 antigen was mapped to a gene on chromosome 19, and Ly2 and Ly3 to two closely linked loci on chromosome 6. Each locus was shown to have two alleles in the mouse population (denoted *Ly1.1, 1.2, Ly2.1, 2.2, Ly3.1, 3.2*),[267] which permitted to raise antisera against the respective antigens by alloimmunization. It was then that a young Polish immunologist, Pavel Kisielow (now the father of immunology in Poland) spending his WHO fellowship at Sloan-Kettering, who first tested these alloantisera on three different T cell functions, namely, help, cytotoxicity, and graft-versus-host reaction. The results that appeared as a relatively inconspicuous *Nature* Letter in January 1975 clearly demonstrated depletion of helper function by anti-Ly1 plus complement treatment, and elimination of cytotoxic activity by anti-Ly2 and complement.[268] Thus the Ly1 and Ly2 antigen appeared to be expressed selectively on two different functional subclasses of T cells.

The initial report was followed half a year later by two very influential papers by Harvey Cantor and Edward Boyse in the *Journal of Experimental Medicine*.[269,270] Their results provided what appeared to be a complete story on the differentiation of functionally distinct T-cell subsets. In terms of Ly antigen expression, T cells were found to fall into three categories, $Ly1^{+}2^{+}3^{+}$, $Ly1^{+}2^{-}3^{-}$, and $Ly1^{-}2^{+}3^{+}$. The Ly2 and Ly3 antigens were always expressed together, and were correctly assumed to represent subunits of the same molecule. Of the three subpopulations, Ly123 cells made up the overwhelming majority of thymocytes, and were also predominant in the spleen and lymph nodes shortly after birth. Ly1 and Ly23 cells, although undetectable in neonatal life, gradually increased in numbers until the tenth week of life. Adult thymectomy reduced selectively the proportion of Ly123 cells, indicating that this subpopulation was dependent on the continued thymic output of T cells. In adult animals, Ly123 cells made up ~50% of total T cells, Ly1 cells were represented with ~30% and Ly23 cells with ~10%. The data also confirmed the exclusive role of Ly1 cells in help, and Ly23 cells in cytotoxicity, whereas Ly123 cells appeared to be inactive. Altogether, the results have suggested that the Ly1 and Ly23 functional subpopulations arise from Ly123 precursors during ontogeny, virtually independent of antigen encounter. The Cantor and Boyse papers acted as a revelation for most immunologists (particularly for those who missed the Kisielow et al. report), and thus 1975 became the year of T-cell subpopulations.

However, as often happens in science, further studies on Ly antigen expression produced data that did not fit into the initial, beautifully simple scheme. The first 'deviant' results came from a rather artificial system, referred to as allohelp, in which the helper activity of T cells was assayed on the in vitro primary anti-sheep erythrocyte response of allogeneic B cells. The data have demonstrated that allohelper T cells activated against class I MHC differences were depleted by both anti-Ly1 and anti-Ly23 plus complement treatment, and that the mixture of the two antibody-treated populations did not restore allohelp, thus indicating that this function was mediated by Ly123 cells.[271] It was also shown that the Ly123 Th cells did not mature into Ly1 Th cells.[272] Similar observations were made in certain Tc responses. For example, Tc generated in wild-type anti-class I mutant strain combinations,[273] or activated against trinitrophenyl-modified syngeneic cells,[274,275] were Ly123. Upon further stimulation, the Ly123 Tc effectors differentiated into Ly23 but not into Ly1 cells.[274,276] These findings challenged the original model at most of its cardinal points, first, the Ly123 subset proved to contain mature effector cells, i.e., it was not merely a precursor population, second, Ly123 cells were shown to mature only to Ly23, but not to Ly1 cells, and third, Ly1 was not an exclusive marker for Th cells. Furthermore, a quantitative analysis of Ly expression on fetal thymocytes has revealed that Ly1 cells appear in the thymus before Ly123 cells, thus these two subsets may represent independent cell lineages.[277] The modified scheme borne out by these studies has proposed that in the thymus two different cell lineages arise, Ly1 (or more correctly Ly23$^-$) and Ly123, the latter further differentiating to Ly23 possibly after antigen encounter.

The biological relevance of these findings, however, remained somewhat dubious in immunologists' minds, owing to the excessive use of alloresponses as experimental models. For it had become increasingly clear by that time that alloreactivity deviated in many respects from normal self-restricted T-cell responses. If one only considered data coming from physiological, self-restricted response models, there was one finding that remained consistent throughout all Ly studies, namely, that class I restricted Tcs were always Ly23$^+$, and class II restricted Th cells Ly23$^-$.

Despite the questionable physiological relevance of the experimental systems, the new data cast serious doubts on the thesis that Ly antigens would mark functional subpopulations of T cells, and thus, a new interpretation for the expression pattern of these markers was sought. It was then proposed by Susan Swain[271,272] that the expression of Ly1 and Ly23, respectively, correlated better with the MHC class recognized by the respective T cells than with the function of the latter. Although the data supporting her hypothesis also came from alloreactive responses,[271,278] the idea itself that Ly antigens may have to do with MHC class recognition, was worth further pursuit.

8.6.2 How T-Cell Surface Markers Became Coreceptors

It is remarkable that in the first 5 years of Ly studies everybody used anti-Ly sera for depleting T-cell subsets in the presence of complement and then tested the surviving T cells for function, instead of investigating the direct effect of these antibodies on T cells without complement.

'The reason for this is something that every immunologist knows but no one talks about, or as Charlie Janeway would have put it: a dirty little secret of immunologists', explains Dr. G. 'This is the notorious unspecific inhibitory activity of mouse antisera. Some of this activity is due to natural antibodies to cell surface molecules, and as such can be removed by appropriate absorption. But even after absorption substantial non-specific inhibition remains that can only be mitigated by diluting the serum. Since most murine alloantisera are relatively low-titered, they cannot be sufficiently diluted without losing also the specific activity. Therefore most immunologists would not even have thought of doing inhibition experiments with such sera. Nevertheless, there was one report from the fathers of anti-Ly sera, in which these sera were used to inhibit the cytolytic function of Tc cells.[279] Obviously, the authors succeeded in producing high-titered alloantisera for this purpose. The results clearly showed that anti-Ly2 and anti-Ly3 sera inhibited cytolysis, whereas anti-Ly1 and a series of other alloantisera failed to do so. They concluded that the Ly23 determinants might have a close spatial relation to the TCR. This was the first indication that Ly23 might act as a coreceptor. However, in general, inhibition studies have been a domain for monoclonal antibodies that can reach extremely high titers, and are amenable to purification procedures.'

Around 1980 monoclonal antibodies (mAbs) to cell surface molecules, including Ly antigens, started to appear, and thus time was ripe for doing antibody inhibition experiments. The first study[280] in this vein compared three mAbs, anti-Ly1, anti-Ly2 and anti-Thy1, all three the same Ig isotype, high-titered and interacting with T cells equally, for their capacity to influence alloresponses. Confirming the previous results of Nakayama et al.[279] with polyclonal antisera, anti-Ly2 mAb was found to inhibit cytolysis. It also blocked partially the mixed lymphocyte reaction (MLR) across full MHC disparity. In contrast to the expectations, however, helper T cells in MLR were not inhibited by anti-Ly1 mAb. Anti-Thy1 was ineffective in both responses. Because the anti-Ly2 mAb inhibited only the alloresponse but did not influence polyclonal T-cell activation, it was assumed that it interfered with T-cell function at the level of antigen recognition. On the contrary, Ly1 did not seem to be involved in antigen recognition of Th cells, and thus failed as candidate receptor for class II MHC. The blocking effect of anti-Ly2 mAb was then shown by Susan Swain[281] to apply to all responses directed against class I MHC, suggesting that Ly2 may selectively interact with class I molecules.

At this point the Ly2 and Ly3 antigens started to establish themselves as subunits of a specific receptor mediating MHC class I recognition, probably by interacting with a monomorphic site shared by all class I, but absent from class II molecules. Logic demanded that another receptor should exist for class II recognition, but the only available candidate, Ly1, failed to satisfy this criterion. Therefore, a chase started for the identification of the putative class II receptor, a project in which human immunology took over the lead. The success followed from a large campaign launched by Stuart Schlossman's group at the Harvard-associated Sidney Farber Cancer Institute in collaboration with Ortho Pharmaceuticals for the production of mAbs against human T-cell surface components.[282] One of the resulting OKT series of mAbs, OKT4, was reported to bind selectively to human Th cells,[283] and subsequent studies confirmed the function of the target molecule (termed Leu-3 or T4) as a receptor for class II MHC recognition.[284,285] A mAb for the murine equivalent was reported 4 years later by Frank Fitch and associates.[286]

'Frank Fitch was "the" immunologist in Chicago', comments Dr. G. 'My first encounter with him was so strange that I cannot resist telling it to you. I was sitting in the cafeteria at some meeting, practically alone, because the session was ongoing, when a rather aged-looking man entered. He obviously did not give a damn to the trendy youthfulness-mania of the time, but let himself age properly or even more. He came straight to my table and sat down beside me. "I am Frank Fitch" he introduced himself. "You know I am an astrophysicist by training, and used to work in New York on the identification of organic material in meteorite samples, a very hot project at that time. Until one day my eyes wandered away from the microscope to the window air condition unit, which was thickly covered with soot. This suggested to me a feasible way of how carbon particles may get into meteorite samples, and so I decided to join immunology." This was all he said, then he stood up and left. I still don't understand today, why he trusted this CV excerpt of his on me.'

The OKT antibodies permitted the identification of a number of additional cell surface molecules on human T cells, most importantly the human equivalent of Ly2 (termed Leu-2 or T8)[284,287] and the signaling molecular complex of TCR (termed T3).[288]

'At this point it may be advisable to take a detour across the jungle of nomenclature', suggests Dr. G. 'The early 1980s experienced an explosion-like increase in the number of mAbs defining cell surface molecules on lymphocytes. This was largely accounted for by mAbs to human lymphoid cells, which held commercial promise to be used as diagnostics and eventually therapeutics. But mouse immunologists were not idle either, for example, Ian McKenzie in Melbourne published almost every week a new anti-Ly mAb. Under these circumstances it was not surprising that the nomenclature of new cell surface molecules went awry. The designation of murine molecules was still relatively straight-forward: Ly plus a serial number. As the numbers became too high Lys were split into Lyt and Lyb, depending on whether the respective molecule was expressed on T or B cells. The nomenclature for human molecules followed a more circuitous path. At the beginning it was Leu plus a serial number, but for T cells it was replaced by T plus the OKT number of the mAb that permitted the identification of the respective molecule, for example Leu-2 became T8, and Leu-3 T4, etc. The mess was almost complete, when a new suggestion came:[289] since each mAb recognizes a single determinant, molecules appear from the serological point of view as clusters of determinants, and should thus be designated as CD. This rather uncommitted nomenclature won the liking of immunologists and has remained final. But the numbers attached to CD were not necessarily serial: at the beginning they were the OKT numbers of the respective mAbs. Thus, T4 became CD4, T8 CD8 and T3 CD3, etc. Murine Ly molecules were also to be renamed CD, and to receive the same CD number as their human homologues.[290] So eventually all these fascinating molecules submerged in a faceless CD database. But one knows at least where to find them!'

The further history of CD4 and CD8 was relatively straight-forward: the genes encoding them were cloned,[291–296] the binding sites for MHC determined by site-directed mutagenesis,[297–300] and finally the molecules were crystallized and their three-dimensional structure determined.[301–303] The gene encoding Ly1 was also cloned,[304] and as expected, the deduced protein sequence did not show homology to CD4, instead, it proved to be related to the human CD5.

The structural information about CD4 and CD8 is briefly summarized as follows (Fig. 8.8). Both molecules consist of a long extracellular region and short transmembrane and intracytoplasmic regions. CD4 is a single polypeptide chain, the extracellular part of which folds into four Ig-like domains (D1 through 4). The two membrane distal domains D1 and D2 form a rigid rod-like structure that is flexibly connected to the two membrane proximal domains. Binding to class II MHC occurs via D1 to a hydrophobic cavity at the basis of the class II molecule, between the β2 and α2 domains. The CD8 molecule, by contrast, is a disulfide-bonded heterodimer of two chains, α and β, that correspond to Ly2 and Ly3 in the mouse. But it can also occur as α-α homodimer. The extracellular parts of both chains have an amino-terminal Ig-like domain and an extended polypeptide region. Both Ig-like domains of CD8 have CDR-like structures that

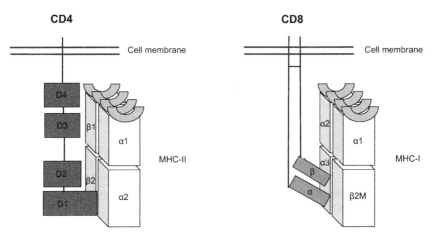

FIGURE 8.8   Schematic representation of the CD4 and CD8 coreceptors and their interaction with MHC molecules. CD4 interacts via its D1 domain with a site between the α2 and β2 domains of MHC class II. Both chains of CD8 interact with a site of the α3 domain of MHC class I. CD4 dark grey, CD8 medium grey, peptide binding site of MHC half circles. Based on References 297–303.

interact with a flexible loop in the α3 domain of class I MHC. One important finding of the structural studies has been that the MHC sites with which the CD4 and CD8 interact are distant from the peptide-binding site. This arrangement permits both TCR and CD4 or CD8 to bind to the same MHC molecule, which is a prerequisite for their proposed coreceptor function.[305,306]

From the ontogenic point of view, CD4 and CD8 behave as it was originally expected for Ly1 and Ly23: thus, both molecules are expressed on early thymocytes (double positive, DP, stage) and later, during repertoire selection, thymocytes become single positive (SP), i.e., they switch off either CD4 or CD8 (see Sections 8.4.1 and 8.4.3). The SP status then remains stable throughout the life of T cells.

Having all important information available on CD4 and CD8, only one critical question remains: what is their true biological function? In the early years of Ly studies, these molecules had been thought to be associated with the function of T-cell subclasses,[268,269] but as our knowledge has progressed, the opinion that they were coreceptors helping the TCR in antigen recognition started to prevail. Therefore, a considerable degree of uncertainty has remained in immunologists' minds as to the question of function.

'As any other biological question, also this one has to be analyzed in an evolutionary context in order to arrive at an acceptable level of understanding', emphasizes Dr. G.

'The first question we may ask: is there an evolutionarily selectable function for coreceptors? What springs immediately to mind is that it should be the stabilization of TCR–ligand interactions. This is indeed necessary and selectable, because TCR–ligand interactions are of low affinity, and they must remain stable until a number of them will be collected that is sufficient to activate the T cell. However, stabilization only makes sense if it sets in *after* the TCR found its ligand. Conversely, "sterile" dockings (i.e., when the TCR does not find a ligand) are not supposed to be stabilized, because this would slow down the screening function of TCR for which evolution can punish. Until now, there is no clear evidence to show that coreceptors really function post-antigen recognition, although some data point in this direction.[307] Another proposed function of coreceptors is to contribute to signaling for T-cell activation after TCR ligation.[308,309] This function, however, may not be easily selectable, because the TCR has its own signaling apparatus (CD3), unless the coreceptors would mediate a qualitatively different signal. Admittedly, I have some difficulties with the identification of easily conceivable evolutionary driving forces for the coreceptor function, which, of course, is not meant to say that such forces do not exist.'

'The next question concerns the biological necessity for MHC class recognition. Clearly, this requirement is independent of antigen recognition, as TCRs cannot tell whether they interact with class I or class II MHC. This information must come from the MHC through CD4 and CD8, respectively. Had antigen recognition been intrinsically associated with MHC class recognition, we would now have two separate sets of TCR *V* genes, one for class I and another for class II, instead of two coreceptors. The evolutionary need for CD4 and CD8 should therefore be sought elsewhere, specifically in antigen presentation. As we know, the presentation of an antigenic peptide by class I or class II, respectively, signals two different types of infectionclass I presentation means intracellular infection (mostly by viruses), whereas the source of antigen presented by class II is mostly extracellular (e.g., bacteria or their products). The defense strategies against these two kinds of invader are fundamentally different: infected cells must be eliminated by cytotoxicity, whereas extracellular pathogens are most effectively rid by antibodies. Consequently, MHC class recognition must be strictly coupled with different effector functions, class I with cytotoxicity and class II with help. This had been proposed at the beginning of T-cell subset studies,[268,269] and has remained ever since the most convincing evolutionary driving force for the development of CD8 and CD4. Decoupling of effector function from MHC class would derange immune defense, and is therefore selected against in nature. Indeed, decoupling occurs only in alloreactivity[284,271] that is not directly under natural selection.'

'What is usually considered as a strong argument against the MHC class association of effector function is the existence of CD4 cytotoxic T cells (Tc). Although most reported examples are alloreactive,[278,284,310] according to my own experience, self-class II restricted peptide-specific T-cell clones can also kill antigen-presenting B cells. However, cytotoxic Th cells are demonstrated, as a rule, in long-term cultured T-cell lines that were repeatedly restimulated with antigen and high concentrations of interleukin-2. These cells are clearly overstimulated, and thus the observed cytotoxic activity is unlikely to occur in vivo, and may not be equivalent to the cytolysis mediated by CD8 cells. In fact, primary Tc specific for allogeneic class II are usually CD8 cells.[238] In my opinion therefore, CD4 class II-specific killers do not constitute a serious argument against the coupling of effector function with MHC class.'

'The true biological function of CD4 and CD8 is thus to ensure proper targeting of the effector response. It cost evolution a lot of effort to make this system work. For example, an extra "learning step" had to be introduced in thymocyte ontogeny that ensures CD8 expression together with class I docking TCR, and CD4 with class II docking TCR, by a mechanism that is still poorly understood. Furthermore, constitutive class II expression was restricted to B cells, and induced expression to inflammatory regions, i.e., to sites where Th cells are needed. I am also convinced that a "confirmatory" signal from MHC through the coreceptor is required for launching the proper response at the effector phase, although there is no experimental evidence for this.'

'Concerning the stage of evolution at which CD4 and CD8 appeared, I can only make assumptions. One possibility may be that they evolved concomitantly from the timepoint of the divergence of class II from class I MHC. But it is also possible that the ancestor of CD8 was already there before the divergence of class II, and served as a coreceptor without influence on the effector function. CD4 and the coupling of coreceptors to the effector function might then have evolved later, simultaneously with the evolution of class II MHC. Studying the ancestors of coreceptors in species more ancient than mouse and man could only shed light on this.'

8.6.3 Th1 and Th2: Functionally Distinct Subsets of T Helper Cells

In this section we will delve into another kind of complexity: the effector functions of T cells, which have turned out to be much more intricate than just help or kill as originally expected. It has all commenced with the observation that the supernatants of in vitro activated T cells contain a variety of miraculous biological activities, collectively termed 'factors'. The factors seemed to affect different kinds of blood cells, and they were named after the cell type on which their activity was assayed, e.g., T-cell growth factor, B-cell stimulatory factor, eosinophil differentiation factor etc.

'At the beginning "factorology" was a rather underrated branch of immunology, mostly because nothing was known about the molecular basis for the observed biological activities', recalls Dr. G 'It was not even known whether a particular factor mediated a single biological activity or several ones, and conversely, whether a particular activity resulted from a single factor or from the interplay of different ones. Nonetheless, factors have proven useful from early on, for example, the discovery of T-cell growth factor (TCGF, now IL-2) in the supernates of T cells activated by concanavalin A or in the mixed lymphocyte reaction enabled the long-term culture and cloning of T cells, a real breakthrough in lymphocyte biology. Later, factors were coined the more respectable "lymphokine" term, and subsequently, as it turned out that they were not only produced by lymphocytes, the more general designation "cytokine". Another very popular name, the godfather for which was Hermann Wagner if I remember correctly, was "interleukin", hinting to the communicative function of these molecules. But named them as you wanted, they have remained unknown for quite a while, because they defied all attempts of protein chemical characterization. Finally molecular biology came to help, and cytokines were then identified very rapidly.'

The detailed history of cytokines is beyond the scope of this discussion. Suffice it to say that they fall into several categories, including hematopoietins (growth and differentiation factors), interferons, tumor necrosis factor (TNF)-related molecules, immunoglobulin superfamily members, and chemokines. Here we will only deal with a few of them in detail, namely with the ones that have already been integrated conceptually into the physiology of immune response.

'But I would not take leave of cytokines so abruptly', intervenes Dr. G 'before at least trying to define briefly what they are good for. From the functional point of view cytokines can be grossly categorized as growth factors and effector molecules. The obvious role of growth factors is to trigger the proliferation of defensive cells, which is the indispensable first step of every immune response.

The proposed driver for this step is the exponential growth of pathogens, which requires the immune response to be also exponential if it is to cope with infections.[311] Certainly, the proliferation of defensive cells is an effective countermeasure, at least in the case where the target of immune attack is an infected host cell. However, it is not sufficient per se, because the proliferation rate of a eukaryotic cell is still far slower than that of a pathogenic microorganism (e.g., lymphocytes divide every 12 hours, bacteria <1 hour, and fungi 1–3 hours). But what the growth of pathogens definitely cannot outpace is the synthesis rate of individual proteins. Therefore the only viable option for the immune system was to use secreted proteins instead of cells as units of effector function against microorganisms. The existence of secreted effector molecules can thus be envisaged as the result of strict evolutionary selection exercised by microorganisms. The mode of action of cytokines also supports this interpretation. Namely, these molecules act at relatively short range, often transmitted upon direct contact to another cell, and thus can function without the need for reaching detectable concentrations in body fluids.'

Cytokines met immunobiology for the first time in a study by Tim Mosmann and colleagues.[312] The authors studied cytokine secretion by a series of different Th cell clones, and were able to identify two different profiles. One group of clones, termed Th1, produced interferon gamma (IFNγ), interleukin-2 (IL-2, formerly TCGF), and TNFβ, and the other, designated Th2, secreted IL-4, IL-5, IL-6, and IL-10. These two cytokine profiles were mutually exclusive, most strikingly for IFNγ and IL-4, and remained unchanged over long-term culture. Thus the Th1 and Th2 phenotypes appeared to be stable. The community received this finding with substantial interest, but not without a critical undertone. Skeptics questioned whether these Th cell subclasses exist also in vivo, and whether this issue can be addressed at all in the absence of distinguishing cell surface markers (specific markers for Th1 and Th2 were identified more than a decade later[313,314]). Furthermore, Th1 and Th2 were only demonstrated in mice, and it took some time to establish their existence in human.[315] Nevertheless, the Th1/Th2 paradigm asserted itself relatively easily, because it made functional sense. Namely, the proinflammatory cytokines IFNγ and TNFβ render the Th1 subset well suited for local inflammatory responses, such as delayed-type hypersensitivity, in which the protective effect is mediated mostly by macrophages. In contrast, Th2 cytokines affect B-cell growth, differentiation and antibody secretion, and thus this subset is more involved in helping antibody responses. The two cytokine profiles could thus be translated into two distinct types of effector response, each being the task for a specialized Th-cell subset (although some overlap in the effector functions of the two subsets was also observed, e.g., both help B cells, and share certain cytokines).

The functional properties of Th1 and Th2 cytokines are summarized in Table 8.3. It is clear from this compilation that a single cytokine can have multiple biological activities depending on the cell type on which it acts, and sometimes even on the very same cell type. Conversely, certain biological

TABLE 8.3 Th1 and Th2 Cytokines and their Functions

Th Type	Cytokine Name	Cytokine Effector Function
Th1	IL-2: interleukin-2	Stimulates T cell growth, costimulates B cell differentiation
Th1	IFNγ: interferon gamma	Induces MHC class II expression and microbicidal activity in macrophages, inhibits viral replication
Th1	TNFβ: tumor necrosis factor beta	Cytotoxic
Th2	IL-4: interleukin-4	Stimulates limited T cell growth, costimulates B cell growth, controls Ig isotype switch from IgM to IgG1, IgG4, and IgE
Th2	IL-5: interleukin-5	Helps B cell differentiation into antibody forming cells, enhances IgA production, helps eosinophil differentiation
Th2	IL-6, IL-10: interleukin-6, -10	Promote Ig secretion
Th1/Th2	IL-3: interleukin-3	Multipotential hematopoietic growth factor, stimulates mast cell growth
Th1/Th2	GMCSF: granulocyte-macrophage colony stimulating factor	Stimulates growth of granulocytes+macrophages from bone marrow progenitor cells

Based on References 316 and 317.

effects, e.g., B-cell help, arise from the cooperative activity of several cytokines. This complex behavior of cytokines causes considerable difficulties in conceiving and conceptualizing the effector functions of Th cells.

Once the existence of Th1 and Th2 cells was firmly established, the next research task was to elucidate how these Th-cell subclasses develop. Important tools in this research were TCR-transgenic mice that provided a source of monospecific naïve T cells, as well as recombinant cytokines and monoclonal antibodies against them. A major conclusion of these studies has been that the Th1 and Th2 profiles, unlike the CD4 and CD8 subsets, are not determined in ontogeny, they develop during the course of immune response. Naïve Th cells upon their first encounter with antigen secret IL-2 only,[318] and give rise to a cell population, termed Th0, producing a mixed set of cytokines.[319–321] Commitment to the Th1 or Th2 cytokine pattern occurs subsequently, but the cytokine profile can convert for some time,[322] until the final commitment takes

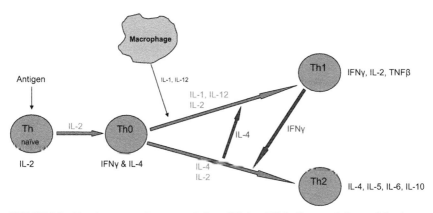

FIGURE 8.9   Development and cross-regulation of Th1 and Th2 effector subclasses. Stimulatory pathways and cytokines in grey, inhibitory pathways and cytokines in dark grey. The initial external source of IL-4 is uncertain. Based on References 317–326.

place after weeks of culture. Analysis of cytokine gene expression at the single-cell level has revealed that each cell produces one or at most two cytokines.[323] Thus, the phenotypes defined by cytokine patterns apply only to cell populations rather than to individual cells.

The most fascinating finding from these studies has been that the Th1 and Th2 subclasses cross-regulate each other (Fig. 8.9). The presence of IL-4 during priming drives Th0 cells toward the Th2 pathway, and simultaneously inhibits the development of IFNγ-producing Th1 cells.[320,321] Conversely, IFNγ inhibits the development of IL-4-producing Th2 cells.[321] However, IFNγ itself does not serve as an autocrine stimulus for Th1 development. The Th1 pathway is driven by macrophage-derived cytokines, IL-12[324,325] and IL-1.[326] The cytokine-driven commitment to the Th1 or Th2 pathway eventually results from a complex transcriptional regulation, which is largely known thanks to the pioneering studies of Laurie Glimcher's group at Harvard Medical School. The reader is referred to her work[327–331] for more detail.

The discovery of Th-cell effector classes has re-raised an old and very important question: how does the immune system choose the proper effector response for the elimination of a certain pathogen?

'The adaptive immune system can only see three-dimensional shapes (epitopes), without regard of other qualities (e.g., chemical) of the antigen.' points out Dr. G. 'Therefore, any additional information on the pathogen should arise from its interaction with the host, most likely via the innate immune system of the latter. A very revealing example for this is provided by studies of experimental infection of mice with *Leishmania major* and *Listeria monocytogenes*. Both pathogens establish intracellular infection of macrophages, and for their clearance macrophage activation by IFNγ is required.[324,332] Thus, protection of the host in these cases is provided by a Th1 response. Th2 cytokines IL-4 and IL-10 interfere with the protective effect of IFNγ.[327] There is evidence that the infected macrophages produce IL-12 and thereby gear the effector response toward Th1, i.e., increased IFNγ production.[324] Thus 'indigestion' of macrophages is obviously one possible signal for Th1 development. Another one is the recognition of microbe-specific nucleotide sequences or bacterial cell wall components by toll-like receptors.[333,334] It is much less clear what stimuli drive the Th2 response. All we know is that an external source of IL-4 is necessary for Th2 commitment, and that infection of mice with extracellular parasites, notably certain nematodes, selectively induces a protective Th2 response.[335] But the link between nematode infection and the initial source of IL-4 has remained unknown. All these examples point at an important role of the host–pathogen interaction (outside the adaptive immune system) in regulating the effector class of Th-cell responses, but many details of how this happens are yet to be learned.'

8.6.4 The Rise and Fall of Suppressor T Cells

One of the most fascinating features of the immune system is that it can mount, under defined conditions (e.g., antigen dose,[336] route of antigen administration,[337] immunological maturity,[337] etc.), specific unresponsiveness to otherwise immunogenic substances. This condition is the exact inverse of acquired immunity and has therefore been referred to as acquired tolerance, although its relatedness to the natural, neonatal tolerance of self molecules has not always been clear.[338] Experimentally induced tolerance looked back upon a long and venerable history including a Nobel Prize for its discovery[339] to Peter Medawar. However, the underlying mechanisms had remained unknown until the results of two groundbreaking studies by Gershon and Kondo appeared in 1970[340] and 1971.[341]

These authors investigated tolerance induction to sheep red blood cells (SRBC). Heterologous erythrocytes were known to be strongly antigenic but poorly tolerogenic,[337] and therefore a complete 're-programming' of the immune system by thymectomy, X-irradiation and bone marrow reconstitution (TXBM) was necessary to induce a short-term (1 month) tolerance by massive doses of SRBC. In the TXBM mice B-cell tolerance was observed, which could be broken by thymocytes injected after the SRBC treatment. The same antigenic treatment induced tolerance also in TXBM mice that had received thymocytes together with the bone marrow inoculum (TXBM+T). But in these mice tolerance could not be broken by later addition of thymocytes. Indeed, the SRBC-tolerized spleen cells of TXBM+T mice prevented the antibody response when transferred into non-tolerized TXBM+T mice. The abrogation of response in the secondary hosts was SRBC specific in that it did not affect the response to horse erythrocytes. The authors coined the term 'infectious immunological tolerance' to this phenomenon. Subsequently Gershon and colleagues[342] showed that thymocytes could directly abrogate the antigen-induced response of other thymocytes, and christened the former suppressor T (Ts) cells.

'Dick Gershon, the father of Ts cells was a very original and amiable person', recalls Dr. G. 'Once I visited Yale University upon Charley Janeway's invitation, and had the opportunity to see him. He received me in his office which reminded me of a luxurious silk-lined shoe carton, with pieces of modern art and pictures of French wineries on the walls attesting his interest in arts and the bright side of life. Perhaps this office served also as a compensation for the bleak surroundings, as the Yale campus was at that time right in the middle of a slum area due to the caprice of economic forces. Dick certainly hated depression, he was always ready for fun, and managed to inspire his people in his humorous, easy-going way. In fact, his group was at the same time his fan club.'

Because of the long-standing interest of immunologists in tolerance, suppressor T cells rapidly gained popularity, and their involvement in responses to a series of different antigens,[343–347] as well as in MHC-controlled unresponsiveness[348–350] was demonstrated. The discovery that Ts cells and their soluble factors carried a serologically detectable MHC-controlled moiety encoded in the newly identified I-J subregion[351–353] lent the data additional weight.

'We should not conceal, however, that Ts cells, popular as they might have been, were not unanimously accepted by the immunological community', stresses Dr. G. 'Skeptics found Ts cells counter-intuitive, and disliked suppressor assays that read out, instead of a response, the lack of it. The latter aversion is conceivable, because the response can have one single cause, the antigen, whereas the failure of a response could occur for a thousand different reasons, many of which might be technical. Skeptics also rejected the argument of Ts proponents, i.e., that the immune system needed "brakes". And they were not quite unright. For a protective response may not need brakes at all, or at most it would need a feedback control to avoid unnecessary overshoot of the response. In contrast, an ineffective response that cannot rid the pathogen does need an immediate brake, because it competes for the antigen with, and thus blocks the function of an effective response. Based on this argument, theoreticians saw a justification for Ts cells only in the regulation of the effector class of response.[338,354,355] However, not a single piece of experimental evidence pointed in this direction. In contrast, many data had to do with tolerance, but theoreticians had good reasons to reject a suppression-based mechanism for self tolerance.[355] Thus the conceptualization of T-cell-mediated suppression was problematic from the beginning, and it has remained so over the entire period of Ts research, despite attempts[356,357] to provide some theoretical foundation for the field.'

'Meanwhile we have learned that the immune system manages to regulate effector responses without Ts cells. Indeed, the effector classes are controlled by Th1 and Th2 cells, and they cross-regulate each other (see Section 8.6.3). Thus the only well-founded argument for the necessity of Ts cells was not supported by reality. By exclusion, one had to assume that Ts cells were required for self tolerance, but a feasible driving force for the evolution of suppression on top of other mechanisms of tolerance (clonal deletion, anergy) has never been proposed. In my opinion, this conceptual insecurity contributed significantly, albeit in a latent manner, to the unfortunate development and demise of the field.'

Perhaps due to the lack of a conceptual framework, immunologists tried feverishly to find solely experimental answers to the outstanding questions. This effort had led to an uncontrolled proliferation of suppressor pathways, factors, and interactions, so that finally not even the participants could overlook the field. At this point a number of negative events shattered Ts research almost simultaneously. First, a putative antigen-specific suppressor factor was identified to be an apolipoprotein.[358] Second, in the molecular map of MHC no gene was found in the region reserved for I-J,[359] and RNA prepared from I-J positive Ts hybridomas did not hybridize with MHC cosmid clones.[360] Third, no TCR β gene rearrangements were found in a number of Ts hybridomas.[361] And finally, Dick Gershon died prematurely in 1983.

Under the concerted attack of these events, the sensitive edifice of suppression collapsed in a tragic way by the mid 1980s. In 2008, a retrospective analysis of these events appeared in a number of reviews[362–364] that marked the fiftieth anniversary of *Immunology*, the journal in which Gershon published his original papers. The authors of these reviews, former players in the Ts arena, all agreed that the collapse was an insecure overreaction caused at least in part by an exaggerated respect for the new molecular technologies which had been used to generate the negative data. More appropriate reaction would have been a thorough re-analysis of some data, instead of 'throwing out the baby with the bathwater'. Indeed, many of the Ts data have now been confirmed in the context of regulatory T cells, to which the next section will be devoted.

8.6.5 Rebirth of the Phoenix: From Ts to Treg

The fall of suppression was followed by a decade of complete silence, during which nothing on Ts cells was published, in fact, most immunologists did not even dare to utter the 's' word. Granting agencies refused to fund Ts research, and most investigators left the field with a ruffled reputation.

'Yet the silence was not complete', adds Dr. G. 'I know of at least one attempt by Ron Schwartz to resuscitate Ts cells.[365] This was all the more surprising because NIH immunologists had not been involved in suppression research before. However, what he eventually found was anergy instead of suppression. When I asked him why he did this study, his answer was the following: "My grandfather who was a stockbroker used to say that nothing in the world is simpler than business. All you have to do is to buy cheap and sell expensive. And I thought I couldn't buy anything cheaper nowadays than suppression." Of course, this was just a joke, but its serious core was that at that time there was no acceptable scientific reason for conducting Ts studies.'

It was clear that repeating and expanding the phenomenology generated by the same or similar experimental systems could not restore the credibility of suppression in the immunological community. The principle had to be approached from a different angle in order to test its validity. As discussed before (Section 8.6.4), suppression was originally borne out by studies of tolerance. And the field where it resurfaced was autoimmunity, the reverse side of self tolerance. The key observation in this respect was that CD4 T-cell populations from which T cells with memory cell markers had been removed were able to induce a wide range of spontaneous autoimmune diseases, when transferred into syngeneic immunodeficient hosts. Addition of the subpopulation with memory markers back to the disease-inducing CD4 cells could prevent disease. The pioneering studies of this type were performed in mice by Shimon Sakaguchi and colleagues[366] in Japan, and subsequently in rats by Powrie and Mason[367] in Oxford. Similar observations were then made in a number of additional autoimmune disease models (reviewed, e.g. in [368–370]).

There were some discrepancies as to the cell surface markers that distinguish between the disease-inducing and disease-preventing CD4 cell subpopulations. In mice the initial studies[366] suggested that the inducer CD4 population was CD5(Ly1)[low], and the inhibitory population CD5[high], but later a better correlation was found with CD25, the α chain of interleukin-2 receptor (IL-2R):[371] the inducer CD4 cells were CD25[−] and the disease-preventing ones CD25[+]. In rats, the two subpopulations were distinguished on the basis of CD45RC (an isotype of the leukocyte common antigen) expression:[367] the disease-inducing CD4 subpopulation was CD45RC[high], and the disease-preventing one CD45RC[low]. Although none of these markers correlated perfectly with the pathogenicity vs. disease-preventing property, the overall conclusion was that the inducer cell corresponded to a naïve T-cell phenotype, while the disease-preventing cell resembled a primed but not activated T cell. A better distinction between the two cell subpopulations was enabled by the discovery that the inhibitory T cells selectively expressed the transcription factor FoxP3, which was also shown to be critical for their function.[372–375]

Perhaps it is worth noting that the results obtained in the diverse autoimmune models can be interpreted in more than one way, but the most straightforward and most favored interpretation has been that within the CD4 T-cell population there are two subsets, one is a self-reactive effector cell, and the other is a regulatory cell that suppresses that activity of the former. A formal but not unimportant element that contributed to the success of this interpretation was that the inhibitory cell was no longer called suppressor, it was rebranded as regulatory T cell or Treg. Although this term was not a happy choice, because regulatory cells should include both Th and Ts cells, it was readily accepted on the basis of its orthographic and acoustic dissimilarity to the 's' word. The demonstration by Ethan Shevach[376] that Treg cells can inhibit the IL-2 production of effector Th cells, in vitro, also helped reinstating suppression in 'respectable' circles of immunology.

From the mid-1990s, Tregs have become a favorite object of investigation, so that the body of information gathered about them by now probably exceeds the size of the old Ts literature. However, this does not necessarily imply that Treg cells are less mysterious than Ts cells used to be. What we know about Tregs, in a nutshell, is the following.

Concerning their origin, two types of Treg cells are distinguished: 'natural' Tregs that arise in the thymus, and 'adaptive' Tregs that differentiate from naïve cells upon antigen encounter at the periphery under certain conditions.[377,378] They both perform suppressive function, and are phenotypically indistinguishable (both are CD4$^+$CD25$^+$FoxP3$^+$). Attention has mostly been devoted to natural Tregs, because of their well established role in preventing experimental autoimmune diseases.[366–370]

Natural Tregs are subject to thymic selection as all other T cells, but their phenotype suggest that they may be, in addition, 'primed' in the thymus[379] with antigens that are by definition self. The way natural Tregs arise is envisaged as a kind of non-lethal negative selection, i.e., certain self reactive T cells, instead of undergoing apoptosis, turn into Tregs.[380] Consequently, the TCR repertoire of natural Tregs should be self reactive.[381] The mechanism that decides between clonal deletion or Treg formation is unknown, although there are some indications that Tregs behave as anergic T cells,[382] and thus their generation may be analogous to the induction of anergy. Despite their self reactivity, Tregs remain harmless to the host, because they do not produce pro-inflammatory cytokines upon antigenic stimulation.

The targets of Treg action are CD4 and CD8 T cells, and possibly also natural killer cells, B cells and dendritic cells. Suppression is manifested in inhibition of activation, proliferation, and effector functions of target cells, but the molecular basis for these actions has remained unclear.[383] The specific problem here is not the absence of information about the mode of action, rather the opposite: there are too many different mechanisms proposed, e.g., inhibition of IL-2 production[376] and/or consumption of IL-2, secretion of immunosuppressive cytokines,[384,385] interaction of the 'co-inhibitory' molecule CTLA-4 expressed on Tregs with its partner molecules CD80/CD86 on the target cell,[386] or downregulation of costimulation,[387] just to mention a few. Data on the involvement of these mechanisms in Treg action have remained somewhat contradictory. However, there seems to be an agreement on the point that the final suppressive mechanism is not antigen specific,[388] which then requires additional assumptions to explain how Tregs can selectively inhibit autoreactive effector cells.

In conclusion, the most robust part of the Treg phenomenology is the demonstration that these cells can prevent autoimmune diseases.[366–371] The strongest backing of this finding is that natural or experimentally induced mutations in the genes encoding some of the implicated molecules, i.e., FoxP3,[375,389,390] CD25,[391] IL-2,[392] and CTLA-4,[393] invariably result in lymphoproliferative and autoimmune-like disorders. In contrast, the identity of Treg as a separate cell lineage, as well as many details of Treg cell biology have still remained unclear. Thus, the existence of a Treg type immunoregulation is beyond any doubt, but the question of how it fits into the 'grand scheme' of the immune system may still be premature to ask.

'Premature or not, it is still worth an attempt!' argues Dr. G 'To my mind the most surprising conclusion from these studies is that the T-cell repertoire, despite negative selection, still appears to harbor a significant proportion of potentially self-destructive cells. A very minor fraction of such cells has been predicted, because this is the substrate on which the evolutionary force of self–non-self discrimination works, but the extent of self reactivity suggested by these studies is astonishing. Taken at face value, this observation almost enforces a paradigm change in self–non-self discrimination. It is widely believed that self–non-self discrimination is achieved by two types of mechanism, first, clonal deletion, and second, anergy and/or suppression, of which the first one is clearly superior, because it physically eliminates autoreactive cells, whereas anergy and suppression are reversible, and thus cannot provide a permanent solution. One would have expected therefore that evolution would favor the deletional mechanism, and would work on it until the fraction of autoreactive cells is diminished to an acceptable minimum. Certainly, evolution did make due efforts, and also had sufficient time to achieve this. But the existence of additional, more risky mechanisms, e.g., Treg and anergy, suggests that it might have been impossible to solve the problem with clonal deletion alone.'

'Why this was impossible is not quite clear, one can only suspect that it had to do with the limited nature of T-cell recognition. As discussed before (Section 8.4.4), the fact that T cells recognize short peptides, limits the theoretical antigenic diversity to the variants of 20 amino acids at ~5 peptide positions, i.e., to ~3.2 million different sequences. Thus T cells see a grossly reduced version of the antigenic universe, and the deletion of self reactive cells should be correspondingly parsimonious, in order to ensure that the defensive potential of the repertoire would not suffer.'

'One could, for example, envisage a model, in which the task for clonal deletion would be limited to the removal of reactivity against peptides of the APC's own proteins, and of proteins in body fluids. It is critical that such peptides must not generate Tregs, because the latter would interfere with the induction of protective responses by the APC. Therefore clonal deletion vs Treg/anergy should be mutually exclusive mechanisms with respect to every single self peptide. The separation of these two types of mechanism may be manageable by the sophisticated signaling mechanism of TCR (see Section 8.3.4), on the basis of affinity and peptide abundance. Natural Tregs arising in the thymus would thus recognize non-APC-derived rare self peptides, including organ-specific ones. At the periphery, such natural Tregs would only be activated, if they localized in, or close to the organ that provides an abundant source of antigen, for example, in a regional lymph node draining the particular organ. Effector T cells recognizing antigens at the same location would then be suppressed. The organ localization would endow suppression with a certain degree of specificity, although the interaction between Tregs and effector T cells is not antigen-specific itself. The lack of a specific interaction between these two cell types may be, to some extent, advantageous, because this way Tregs of a single specificity could inhibit a whole array of effector T cells recognizing different antigens of that particular organ, including antigens not presented in the thymus. But the price to be paid for this advantage is high: responses to pathogens at the same locations would also be suppressed.'

'This little sketch of a model is based on the current interpretation of the Treg phenomenology, and thus, it would presumably meet the agreement of most tregologists. However, for fairness' sake, I must admit that upon closer scrutiny the model reveals a number of weaknesses.'

'First, evolutionary tinkering necessitated by the limits of the pentapeptide universe is given as a cause for the existence of Tregs. While this might have been the case, it fails to convince as a clear-cut evolutionary driving force.'

'Second, the TCR repertoire of Tregs, to be able to make self–non-self discrimination, must be per force anti-self. As we know the receptor repertoires of T and B cells are randomly generated and purged of anti-self, so that the remainder becomes anti-non-self. The Treg repertoire, in contrast, is assumed to be anti-self and not purged of anti-non-self (the latter would be impossible). Consequently, Tregs would not be able to make self–non-self discrimination, i.e., pathogen-derived peptides that crossreact with self would induce suppression of protective responses with potentially fatal consequences.'

'Third, there is no evolutionary driving force for maintaining the diverse TCR repertoire of Tregs. This follows from the statement that the interaction between Tregs and effector Th cells is not antigen-specific. Thus the role of Treg-TCR is reduced to navigating the Treg cell to a particular organ that provides the autoantigen. This function does not require TCRs; it could be performed by a few organ-specific homing receptors.'

'Fourth, although not stated explicitly, the model does not distinguish between Tregs and anergic Th cells,[382,394] which is equivalent to claiming that Treg as a separate cell lineage does not exist. There would thus be one single regulatory cell type, the Th cell, that regulates in both directions: up and down. Although this possibility has not been ruled out, a model of Treg cells that denies their very existence is not a happy choice.'

'So I am afraid I'd better stop at this point, and admit that I could not formulate a convincing model based on the present interpretation of Treg data.'

Finally it is worth mentioning that a recent analysis by Mel Cohn[395] places the Treg phenomenology into a completely different light. His salient point of argument is that histological evidence of immunopathology does not necessarily imply a disease of autoimmune origin. The conclusion that the pathology observed in Treg-deficient mice[371] is autoimmune, i.e., due to breaking of self-tolerance, is justified only if the disease is demonstrated to be induced by a self antigen. In the absence of such evidence, one may as well assume that the observed immunopathology is 'collateral damage' due to an uncontrolled overshoot of effector Th cell responses to *foreign antigens*, since the effector mechanisms may be identical whether the antigen is self or foreign. He proposes therefore that the role of Tregs is to provide feedback inhibition of effector

Th-cell responses to foreign antigens. Such a mechanism would be biologically relevant: its evolutionary driver would be the requirement to confine the effector response to the pathogen, and to avoid or at least minimize innocent bystander damage. The model he has put forward is consistent with the experimental data, and it avoids the pitfalls associated with a proposed role of Tregs in self–non-self discrimination. However, it has a problem too: the proposed function of Treg is not sufficiently distinct from the function of the 'co-inhibitory' molecule CTLA-4 expressed on Th cells (see Section 8.7.2). And there seems to be not much need for Treg, if Th cells can themselves control their own expansion.

'A possible way out of the conceptual deadlock is offered by proposing that Treg cells are indeed anergic Th cells', adds Dr. G. 'This idea is not as far-fetched as it appears at first sight, because anergic Th cells (see Section 9.3.3) are metabolically inactive, mostly self-specific, and are likely to localize at the source of antigen, where they could compete with autoreactive Th cells for antigen or cytokines[396] or both. At present there is no experimental support for this idea, but it would be of interest to learn, for example, whether anergic Th cells express FoxP3 or not.'

8.7 CELL ADHESION, COSTIMULATION, CO-INHIBITION

In sharp contrast to other sub-disciplines of immunology, the research that led to the discovery of cell adhesion and costimulatory molecules had not been driven by either a well-defined conceptual need or a long-standing puzzle. Indeed, most of these molecules were identified by the pragmatic use of subtractive gene libraries or monoclonal antibodies, i.e., the discoveries resulted directly from technological progress. However, subsequent characterization has revealed that these molecules have fundamentally important functions in lymphocyte physiology, which facilitated their rapid integration into the immune system.

8.7.1 Cell Adhesion Receptors of the Immune System

Cell-to-cell and cell-to-matrix interactions have long been recognized by cell biologists as major mechanisms in the development of tissues and organs. But immunology, focussing on antigen-specific cell interactions, has not dealt with the idea of tissue-specific cell adhesion until the discovery of cell surface molecules that mediate antigen-independent adherence between cells of the immune system.

Immunology and cell adhesion have first intersected in studies of conjugate formation between cytotoxic T lymphocytes (Tc) and their target cells. The key finding has been that conjugates can form even with target cells that do not carry the antigen to which the Tc are specific,[397,398] suggesting that an antigen-independent process of cell adhesion should take place simultaneously with or prior to antigen recognition. These experiments, championed by Tim Springer and his colleagues at Harvard Medical School, have identified cell adhesion molecules that have been termed lymphocyte function-associated antigens (LFA),[399] because monoclonal antibodies directed against them inhibited the killing of target cells by Tc cells. LFA-1, a member of the integrin family,[400,401] was found to be expressed on T cells (and leukocytes in general). Its counter-receptor on the target cell was shown to be ICAM-1 or ICAM-2 (for intercellular adhesion molecule), both members of the immunoglobulin family.[402,403] A second pair of adhesion receptors consisting of two further members of the immunoglobulin family, LFA-2 (or CD2) on T cells and LFA-3 on the target cells, was also identified.[404] In addition to the Tc–target-cell interaction, the same adhesion receptor pairs were shown to be involved also in T–B-cell and T-cell–antigen-presenting-cell (APC) interactions.[405]

Because the necessity for adhesion receptors in lymphocyte interactions has been self-evident, these findings belong to those few in immunology that have never incited any conceptual debate. However, much less self-evident has been to find out how these receptors 'know' when and where to adhere. Obviously, lymphocytes circulating in the blood should be non-adherent, but the very same cells when migrating through tissues and lymphoid organs are supposed to express the proper adhesion receptors that permit crossing the endothelium and basement membranes, aggregating at sites of infection, or binding to cells bearing foreign antigen. A rapid transition between adherent and non-adherent states is therefore of key importance for lymphocyte function.

The principle nature chose for the regulation of lymphocyte adhesion was to subordinate adherence to cell activation. This principle was translated into a number of mechanisms, of which the regulation of LFA-1 function is a particularly elegant one. As shown by Dustin and Springer,[406] the crosslinking of TCR converts LFA-1 from a low to a high avidity state at unchanged expression level. This change occurs within a few minutes, the avidity then returns to low, resting values after 30 minutes, providing a mechanism for rapid adhesion and detachment. Thus the high-avidity, functional state of LFA-1 is an immediate consequence of antigen recognition by TCR on the target cell or APC. In contrast, ICAM-1, the counter-receptor of LFA-1 is regulated through expression: in the resting state it is only expressed on a few cell types (e.g., dendritic cells[407]), but it is strongly induced by inflammatory mediators in a wide variety of tissues.[399] Yet another mechanism is used for the regulation of cell adhesion through the CD2-LFA-3 receptor pair. Adhesion via these receptors also increases upon T-cell activation, but this is achieved by the regulation of negative charge of the T-cell surface, which is mostly due to sialic acid.[408] Circulating T cells are highly sialylated, and thus their contact is opposed by charge repulsion.[409] Activated T cells have much less sialic acid than resting T cells,[410] and the decreased negative charge permits the cells to engage in CD2–LFA-3 interactions.

Another set of adhesion molecules, collectively called 'homing' receptors, facilitates the recirculation of lymphocytes from blood to lymph. In contrast to the adhesion receptors discussed above, homing receptors are not directly controlled by antigen recognition. Their best known representative is Mel-14/ LAM-1, a member of the selectin family, which mediates the adherence of naïve lymphocytes to specialized high endothelial cells lining the venules of lymph nodes.[411,412] Alternatively to naïve cells, memory T cells emigrate from the blood through tissue endothelium in order to patrol different organs for the presence of antigen and enter the lymph node through afferent lymph.[412] Accordingly, memory cells express different homing receptors (e.g., VLA-4 and CD44).[413]

The multitude of receptors and mechanisms involved in lymphocyte adhesion illustrates well the evolutionary/physiological importance of this process for the immune system.

8.7.2 Costimulation, Co-Inhibition

The simple biological definition of costimulation is the enhancement of a suboptimal proliferative response of T cells. The primary stimulus must be provided through the TCR by peptide-MHC or anti-CD3 antibody. Costimulation should only occur in conjunction with the primary stimulus, not alone. The molecular nature of costimulation, however, has been difficult to define on the basis of bioassays, because many different stimuli can enhance a suboptimal response, including nutrients, hormones, cytokines, cell adhesion molecules, etc., and yet these do not qualify as costimulatory molecules.

Costimulatory molecules are defined more strictly, as a unique set of molecules required for optimal production interleukin-2 (IL-2), the major growth factor for activated T cells. Signalling of T cells via TCR is known to activate transcription of the IL-2 gene, yet very little IL-2 is produced when this signal is given alone. For full-blown IL-2 production an additional signal is required that is provided through CD28, a transmembrane glycoprotein of the immunoglobulin superfamily, expressed constitutively on the surface of most T cells.[414] Crosslinking of CD28 with antibody results in a ~30 fold augmentation of IL-2 production by T helper (Th) cells triggered through their TCR.[414,415] The enhancement of IL-2 production is largely the consequence of IL-2 mRNA stabilization by the CD28 signal.[415]

The natural ligands of CD28 are B7-1 (CD80)[416,417] and B7-2 (CD86),[418–420] two further members of the immunoglobulin superfamily. Interaction of either molecule with CD28 induces costimulation of IL-2 production in T cells.[416,418] B7-1, the ligand discovered first, is expressed poorly on 'professional' antigen presenting cells (APC, i.e., dendritic cells and macrophages), and its expression increases several days after interaction with T cells. In contrast, B7-2 is expressed constitutively on professional APC, and its level of expression increases rapidly after presenting antigen to T cells.[418] Therefore, B7-2 appears to be the primary costimulatory ligand for the initiation of a T-cell response, whereas B7-1 is probably important for sustaining T-cell expansion at later stages of the response.

A rather interesting participant of the costimulation process is CTLA-4 (CD152), yet another member of the immunoglobulin superfamily. It was discovered by screening of cytotoxic-T-cell-derived cDNA libraries,[421] but it is expressed on the surface of both CD4 and CD8 T cells. It has a high degree of homology (~75%) with CD28, and the genes encoding these two molecules are closely linked, suggesting that they arose by gene duplication.[422] CTLA-4 binds to B7 molecules[423] with a 20–50-fold higher affinity than CD28. Unlike CD28, which is constitutively expressed on the surface of T cells, CTLA-4 is induced upon activation, reaching maximal levels 1–2 days later.[424] Thus, naïve T cells express two receptors for B7, CD28 with high abundance and low affinity, and CTLA-4 with low abundance and high affinity. Not surprisingly, the relative roles of these two receptors in costimulation had remained enigmatic for some time, until it was demonstrated that CTLA-4 is indeed an inhibitor of IL-2 synthesis,[425,426] i.e., a functional antagonist of CD28. Studies with CTLA-4-deficient mice have revealed an important physiological role of this molecule in preventing excessive T-cell proliferation.[427,428] CTLA-4 is thus a counter-costimulatory or co-inhibitory molecule.

Another pair of molecules implicated in costimulation consists of CD40 expressed on B cells and APC, and CD40 ligand (CD40L or CD154)) expressed on T cells. CD40L appears to perform multiple functions. In the first place, it induces B7 expression on B cells and APC and thus costimulation via CD28-B7 interaction.[429,430] In addition, other, CD28-independent costimulatory pathways (involving e.g., CD44H or ICAM-1)[431] may also be induced by CD40L. Thus this molecule acts as a general promoter for costimulation, but is not per se a costimulation receptor. Furthermore, CD40L seems to be responsible for delivering 'help' of Th cells to B cells[432] and to cytotoxic T cells.[433,434]

More recently a number of additional molecules have been identified as potential costimulatory receptors and ligands, but their biological roles have not been clarified to an extent comparable to that of the CD28–CTLA-4–B7 system.

In summary, the first phase of immune responses, antigen-induced T-cell proliferation, appears to be controlled by one major costimulatory pathway triggered by the CD28–B7 interaction and negatively regulated by CTLA-4. There may exist a couple of additional, minor or auxiliary costimulatory pathways, but some molecules involved in the latter, e.g., ICAM-1, cross the border between cell adhesion and costimulation, and thus it is difficult to assign a clear costimulatory role to these pathways.

This brief account was meant to give an overview of the facts known about costimulation. However, the biological questions, which have arisen in connection with these facts and without which the topic of costimulation would remain incomplete, are yet to be dealt with.

The first and most obvious question concerns the biological necessity of costimulation.

'The question may be obvious, but this does not warrant a simple answer', replies Dr. G. 'It may be useful to reemphasize in this context that T-cell activation and

IL-2 production can occur also in the absence of CD28 signaling, for example, in CD28-deficient mice,[435] under CD28 blockade,[436] or when high numbers of TCR are ligated.[437] Thus neither CD28 nor any other costimulatory receptor is an exclusive IL-2 switch. Costimulation serves solely to amplify antigen-induced IL-2 production, as also indicated by the "co" syllable in this unusually apt term.'

'The answer as to why "co"-s are needed should probably be sought for in the nature of antigen presentation. As discussed before (Section 7.5), the presentation of foreign peptides is a rather inefficient process, damped by competition of abundant self peptides and also by mutations of pathogens aimed at escaping presentation. As a result foreign antigenic peptides are usually represented in small copy numbers on the surface of APC. For the same reason the number and abundance of presented foreign peptides are not necessarily related to the severity of infection. Thus it would be dangerous for the host, if the magnitude of response were placed under the direct control of antigen. Probably this is why costimulation, a kind of signal amplification mechanism, has evolved that enables the immune system to give due attention to every foreign peptide. In the case of poor peptide presentation more costimulation is provided, and at high-density presentation less costimulation occurs. As a result, the initial proliferative phase that is crucial for the success of T-cell responses is amplified and equalized.'

An often heard concern about costimulation is that it may compromise self–non-self discrimination. Could that really be the case?

'This is unlikely in my opinion. But in principle, costimulation could endanger self–non-self discrimination in two ways, namely by allowing T-cell activation through self ligands of low affinity and high abundance, or higher affinity and very low abundance. As pointed out earlier (Section 8.4.3), elimination of self-reactive T cells (negative selection) occurs in the thymus, when the affinity of TCR for its ligand exceeds a precisely defined limit. Thus the option of becoming activated by either a high-affinity low-abundance ligand or a low-affinity high-abundance ligand does not exist for mature T cells. Since affinity is a major instrument of self–non-self discrimination, costimulation could not fumble with it unpunished. The second possibility, i.e., activation by low-abundance self ligands, is a more viable one, but this is what CTLA-4 is likely to control. Indeed, the concern of costimulation-induced autoreactivity is based on the phenotype of CTLA-4-deficient mice that is characterized by a severe lymphoproliferative disorder with early lethality.[427] Although it has remained unclear whether this disorder displays autoimmune characteristics or not, the data have demonstrated that costimulation without CTLA-4 would be life-threatening, and this fact must have provided the selective pressure in the evolution of CTLA-4.'

The final question is why costimulation is interpreted almost unanimously as evidence for the two-signal model of lymphocyte activation.

'The two-signal theory[52] (discussed in detail in Section 9.2.4) was proposed by Peter Bretscher and Mel Cohn in 1970, and it has remained largely unchallenged ever since. Its basic postulate is that Signal 1, the recognition of a single epitope of any antigen, is tolerogenic; to turn antigen recognition into activation, an additional Signal 2 is required that is provided by a helper T cell recognizing another epitope of the same antigen. The theory implies that each antigen recognition event is subject to self–non-self discrimination: a Th cell (Signal 2) must confirm the antigen to be non-self, and if this does not happen, the antigen is considered by default as self.'

'What brought the two-signal concept in connection with costimulation was a series of studies on T-cell anergy championed by Ron Schwartz[438] and colleagues in the NIH. Anergy, a state of unresponsiveness characterized by the lack of IL-2 production was shown to be inducible in Th1 clones in many different ways, the common denominator of which seemed to be the stimulation through TCR in the absence of costimulation. This situation bore some resemblance to the Bretscher-Cohn model, in that the antigen signal (Signal 1) appeared tolerogenic, and a second signal provided by costimulation was required for activation. However, this resemblance is delusive for several reasons. First, anergy cannot be considered equivalent with tolerance. Second, in contrast to Th1 clones, normal unprimed T cells may not become anergic when stimulated with antigen in the absence of costimulation.[437] Third, and most importantly, it is difficult to envisage how antigen-non-specific costimulation could replace Signal 2, since it is unable to make self–non-self discrimination.[439] And the two-signal mode of activation would lose most of its biological sense, were it not for self–non-self discrimination.'

'Nevertheless, immunologists love to draw a parallel between costimulation and the two-signal model, only Peter Bretscher and Mel Cohn protest against this – in vain.'

REFERENCES

1. Kindred B, Shreffler DC. *J. Immunol.* 1972;**109**:940.
2. Katz DH, Hamaoka T, Benacerraf B. *J. Exp. Med.* 1973;**137**:1405.
3. Katz DH, Hamaoka T, Dorf MD, Benacerraf B. *Proc. Natl. Acad. Sci. USA* 1973;**70**:2624.
4. Katz DH, Graves M, Dorf ME, Dimuzio H, Benacerraf B. *J. Exp. Med.* 1975;**141**:263.
5. Zinkernagel RM, Doherty PC. *Nature* 1974;**248**:701.
6. Zinkernagel RM, Doherty PC. *Nature* 1974;**251**:547.
7. Zinkernagel RM, Doherty PC. *J. Exp. Med.* 1975;**141**:1427.
8. von Boehmer H, Hudson L, Sprent J. *J. Exp. Med.* 1975;**142**:989.
9. von Boehmer H, Haas W. *Nature* 1976;**261**:141.
10. Pfizenmaier K, Starzinski-Powitz A, Rodt H, Röllinghof M, Wagner H. *J. Exp. Med.* 1976;**143**:999.
11. Zinkernagel RM. *Nature* 1976;**261**:139.
12. Gardner ID, Bowern NA, Blanden RV. *Eur. J. Immunol.* 1974;**4**:63.
13. Wainberg MA, Markson Y, Weiss DW, Donjanski F. *Proc. Natl. Acad. Sci. USA* 1974;**71**:3565.
14. Shearer GM. *Eur. J. Immunol.* 1974;**4**:527.
15. Shearer GM, Lozner EC, Rehn TG, A-M Schmitt-Verhulst. *J. Exp. Med.* 1975;**141**:930.
16. Forman J. *J. Exp. Med.* 1975;**142**:403.
17. Bevan MJ. *Nature* 1975;**256**:419.
18. Bevan MJ. *J. Exp. Med.* 1975;**142**:1349.
19. Gordon RD, Simpson E, Samelson LE. *J. Exp. Med.* 1975;**142**:1108.
20. Marshak A, Doherty PC, Wilson DB. *J. Exp. Med.* 1977;**146**:1773.
21. McMichael AJ, Ting A, Zweerink HJ, Askonas BA. *Nature* 1977;**270**:524.

22. Bevan MJ, Cohn M. *J. Immunol.* 1975;**114**:559.

23. Blanden RV, Doherty PC, Dunlop MB, Gardner ID, Zinkernagel RM, David CS. *Nature* 1975;**254**:269.

24. Erb P, Feldmann M. *J. Exp. Med.* 1975;**142**:460.

25. Swierkosz JE, Rock K, Marrack P, Kappler JW. *J. Exp. Med.* 1978;**147**:554.

26. Yamashita U, Shevach EM. *J. Exp. Med.* 1978;**148**:1171.

27. McDougal JS, Cort SP. *J. Immunol.* 1978;**120**:445.

28. Sprent J. *J. Exp. Med.* 1978;**147**:1142.

29. Sprent J. *J. Exp. Med.* 1978;**147**:1159.

30. Sprent J. *J. Exp. Med.* 1978;**148**:478.

31. Erb P, Meier B, Matsunaga T, Feldmann M. *J. Exp. Med.* 1979;**149**:686.

32. Singer A, Hathcock KS, Hodes RJ. *J. Exp. Med.* 1979;**149**:1208.

33. Shih WW, Matzinger PC, Swain SL, Dutton RW. *J. Exp. Med.* 1980;**152**:1311.

34. Rajewsky K, Schirrmacher V, Nase S, Jerne NK. *J. Exp. Med.* 1969;**129**:1131.

35. Mitchison NA. *Eur. J. Immunol.* 1971;**1**:18.

36. Rosenthal AS, Shevach EM. *J. Exp. Med.* 1973;**138**:1194.

37. Yano A, Schwartz RH, Paul WE. *J. Exp. Med.* 1977;**146**:828.

38. Lanzavecchia A. *Nature* 1985;**314**:537.

39. Cunningham AJ, Lafferty KJ. *Scand. J. Immunol.* 1977;**6**:1.

40. Matzinger P, Bevan MJ. *Cell. Immunol.* 1977;**29**:1.

41. Matzinger P. *Nature* 1981;**292**:497.

42. Zinkernagel RM, Doherty PC. *Cold Spring Harbor Symp. Quant. Biol.* 1976;**41**:505.

43. Doherty PC, Götze D, Trinchieri G, Zinkernagel RM. *Immunogenet* 1976;**3**:517.

44. Janeway Jr CA, Wigzell H, Binz H. *Scand. J. Immunol.* 1976;**5**:993.

45. Blanden RV, Ada GL. *Scand. J. Immunol.* 1978;**7**:181.

46. Langman RE. *Rev. Physiol. Biochem. Pharmacol.* 1978;**81**:1.

47. Cohn M, Epstein R. *Cell. Immunol.* 1978;**39**:125.

48. Cohn M, Langman R. *Behring Inst. Mitt.* 1982;**70**:219.

49. Cohn M. *Cell* 1983;**33**:657.

50. Langman RE, Cohn M. *Cell. Immunol.* 1985;**94**:598.

51. Matzinger P, Mirkwood G. *J. Exp. Med.* 1978;**148**:84.

52. Bretscher P, Cohn M. *Science* 1970;**169**:1042.

53. Langman RE, Cohn M. *Mol. Immunol.* 1987;**24**:675.

54. Langman RE, Cohn M. *Scand. J. Immunol.* 1999;**49**:570.

55. Langman RE, Cohn M. *Immunol. Rev.* 2000;**159**:214.

56. Cohn M, Langman RE, Mata JJ. *Int. Immunol.* 2002;**14**:1105.

57. Crone M, Koch C, Simonsen M. *Transplant. Rev.* 10:36(19872).

58. Williams AF. *Nature* 1984;**308**:108.

59. Burnet FM. *The Clonal Selection Theory of Acquired Immunity.* London: Cambridge Univ. Press; 1959.

60. Raff MC, Feldmann M, de Petris S. *J. Exp. Med.* 1973;**137**:1024.

61. Marchalonis JJ, Cone RE, Atwell JL. *J. Exp. Med.* 1972;**135**:956.

62. Vitetta ES, Bianco C, Nussenzweig V, Uhr JW. *J. Exp. Med.* 1972;**136**:81.

63. Hudson L, Thantrey N, Roitt IM. *Immunol.* 1975;**28**:151.

64. Sprent J, Hudson L. *Transplant. Proc.* 1973;**5**:1731.

65. Pernis B, Miller JFAP, Forni L, Sprent J. *Cell. Immunol.* 1974;**10**:476.

66. Goldschneider I, Cogen RB. *J. Exp. Med.* 1973;**138**:163.

67. Perkins WD, Robson LC, Schwarz MR. *Science* 1975;**188**:365.

68. Hudson L, Sprent J, Miller JFAP, Playfair JHL. *Nature* 1974;**251**:60.

69. Hudson L, Sprent J. *J. Exp. Med.* 1975;**143**:444.

70. Krammer PH, Hudson L, Sprent J. *J. Exp. Med.* 1975;**142**:1403.

71. Julius MH, Simpson E, Herzenberg LA. *Eur. J. Immunol.* 1973;**3**:645.

72. Nagy Z, Elliott BE, Nabholz M, Krammer PH, Pernis B. *J. Exp. Med.* 1976;**143**:648.

73. Nagy Z, Elliott BE, Nabholz M. *J. Exp. Med.* 1976;**144**:1545.

74. Oudin J, Michel M, . Hebd CR. *Seances Acad. Sci.* 1963;**257**:805.

75. Gell PGH, Kelus A. *Nature (London)* 1964;**201**:687.

76. Ramseier H. *Cell. Immunol.* 1973;**8**:177.

77. Binz H, Wigzell H. *J. Exp. Med.* 1975;**142**:197.

78. Krammer PH, Eichmann K. *Nature* 1977;**270**:733.

79. Kees UR. *J. Exp. Med.* 1981;**153**:1562.

80. Eichmann K, Rajewsky K. *Eur. J. Immunol.* 1975;**5**:661.

81. Rubin B, Hertel-Wulff B, Kimura A. *J. Exp. Med.* 1979;**150**:307.

82. Fathman CG, Hengartner H. *Proc. Natl. Acad. Sci. USA* 1979;**76**:5863.

83. von Boehmer H, Hengartner H, Nabholz M, Lernhardt W, Schreier MH, Haas W. *Eur. J. Immunol.* 1979;**9**:592.

84. Glasebrook AL, Fitch FW. *J. Exp. Med.* 1980;**151**:876.

85. Sredni B, Tse HY, Schwartz RH. *Nature* 1980;**283**:581.

86. Kappler JW, Skidmore B, White J, Marrack P. *J. Exp. Med.* 1981;**153**:1198.

87. Meuer SC, Fitzgerald KA, Hussey RE, Hongdon JC, Schlossman SF, Reinherz EL. *J. Exp. Med.* 1983;**157**:705.

88. Reinherz EL, Meuer S, Fitzgerald KA, Hussey RE, Levine H, Schlossman SF. *Cell* 1982;**30**:735.

89. Haskins K, Kubo R, White J, Pigeon M, Kappler J, Marrack P. *J. Exp. Med.* 1983;**157**:1149.

90. Lancki DW, Lorber MI, Loken MR, Fitch FW. *J. Exp. Med.* 1983;**157**:921.

91. JKaye S, Porcelli J, Tite B, Jones Janeway Jr CA. *J. Exp. Med.* 1983;**158**:836.

92. Meuer SC, Acuto O, Hussey RE, Hodgdon JC, Fitzgerald KA, Schlossman SF, et al. *Nature* 1983;**303**:808.

93. Samelson LE, Germain RN, Schwartz RH. *Proc. Natl. Acad. Sci. USA* 1983;**80**:6972.

94. Staerz UD, Pasternack MS, Klein JR, Benedetto JD, Bevan MJ. *Proc. Natl. Acad. Sci. USA* 1984;**81**:1799.

95. Infante AJ, Infante PD, Gillis S, Fathman CG. *J. Exp. Med.* 1982;**155**:1100.

96. Haskins K, Hannum C, White J, Roehm N, Kubo R, Kappler J, et al. *J. Exp. Med.* 1984;**160**:452.

97. Kubo RT, Born W, Kappler JW, Marrack P, Pigeon M. *J. Immunol.* 1989;**142**:2736.

98. Allison JP, MacIntyre BW, Block D. *J. Immun.* 1982;**129**:2293.

99. Behlke MA, Chou HS, Huppi K, Loh DY. *Proc. Natl. Acad. Sci. USA* 1986;**83**:767.

100. Staerz UD, Rammensee HG, Benedetto JD, Bevan MJ. *J. Immunol.* 1985;**134**:3994.

101. Hedrick SM, Cohen DI, Nielsen EA, Davis MM. *Nature* 1984;**308**:149.

102. Hedrick SM, Nielsen EA, Kavaler J, Cohen DI, Davis MM. *Nature* 1984;**308**:153.

103. Yanagi Y, Yoshikai Y, Leggett K, Clark SP, Aleksander I, Mak TW. *Nature* 1984;**308**:145.

104. Chien Y, Becker DM, Lindsten T, Okamura M, Cohen DI, Davis MM. *Nature* 1984;**312**:31.

105. Saito H, Kranz DM, Takagaki Y, Hayday AC, Eisen HN, Tonegawa S. *Nature* 1984;**312**:36.

106. Sim GK, Yagüe J, Nelson J, Marrack P, Palmer E, Augustin A, Kappler J. *Nature* 1984;**312**:771.

107. Kranz DM, Saito H, Heller M, Takagaki Y, Haas W, Eisen HN, Tonegawa S. *Nature* 1985;**313**:752.

108. Lefranc MP, Rabbitts TH. *Nature* 1985;**316**:464.

109. Murre C, Waldmann RA, Morton CC, Bongiovanni KF, Waldmann TA, Shows TB, et al. *Nature* 1985;**316**:549.

110. Brenner MB, McLean J, Dialynas DP, Strominger JL, Smith JA, Owen FL, et al. *Nature* 1986;**322**:145.

111. Goettrup M, Ungewiss K, Azogui O, Palacios R, Owen MJ, Hayday AC, et al. *Cell* 1993;**75**:283.

112. von Boehmer H, Fehling HJ. *Ann. Rev. Immunol.* 1997;**15**:433.

113. Kudo A, Melchers F. *EMBO J* 1987;**6**:2267.

114. Gascoigne NRJ, Chien Y, Becker DM, Kavaler J, Davis MM. *Nature* 1984;**310**:387.

115. Lai F, Barth RK, Hood L. *Proc. Natl. Acad. Sci. USA* 1987;**84**:3846.

116. Winoto A, Mjolsness S, Hood L. *Nature* 1985;**316**:832.

117. Davis MM, Bjorkman PJ. *Nature* 1988;**334**:395.

118. Wilson RK, Lai E, Concannon P, Barth RK, Hood LE. *Immunol. Rev.* 1988;**101**:149.

119. Leiden JM, Strominger JL. *Proc. Natl. Acad. Sci. USA* 1986;**83**:4456.

120. Kimura N, Toyonaga B, Yoshikai Y, Triebel F, Debre P, Minden MD, et al. *J. Exp. Med.* 1986;**164**:739.

121. Rowen L, Koop BF, Hood L. *Science* 1996;**272**:1755.

122. LeFranc MP, Forster A, Baer R, Stinson MA, Rabbitts TH. *Cell* 1986;**45**:237.

123. Griesser H, Champagne E, Tkachuk D, Takihara Y, Lalande M, Baillie E, et al. *Eur. J. Immunol.* 1988;**18**:641.

124. Vidovic D, Roglic M, McKune K, Guerder S, MacKay C, Dembic Z. *Nature* 1989;**340**:646.

125. Tanaka Y, Morita CT, Tanaka Y, Nieves E, Brenner MB, Bloom BR. *Nature* 1995;**375**:155.

126. Bukowski JF, Morita CT, Brenner MB. *Immunity* 1999;**11**:57.

127. Russano AM, Bassotti G, Agea E, Mazzocchi A, Morelli A, Porcelli SA, et al. *J. Immunol.* 2007;**178**:3620.

128. Garman RD, Ko JL, Vulpe CD, Raulet DH. *Proc. Natl. Acad. Sci. USA* 1986;**83**:3987.

129. Kappler JW, Wade T, White J, Kushnir E, Blackman M, Bill J, et al. *Cell* 1987;**49**:263.

130. Jorgensen JL, Esser U, Fazekas de St. Groth B, Reay PA, Davis MM. *Nature* 1992;**355**:224.

131. Fields BA, Ober B, Malchiodi EL, Lebedeva MI, Branden BC, Ysern X, et al. *Science* 1995;**270**:1821.

132. Bentley GA, Boulot G, Karjalainen K, Mariuzza RA. *Science* 1995;**267**:1984.

133. Garcia KC, Degano M, Stanfield RL, Brunmark A, Jackson MR, Peterson PA, et al. *Science* 1996;**274**:209.

134. Garboczi DN, Ghosh P, Utz U, Fan QR, Biddison WE, Wiley DC. *Nature* 1996;**384**:134.

135. Garcia KC, Degano M, Pease LR, Huang M, Peterson PA, Teyton L, et al. *Science* 1998;**279**:1166.

136. Teng MK, Smolyar A, Tse AG, Liu JH, Hussey RE, Nathenson SG, et al. *Curr. Biol.* 1998;**8**:409.

137. Ding YH, Smith KJ, Garboczi DN, Utz U, Biddison WE, Wiley DC. *Immunity* 1998;**8**:403.

138. Reinherz EL, Tan K, Tang L, Kern P, Liu JH, Xiong Y, et al. *Science* 1999;**286**:1913.

139. Hennecke J, Carfi A, Wiley DC. *EMBO J* 2000;**19**:5611.

140. Bill J, Appel VB, Palmer E. *Proc. Natl. Acad. Sci. USA* 1988;**85**:9184.

141. Gulwani-Akolkar B, Posnett DN, Janson CH, Grunewald J, Wigzell H, Akolkar P, et al. *J. Exp. Med.* 1991;**174**:1139.

142. Morel PA, Livingstone AM, Fathman CG. *J. Exp. Med.* 1987;**166**:583.

143. Sim BC, Zerva L, Greene MI, NRJ Gascoigne. *Science* 1996;**273**:963.

144. Matsui K, Boniface JJ, Reay PA, Schild H, Fazekas de St. Groth B, Davis MM. *Science* 1991;**254**:1788.

145. Garcia KC, Tallquist MD, Pease LR, Brunmark A, Scott CA, Degano M, et al. *Proc. Natl. Acad. Sci. USA* 1997;**94**:13838.

146. Nagy ZA. *Scand J. Immunol.* 2008;**67**:313.

147. Gleimer N, Parham P. *Immunity* 2003;**19**:469.

148. Siu G, Kronenberg M, Strauss E, Haars R, Mak TW, Hood L. *Nature* 1984;**311**:344.

149. Huseby ES, White J, Crawford F, Vass T, Becker D, Pinilla C, et al. *Cell* 2005;**122**:247.

150. Dai S, Huseby ES, Rubtsova K, Scott-Browne J, Crawford F, Macdonald WA, et al. *Immunity* 2008;**28**:324.

151. Harding CV, Unanue ER. *Nature* 1990;**346**:574.

152. Demotz S, Grey HM, Sette A. *Science* 1990;**249**:1028.

153. Butz EA, Bevan MJ. *Immunity* 1998;**8**:167.

154. Alam SM, Travers PJ, Wung JL, Nasholds W, Redpath S, Jameson SC, et al. *Nature* 1996;**381**:616.

155. Viret C, Wong FS, Janeway CS. *Immunity* 1999;**10**:559.

156. Ernst B, Lee D, Chang JM, Sprent J, Surh CD. *Immunity* 1999;**11**:173.

157. Sloan-Lancaster J, Allen PM. *Ann. Rev. Immunol.* 1996;**14**:1.

158. Sloan-Lancaster J, Shaw AS, Rothbard JB, Allen PM. *Cell* 1994;**79**:913.

159. Madrenas J, Wange RL, Wang JL, Isakov N, Samelson LE, Germain RN. *Science* 1995;**267**:515.

160. Neumeister-Kersh E, Shaw AS, Allen PM. *Science* 1998;**281**:572.

161. Beddoe T, Chen Z, Clements CS, Ely LK, Bushell SR, Vivian JP, et al. *Immunity* 2009;**30**:777.

162. Miller JFAP. *Lancet* 1961;**II**:748.

163. Shortman K, Wu L. *Ann. Rev. Immunol.* 1996;**14**:29.

164. Mombaerts P, Clarke AR, Rudnicki MA, Iacomini J, Itohara S, Lafaille JJ, et al. *Nature* 1992;**360**:225.

165. Havran WL, Allison JP. *Nature* 1988;**335**:443.

166. Irving BA, Alt FW, Killeen N. *Science* 1998;**280**:905.

167. Jerne NK. *Eur. J. Immunol.* 1971;**1**:1.

168. Simonsen M. *Cold Spring Harbor Symp. Quant. Biol.* 1967;**32**:517.

169. Wilson DB, Nowell PC. *J. Exp. Med.* 1970;**131**:391.

170. Cohn M. *Immunol.Res.* 2011;**50**:49.

171. Vidovic D, Boulanger N, Kuye O, Toral J, Ito K, Guenot J, et al. *Immunogenet* 1997;**45**:325.

172. Zerrahn J, Held W, Raulet DH. *Cell* 1997;**88**:627.

173. von Boehmer H, Sprent J, Nabholz M. *J. Exp. Med.* 1975;**141**:322.

174. Zinkernagel RM, Callahan GN, Althage A, Cooper S, Klein PA, Klein J. *J. Exp. Med.* 1978;**147**:882.

175. Fink PJ, Bevan MJ. *J. Exp. Med.* 1978;**148**:766.

176. Chan S, Cosgrove D, Waltzinger C, Benoist C, Mathis D. *Cell* 1993;**73**:225.

177. Grusby M, Auchincloss H, Lee R, Johnson R, Spencer J, Ziljstra M, et al. *Proc. Natl. Acad. Sci. USA* 1993;**90**:3913.

178. Philpott KL, Viney JL, Kay G, Rastan S, Gardiner EM, Chae S, et al. *Science* 1992;**256**:1448.

179. Kisielow P, Blüthmann H, Staerz UD, Steinmetz M, von Boehmer H. *Nature* 1988;**333**:742.

180. Teh HS, Kisielow P, Scott B, Kishi H, Uematsu Y, Blüthmann H, et al. *Nature* 1988;**335**:229.

181. Ignatowicz L, Kappler J, Marrack P. *Cell* 1996;**84**:521.

182. Myazaki T, Wolf P, Tourne S, Waltzinger C, Dierich A, Barois N, et al. *Cell* 1996;**84**:531.

183. Nikolic-Zugic J, Bevan MJ. *Nature* 1990;**344**:65.

184. Ashton-Rickardt PG, van Kaer L, Schumacher TN, Ploegh HL, Tonegawa S. *Cell* 1993;**73**:1041.

185. Hogquist KA, Jameson SC, Heath WR, Howard JL, Bevan MJ, Carbone FR. *Cell* 1994;**76**:17.

186. Sebzda E, Kündig TM, Thomson CT, Aoki K, Mak SY, Mayer SP, et al. *J. Exp. Med.* 1996;**183**:1093.

187. Hunt DF, Michel H, Dickinson TA, Shabanowitz J, Cox AL, Sakaguchi K, et al. *Science* 1992;**256**:1817.

188. Correia-Neves M, Waltzinger C, Mathis D, Benoist C. *Immunity* 2001;**14**:21.

189. Matzinger P. *Immunol. Rev.* 1993;**135**:81.

190. Naeher D, Daniels MA, Hausmann B, Guillaume P, Luescher I, Palmer E. *J. Exp. Med.* 2007;**204**:2553.

191. Miceli MC, von Hoegen P, Parnes JR. *Proc. Natl. Acad. Sci. USA* 1991;**88**:2623.

192. Park JH, Adoro S, Guinter T, Erman B, Alag AS, Catalfamo M, et al. *Nat. Immunol.* 2010;**11**:257.

193. Huesmann M, Scott B, Kisielow P, von Boehmer H. *Cell* 1991;**66**:533.

194. Daniels MA, Teixeiro E, Gill J, Hausmann B, Roubaty D, Holmberg K, et al. *Nature* 2006;**444**:724.

195. Huseby ES, Crawford F, White J, Kappler J, Marrack P. *Proc. Natl. Acad. Sci. USA* 2003;**100**:11565.

196. Kosmrlj A, Jha AK, Huseby ES, Kardar M, Chakraborty AK. *Proc. Natl. Acad. Sci. USA* 2008;**105**:16671.

197. Huseby ES, Crawford F, White J, Marrack P, Kappler JW. *Nat. Immunol.* 2006;**7**:1191.

198. Feng D, Bond CJ, Ely LK, Maynard J, Garcia KC. *Nat. Immunol.* 2007;**8**:975.

199. Cohn M. *Mol. Immunol.* 2005;**42**:1419.

200. Bowerman NA, Colf LA, Garcia KC, Kranz DM. *J. Biol. Chem.* 2009;**284**:32551.

201. Mannie MD. *J. Theoret. Biol.* 1991;**151**:169.

202. Detours V, Mehr R, Perelson AS. *J. Theoret. Biol.* 1999;**200**:389.

203. Kosmrlj A, Chakraborty AK, Kadar M, Shakhnovich EI. *Phys. Rev. Lett.* 2009;**103**:068103.

204. Mason D. *Immunol. Rev.* 2001;**182**:80.

205. Hunt DF, Henderson RA, Shabanowitz J, Sakaguchi K, Michel H, Sevilir N, et al. *Science* 1992;**255**:1261.

206. Chicz RM, Urban RG, Gorga JC, Vignali DAA, Lane WS, Strominger JL. *J. Exp. Med.* 1993;**178**:27.

207. Rammensee HG, Friede T, Stevanovic S. *Immunogenet* 1995;**41**:178.

208. Zhong W, Reche PA, Lai CC, Reinhold B, Reinherz EL. *J. Biol. Chem.* 2003;**278**:45135.

209. Selin LK, Nahill SR, Welsh RM. *J. Exp. Med.* 1994;**179**:1933.

210. Percus JK, Percus OE, Perelson AS. *Proc. Natl. Acad. Sci. USA* 1993;**90**:1691.

211. Warren RL, Freeman JD, Zeng T, Choe G, Munro S, Moore R, et al. *Genome Res.* 2011 in press.

212. Price DA, West SM, Betts MR, Ruff LE, Brenchley JM, Ambrozak DR, et al. *Immunity* 2004;**21**:793.

213. Turner SJ, Kedzierska K, Komodromou H, La Gruta NL, Dunstone MA, Webb AI, et al. *Nat. Immunol.* 2005;**6**:382.

214. Wucherpfennig KW, Allen PM, Celada F, Cohen IR, De Boer R, Garcia KC, et al. *Semin. Immunol.* 2007;**19**:216.

215. Medawar PB. *J. Anat.* 1944;**78**:176.

216. Mitchison NA. *Proc. R. Soc. London Ser. B* 1954;**142**:72.

217. Billingham RE, Brent L, Medawar PB. *Proc. R. Soc. London Ser. B* 1954;**143**:43.

218. Carosella ED, Moreau P, Le Maoult J, Discorde M, Dausset J, Rouas-Freiss N. *Adv. Immunol.* 2003;**81**:199.

219. Simonsen M. *Progr. Allergy* 1962;**6**:349.

220. Hirschhorn K, Bach FH, Kolodny RL, Firschein IL, Hashem N. *Science* 1963;**142**:1185.
221. Cerottini JC, Brunner KT. *Adv. Immunol* 1974;**18**:67.
222. Simonsen M. *Cold Spring Harbor Symp. Quant. Biol.* 1967;**32**:517.
223. Bevan MJ. *Proc. Natl. Acad. Sci. USA* 1977;**74**:2094.
224. Finberg R, Burakoff SJ, Cantor H, Benacerraf B. *Proc. Natl. Acad. Sci. USA* 1978;**75**:5145.
225. Lemonnier F, Burakoff SJ, Germain RG, Benacerraf B. *Proc. Natl. Acad. Sci. USA* 1977;**74**:1229.
226. von Boehmer H, Hengartner H, Nabholz M, Lernhardt W, Schreier MH, et al. *Eur. J. Immunol* 1979;**9**:592.
227. Sredni B, Schwartz RH. *Nature* 1980;**287**:855.
228. Braciale TJ, Andrew ME, Braciale VL, Exp J. *Med* 1981;**153**:1371.
229. Guimezanes A, Albert F, Schmitt-Verhulst AM. *Eur. J. Immunol* 1982;**12**:195.
230. Marrack P, Shimonkevitz R, Hannum C, Haskins K, Kappler J. *Exp. J. Med* 1983;**158**:1635.
231. Naquet P, Pierres A, Pierres M. *Immunogenet* 1983;**18**:475.
232. Fischer Lindahl K, Wilson DB. *J. Exp. Med.* 1977;**145**:508.
233. Simpson E, Mobraaten L, Chandler P, Hetherington C, Hurme M, Brunner C, et al. *J. Exp. Med.* 1978;**148**:1478.
234. Fathman CG, Collavo D, Davies S, Nabhloz M. *J. Immunol.* 1977;**118**:1232.
235. Wagner H, Götze D, Ptschelinzew L, Röllinghof M. *J. Exp. Med.* 1975;**142**:1477.
236. Juretic A, Nagy ZA, Klein J. *Nature* 1981;**289**:308.
237. Swain SL, Panfili PR. *J. Immunol.* 1979;**122**:383.
238. Vidovic D, Juretic A, Nagy ZA, Klein J. *Eur. J. Immunol.* 1981;**11**:499.
239. Vidovic D, Simon MM, Nagy ZA, Klein J. *Scand. J. Immunol.* 1983;**17**:583.
240. Nathenson SG, Geliebter J, Pfaffenbach GM, Zeff RA. *Annu. Rev. Immunol.* 1986;**4**:471.
241. Nabholz M, Young H, Meo T, Miggiano V, Rijnbeek A, Shreffler DC. *Immunogenet* 1975;**1**:457.
242. Forman J, Klein J. *Immunogenet* 1975;**1**:469.
243. Melief CJM, Schwartz RS, Kohn HI, Melvold RW. *Immunogenet* 1975;**2**:337.
244. Widmer MB, MacDonald HR. *J. Immunol.* 1980;**124**:48.
245. Bjorkman PJ, Saper MA, Samraoui B, Bennett WS, Strominger JL, Wiley DC. *Nature* 1987;**329**:512.
246. Chattopadhyay S, Theobald M, Biggs J, Sherman LA. *J. Exp. Med.* 1994;**179**:213.
247. Song ES, Linsk R, Olson CA, McMillan M, Goodenow RS. *Proc. Natl. Acad. Sci. USA* 1988;**85**:1927.
248. Mattson DH, Shimojo N, Cowan EP, Baskin JJ, Turner RV, Shvetsky BD, et al. *J. Immunol.* 1989;**143**:1101.
249. Olson CA, Williams LC, McLaughlin-Taylor E, McMillan M. *Proc. Natl. Acad. Sci. USA* 1989;**86**:1031.
250. Heath WR, Hurd ME, Carbone FR, Sherman LA. *Nature* 1989;**341**:749.
251. Elliott TJ, Eisen HN. *Proc. Natl. Acad. Sci. USA* 1990;**87**:5213.
252. Smith PA, Brunmark A, Jackson MR, Potter TA. *J. Exp. Med.* 1997;**185**:1023.
253. Rötzschke OR, Falk K, Faath S, Rammensee HG. *J. Exp. Med.* 1991;**174**:1059.
254. Obst R, Netuschil N, Klopfer K, Stevanovic S, Rammensee HG. *J. Exp. Med.* 2000;**191**:805.
255. Guimezanes A, Albert F, Schmitt-Verhulst AM. *Eur. J. Immunol.* 1982;**12**:195.
256. Marrack P, Shimonkevitz R, Hannum C, Haskins K, Kappler J. *J. Exp. Med.* 1983;**158**:1635.
257. Naquet P, Pierres A, Pierres M. *Immunogenet* 1983;**18**:475.
258. Nagy ZA, Servis C, Walden P, Klein J, Goldberg E. *Eur. J. Immunol.* 1985;**15**:814.

259. Speir JA, Garcia KC, Brunmark A, Degano M, Peterson PA, Teyton L, et al. *Immunity* 1998;**8**:553.

260. Cohn M. *Immunol. Res.* 2011;**50**:49.

261. Reiser JB, Darnault C, Guimezanes A, Gregoire C, Mosser T, Schmitt-Verhulst AM, et al. *Nat. Immunol.* 2000;**1**:291.

262. Naeher D, Daniels MA, Hausmann B, Guillaume P, Luescher I, Palmer E. *J. Exp. Med.* 2007;**204**:2553.

263. Schneck J, Maloy WL, Coligan JE, Margulies DH. *Cell* 1989;**56**:47.

264. Sykulev Y, Brunmark A, Tsomides TJ, Kageyama S, Jackson M, Peterson PA, et al. *Proc. Natl. Acad. Sci. USA* 1994;**91**:11487.

265. Nagy ZA. *Scand. J. Immunol.* 2012;**75**:463.

266. Bux E, Matsunaga K, Nagatani T, Walden P, Nagy ZA, Klein J. *Immunogenet* 1985;**22**:189.

267. Itakura K, Hutton JJ, Boyse EA, Old LJ. *Transplantation* 1972;**13**:239.

268. Kisielow P, Hirst JA, Shiku H, Beverley PCL, Hoffmann MK, Boyse EA, Oettgen HF. *Nature* 1975;**253**:219.

269. Cantor H, Boyse EA. *J. Exp. Med.* 1975;**141**:1376.

270. Cantor H, Boyse EA. *J. Exp. Med.* 1975;**141**:1390.

271. Swain SL, Panfili PR. *J. Immunol.* 1979;**122**:383.

272. Swain SL, Bakke A, English M, Dutton RW. *J. Immunol.* 1979;**123**:2716.

273. Wettstein PJ, Bailey DW, Mobraaten LE, Klein J, Frelinger JA. *Proc. Natl. Acad. Sci. USA* 1979;**76**:3455.

274. Hardt C, Pfizenmaier K, Röllinghof M, Klein J, Wagner H. *J. Exp. Med.* 1980;**152**:1413.

275. Teh HS, Teh SJ. *J. Immunol.* 1980;**125**:1977.

276. Nagy ZA, Kusnierczyk P, Klein J. *Eur. J. Immunol.* 1981;**11**:167.

277. Mathieson BJ, Sharrow SO, Rosenberg Y, Hämmerling U. *Nature* 1981;**289**:179.

278. Swain SL, Dennert G, Wormsley S, Dutton RW. *Eur. J. Immunol.* 1981;**11**:175.

279. Nakayama E, Shiku H, Stockert E, Oettgen HF, Old LJ. *Proc. Natl. Acad. Sci. USA* 1979;**76**:1977.

280. Hollander N, Pillemer E, Weissman IL. *J. Exp. Med.* 1980;**152**:674.

281. Swain SL. *Proc. Natl. Acad. Sci. USA* 1981;**78**:7101.

282. Kung PC, Goldstein G, Reinherz EL, Schlossman SF. *Science* 1979;**206**:347.

283. Reinherz EL, Kung PC, Goldstein G, Schlossman SF. *Proc. Natl. Acad. Sci. USA* 1979;**76**:4061.

284. Meuer SC, Schlossman SF, Reinherz EL. *Proc. Natl. Acad. Sci. USA* 1982;**79**:4395.

285. Meuer SC, Hussey RE, Hogdon JC, Hercend T, Schlossman SF, Reinherz EL. *Science* 1982;**218**:471.

286. Dialynas DP, Quan ZS, Wall KA, Pierres A, Quintans J, Loken MR, et al. *J. Immunol.* 1983;**131**:2445.

287. Landgren U, Ramstedt U, Axberg I, Ullberg M, Jondal M, Wigzell H. *J. Exp. Med.* 1982;**155**:1579.

288. Reinherz EL, Meuer S, Fitzgerald KA, Hussey RE, Levine H, Schlossman SF. *Cell* 1982;**30**:735.

289. Knapp W, Rieber P, Dörken B, Schmidt RE, Stein H. *AEGKr Van Den Borne, Immunol. Today* 1989;**10**:253.

290. Morse III HC. *J. Immunol.* 1992;**149**:3129.

291. Maddon PJ, Littman DR, Godfrey M, Maddon DE, Chess L, Axel R. *Cell* 1985;**42**:93.

292. Tourvielle B, Gorman SD, Field EH, Hunkapiller T, Parnes JR. *Science* 1986;**234**:610.

293. Littman DR, Thomas Y, Maddon PJ, Chess L, Axel R. *Cell* 1985;**40**:237.

294. Johnson P. *Immunogenet* 1987;**26**:174.
295. Zamoyska R, Vollmer AC, Sizer KC, Liaw CW, Parnes JR. *Cell* 1985;**43**:153.
296. Nakauchi H, Shinkai Y, Okamura K. *Proc. Natl. Acad. Sci. USA* 1987;**84**:4210.
297. König R, Huang LY, Germain R. *Nature* 1992;**356**:796.
298. Camarola G, Schierle A, Takacs B, Doran D, Knorr R, Bannworth W, et al. *Nature* 1992;**356**:799.
299. Salter RD, Benjamin RJ, Wesley PK, Buxton SE, Garrett TPJ, Clayberger C, et al. *Nature* 1990;**345**:41.
300. Potter TA, Rajan TV, Dick II RF, Bluestone JA. *Nature* 1989;**337**:73.
301. Wu H, Kwong PD, Hendrickson WA. *Nature* 1997;**387**:527.
302. Gao GF, Tormo J, Gerth UC, Wyer JR, McMichael AJ, Stuart DI, et al. *Nature* 1997;**387**:630.
303. Kern PS, Teng MK, Smolyar A, Liu JH, Hussey RE, Spoerl R, et al. *Immunity* 1998;**9**:519.
304. Huang HJS, Jones NH, Strominger JL, Herzenberg LA. *Proc. Natl. Acad. Sci. USA* 1987;**84**:204.
305. Kupfer A, Singer SJ, Janeway Jr CA, Swain SL. *Proc. Natl. Acad. Sci. USA* 1987;**84**:5888.
306. Miceli MC, von Hoegen P, Parnes JR. *Proc. Natl. Acad. Sci. USA* 1991;**88**:2623.
307. O'Rouke A, Mescher M. *Immunol. Today* 1993;**14**:183.
308. Veillette A, Bookman MA, Horak EM, Bolen JB. *Cell* 1988;**55**:301.
309. Janeway CJ. *Annu. Rev. Immunol.* 1992;**10**:645 W.
310. Krensky AM, Reiss CS, Mier JW, Strominger JL, Burakoff SJ. *Proc. Natl. Acad. Sci. USA* 1982;**79**:2365.
311. Cohn M. *Lymphokines* 1985;**10**:201.
312. Mosmann TR, Cherwinski H, Bond mw, Giedlin MA, Coffman RL. *J. Immunol* 1986;**136**:2348.
313. Xu D, Chan WL, Leung BP, Hunter D, Schulz K, Carter RW, et al. *J. Exp. Med.* 1998;**188**:1485.
314. Löhning ML, Stroehmann A, Coyle AJ, Grogan JL, Lin S, Guiterrez-Ramos JC, et al. *Proc. Natl. Acad. Sci. USA* 1998;**95**:6930.
315. Romagnani S. *Immunol. Today* 1991;**12**:256.
316. Mosmann TR, Coffman RL. *Immunol. Today* 1987;**8**:223.
317. Paul WE, Seder RA. *Cell* 1994;**76**:241.
318. Swain S, Bradley LM, Croft M, Tonkonogy S, Atkins G, Weinberg AD, et al. *Immunol. Rev.* 1991;**123**:115.
319. Firestein GS, Roeder WD, Laxer JA, Townsend KS, Weaver CT, Hom JT, et al. *J. Immunol.* 1989;**143**:518.
320. Hsieh CS, Heimberger AB, Gold JS, O'Garra A, Murphy KM. *Proc. Natl. Acad. Sci. USA* 1992;**89**:6065.
321. Seder RA, Paul WE, Davis MM, Fazekas de St. Groth B. *J. Exp. Med.* 1992;**176**:1091.
322. Murphy E, Shibuya K, Hosken N, Openshaw P, Maino V, Murphy K, et al. *J. Exp. Med.* 1996;**183**:901.
323. Bucy RP, Karr L, Huang G-Q, Li J, Carter D, Honjo K, et al. *Proc. Natl. Acad. Sci. USA* 1995;**92**:7565.
324. Hsieh CS, Macatonia SE, Tripp CS, Wolf SF, O'Garra A, Murphy KM. *Science* 1993;**260**:547.
325. Seder RA, Gazinelli R, Sher A, Paul WE. *Proc. Natl. Acad. Sci. USA* 1993;**90**:10188.
326. Schmitz J, Assenmacher M, Radbruch A. *Eur. J. Immunol.* 1993;**23**:191.
327. Ho IC, Hodge MR, Rooney JW, Glimcher LH. *Cell* 1996;**85**:973.
328. Ranger AM, Oukka M, Rengarajan J, Glimcher LH. *Immunity* 1998;**9**:627.
329. Ho IC, Lo D, Glimcher LH. *J. Exp. Med.* 1998;**188**:1859.
330. Szabo SJ, Kim ST, Costa GL, Zhang X, Fathman CG, Glimcher LH. *Cell* 2000;**100**:655.
331. Rengarajan J, Szabo SJ, Glimcher LH. *Immunol. Today* 2000;**21**:479.

332. Liew FY, Millott S, Lelchuk R, Chan WL, Ziltener H. *Eur. J. Immunol.* 1989;**19**:1227.
333. Mezhitov R, Preston-Hurlburt P, Janeway Jr CA. *Nature* 1997;**388**:394.
334. Yang RB, Mark MR, Gray A, Huang A, Xie MH, Zhang M, et al. *Nature* 1998;**395**:284.
335. Urban JJ, Katona I, Paul WE, Finkelman FD. *Proc. Natl. Acad. Sci. USA* 1991;**88**:5513.
336. Mitchison NA. *Proc. Roy. Soc. Ser. B* 1964;**161**:275.
337. Weigle WO. *Adv. Immunol.* 1973;**16**:61.
338. Bretscher PA. *Federation Proc.* 1981;**40**:1473.
339. Billingham RE, Brent L, Medawar PB. *Nature* 1953;**172**:603.
340. Gershon RK, Kondo K. *Immunol.* 1970;**18**:723.
341. Gershon RK, Kondo K. *Immunol.* 1971;**21**:903.
342. Gershon RK, Cohen P, Hencin R, Liebhaber SA. *J. Immunol* 1972;**108**:586.
343. Basten A, Miller JF, Johnson P. *Transplant. Rev.* 1975;**26**:130.
344. Herzenberg LA, Okumura K, Metzler CM. *Transplant. Rev.* 1975;**27**:57.
345. Greene MI, Perry LL, Benacerraf B. *Am. J. Pathol.* 1979;**95**:159.
346. Claman HN, Miller SD, Sy MS, Moorhead JW. *Immunol. Rev.* 1980;**50**:105.
347. Greene MI, Nelles MJ, Sy MS, Nisonoff A. *Adv. Immunol.* 1982;**32**:253.
348. Kapp JA, Pierce CW, Schlossman S, Benacerraf B. *J. Exp. Med.* 1974;**140**:648.
349. Debre P, Kapp JA, Benacerraf B. *J. Exp. Med.* 1975;**142**:1436.
350. Baxevanis CN, Nagy ZA, Klein J. *Proc. Natl. Acad. Sci. USA* 1981;**78**:3809.
351. Okumura K, Herzenberg LA, Murphy DB, McDevitt HO. *J. Exp. Med.* 1976;**144**:685.
352. Murphy DB, Herzenberg LA, Okumura K, McDevitt HO. *J. Exp. Med.* 1976;**144**:699.
353. Tada T, Taniguchi M, David CS. *J. Exp. Med.* 1976;**144**:713.
354. Cohn M, et al. Neural Modulation of Immunity. In: Guillemin R, editor. New York: Raven Press; 1985. p. 3.
355. Langman RE. *Cell. Immunol.* 1987;**108**:214.
356. Benacerraf B, Germain RN. *Scand. J. Immunol.* 1981;**13**:1.
357. Sercarz EE, Yowell RL, Turkin D, Miller A, Araneo BA, Adorini L. *Immunol. Rev.* 1978;**39**:108.
358. Breslow JL, Ross D, McPherson J, Williams H, Kurnit D, Nussbaum AL, et al. *Proc. Natl. Acad. Sci. USA* 1983;**79**:6861.
359. Steinmetz M, Minard K, Horvath S, McNicholas J, Frelinger J, Wake C, et al. *Nature* 1982;**300**:35.
360. Kronenberg M, Steinmetz M, Kobori J, Kraig E, Kapp JA, Pierce CW, et al. *Proc. Natl. Acad. Sci. USA* 1983;**80**:5704.
361. Hedrick SM, Germain RN, Bevan MJ, Dorf M, Engel I, Fink P, et al. *Proc. Natl. Acad. Sci. USA* 1985;**82**:531.
362. Germain RN. *Immunol.* 2008;**123**:20.
363. Kapp JA. *Immunol.* 2008;**123**:28.
364. Basten A, Fazekas de St Groth B. *Immunol.* 2008;**123**:33.
365. Jenkins MK, Schwartz RH. *J. Exp. Med.* 1987;**165**:302.
366. Sakaguchi S, Fukuma K, Kuribayashi K, Masuda T. *J. Exp. Med.* 1985;**161**:72.
367. Powrie F, Mason D. *J. Exp. Med.* 1990;**172**:1701.
368. Saoudi A, Seddon B, Heath V, Powell D, Mason D. *Immunol. Rev.* 1996;**149**:195.
369. Shevach EM. *Annu. Rev. Immunol.* 2000;**18**:423.
370. Sakaguchi S, Ono M, Setoguchi R, Hori S, Fehervari Z, Shimizu J, et al. *Immunol. Rev.* 2006;**212**:8.
371. Sakaguchi S, Sakaguchi N, Asano M, Itoh M, Toda M. *J. Immunol.* 1995;**155**:1151.
372. Hori S, Nomura T, Sakaguchi S. *Science* 2003;**299**:1057.
373. Fontenot JD, Gavin MA, Rudensky AY. *Nat. Immunol.* 2003;**4**:330.

374. Khattri R, Cox T, Yasako SA, Ramsdell F. *Nat. Immunol.* 2003;**4**:337.
375. Brunkow ME, Jeffery EW, Hjerrild KA, Paeper B, Clark LB, Yasayko SA, et al. *Nat. Genet.* 2001;**27**:68.
376. Thornton AM, Shevach EM. *J. Exp. Med.* 1998;**188**:287.
377. Chen W, Jin W, Hardegen N, Lei KJ, Li L, Marinos N, McGrady G, Wahl SM. *J. Exp. Med.* 2003;**198**:1875.
378. Apostolou I, von Boehmer H. *J. Exp. Med.* 2004;**199**:1401.
379. Itoh M, Takahashi T, Sakaguchi N, Kuniyasu Y, Shimizu J, Otsuka F, Sakaguchi S. *J. Immunol.* 1999;**162**:5317.
380. Jordan MS, Boesteanu A, Reed AJ, Petrone AL, Holenbeck AE, Lerman MA, Naji A, Caton AJ. *Nat. Immunol.* 2001;**2**:301.
381. Hsieh CS, Zheng Y, Liang Y, Fontenot JD, Rudensky AY. *Nat. Immunol.* 2006;**7**:401.
382. Takahashi T, Kuniyasu Y, Toda M, Sakaguchi N, Itoh M, Iwata M, et al. *Int. Immnol.* 1998;**10**:1969.
383. von Boehmer H. *Nat. Immunol.* 2005;**6**:338.
384. Powrie F, Carlino J, Leach mw, Mauze S, Coffman RL. *J. Exp. Med* 1996;**183**:2669.
385. Seddon B, Mason D. *J. Exp. Med.* 1999;**189**:877.
386. Paust S, Lu L, McCarty N, Cantor H. *Proc. Natl. Acad. Sci. USA* 2004;**101**:10398.
387. Cederbom L, Hall H, Ivars F. *Eur. J. Immunol.* 2000;**30**:1538.
388. Thornton AM, Shevach EM. *J. Immunol.* 2000;**164**:183.
389. Bennett CL, Christie J, Ramsdell F, Brunkow ME, Ferguson PJ, Whitesell L, et al. *Nat. Genet.* 2001;**27**:20.
390. Fontenot JD, Gavin MA, Rudensky AY. *Nat. Immunol.* 2003;**4**:330.
391. Sharfe N, Dadi HK, Shahar M, Roifman CM. *Proc. Natl. Acad. Sci. USA* 1997;**94**:3168.
392. Horak I, Lohler J, Ma A, Smith KA. *Immunol. Rev.* 1995;**148**:35.
393. Tivol EA, Gorski J. *J. Immunol.* 2002;**169**:1852.
394. Shevach EM. *J. Exp. Med.* 2001;**193**:F41.
395. Cohn M. *Int. Immunol.* 2008;**20**:1107.
396. Günther J, Haas W, von Boehmer H. *Eur. J. Immunol.* 1982;**12**:247.
397. Spits H, van Schooten W, Keizer H, van Seventer G, van de Rijn M, Terhorst C, et al. *Science* 1986;**232**:403.
398. Shaw S, Luce GE, Quinones R, Gress RE, Springer TA, Sanders ME. *Nature* 1986;**323**:262.
399. Springer TA, Dustin ML, Kishimoto TK, Marlin SD. *Annu. Rev. Immunol.* 1987;**5**:223.
400. Kishimoto TK, O'Connor K, Lee A, Roberts TM, Springer TA. *Cell* 1987;**48**:681.
401. Larson RS, Corbi AL, Berman L, Springer T. *J. Cell Biol.* 1989;**108**:703.
402. Staunton DE, Marlin SD, Stratowa C, Dustin ML, Springer TA. *Cell* 1988;**52**:925.
403. Staunton DE, Dustin ML, Springer TA. *Nature* 1989;**339**:61.
404. Selvaraj P, Plunkett ML, Dustin M, Sanders ME, Shaw S, Springer TA. *Nature* 1987;**326**:400.
405. Springer TA. *Nature* 1990;**346**:425.
406. Dustin ML, Springer TA. *Nature* 1989;**341**:619.
407. Dustin ML, Rothlein R, Bhan AK, Dinarello CA, Springer TA. *J. Immunol.* 1986;**137**:245.
408. Wigzell H, Hayry P. *Curr. Topics Microbiol. Immunol.* 1974;**67**:1.
409. Bell GI, Dembo M, Bongrand P. *Biophys. J.* 1984;**45**:1051.
410. Despont JP, Abel CA, Grey HM. *Cell. Immunol.* 1975;**17**:487.
411. Tedder TF, Isaacs CM, Ernst TJ, Demetri GD, Adler DA, Disteche CM. *J. Exp. Med.* 1989;**170**:123.
412. Mackay CR, Marston WL, Dudler L. *J. Exp. Med.* 1990;**171**:801.
413. Stoolman LM. *Cell* 1989;**56**:907.

414. Hara T, Fu SM, Hansen JA. *J. Exp. Med.* 1985;**161**:1513.
415. Lindstein T, June CH, Ledbetter JA, Stella G, Thompson CB. *Science* 1989;**244**:339.
416. Linsley PS, Brady W, Grosmaire L, Aruffo A, Damle NK, Ledbetter JA. *J. Exp. Med.* 1991;**173**:721.
417. Linsley PS, Clark EA, Ledbetter JA. *Proc. Natl. Acad. Sci. USA* 1990;**87**:5031.
418. Lenschow DJ, Su GH, Zuckerman LA, Nabavi N, Jellis CL, Gray GS, et al. *Proc. Natl. Acad. Sci. USA* 1993;**90**:11054.
419. Hathcock KS, Laszlo G, Dickler HB, Bradshaw J, Linsley P, Hodes RJ. *Science* 1993;**262**:905.
420. Freeman GJ, Gribben JG, Boussiotis VA, Ng JW, Restivo Jr VA, Lombard LA, et al. *Science* 1993;**262**:909.
421. Brunet JF, Denizot F, Luciani MF, Roux-Dosseto M, Suzan M, Mattei MG, Goldstein P. *Nature* 1987;**328**:267.
422. Harper K, Balzano C, Rouvier E, Mattei MG, Luciani MF, Goldstein P. *J. Immunol.* 1991;**147**:1037.
423. Linsley PS, Brady W, Urnes M, Grosmaire LS, Damle NK, Ledbetter JA. *J. Exp. Med.* 1991;**174**:561.
424. Freeman GJ, Lombard DB, Gimmi CD, Brod SA, Lee K, Laning JC, et al. *J. Immunol.* 1992;**149**:3705.
425. Krummel MF, Allison JP. *J. Exp. Med.* 1995;**182**:459.
426. Krummel MF, Allison JP. *J. Exp. Med.* 1996;**183**:2533.
427. Waterhouse P, Penninger JM, Timms E, Wakeham A, Shahinian A, Lee KP, et al. *Science* 1995;**270**:985.
428. Tivol EA, Borriello F, Schweitzer AN, Lynch WP, Bluestone JA, Sharpe AH. *Immunity* 1995;**3**:541.
429. Holländer GA, Castigli E, Kulbacki R, Su M, Burakoff SJ, Guiterrez-Ramos JC, et al. *Proc. Natl. Acad. Sci. USA* 1996;**93**:4994.
430. Grewal IS, Foellmer HG, Grewal KD, Xu J, Hardardottir F, Baron JL, et al. *Science* 1996;**273**:1864.
431. Shinde S, Wu Y, Guo Y, Niu Q, Xu J, Grewal IS, et al. *J. Immunol.* 1996;**157**:2764.
432. Noelle RJ, Roy M, Shepherd DM, Stamenkovic I, Ledbetter JA, Aruffo A. *Proc. Natl. Acad. Sci. USA* 1992;**89**:6550.
433. Bennett SRM, Carbone FR, Karamalis F, Flawell RA, Miller JFAP, Heath WR. *Nature* 1998;**393**:478.
434. Schoenberger SP, Toes REM, EIH van der Voort, Offringa R, CJM Melief. *Nature* 1998;**393**:480.
435. Green JM, Noel PJ, Sperling AI, Walunas TL, Gray GS, Bluestone JA, et al. *Immunity* 1994;**1**:155.
436. Chen C, Faherty DA, Gault A, Connaughton SE, Powers GD, Godfrey DI, et al. *J. Immunol.* 1994;**152**:2105.
437. Bluestone JA. *Immunity* 1995;**2**:555.
438. Schwartz RH. *Science* 1990;**248**:1349.
439. Bretscher PA. *Proc. Natl. Acad. Sci. USA* 1999;**96**:185.

Chapter 9

Acquired Immunological Tolerance

The adaptive immune system has evolved to provide long-lived and not very prolific vertebrates with a fair chance of survival in the battle against fast-growing and constantly changing microbial pathogens. Obviously, the short generation times of pathogenic microorganisms allow the pathogens to change much faster by mutation than any germ-line-encoded defense system of higher organisms could do. Therefore microbes are expected to evade the innate (i.e., germ-line-encoded) immune system, and thus drive the evolution of the adaptive immune system that is free from 'mutational race'. As already discussed (Sections 5.2, 5.3, 8.2.3), the adaptive immune system generates somatically a vast number of receptor specificities at random, covering thereby also future changes of pathogens. While this solution eliminates the problem of pathogen escape, it creates another: namely, a fraction of the random specificities will inevitably recognize self structures of the host and trigger autoimmune damage. Therefore an additional somatic process is required that eliminates self reactivity from the receptor repertoire. This somatic process is referred to as acquisition of self tolerance.

Because self tolerance is the property of the immune system and not that of individual lymphocytes, and because it is largely established in embryonic age, experimental approaches to its study have proven troublesome. This explains why a 34-year gap separates the discovery of immune tolerance[1] from the first experimental evidence for its mechanism.[2] In the long intermission, theoreticians took over the lead and constructed hypothetical models of how the immune system could discriminate between self and non-self, or as Mel Cohn used to put it: tried 'reconstructing a cabbage from sauerkraut'.[3] As a result of this historical development, our understanding of self tolerance has become a mosaic of concepts and scattered experimental evidence, and it has remained incomplete with elements of mysticism up to now.

9.1 DISCOVERY

The key observation leading to the discovery of self tolerance was made by Ray Owen[4] in 1945. Owen found that dizygotic (genetically distinct) twin

A History of Modern Immunology. http://dx.doi.org/10.1016/B978-0-12-416974-6.00009-0

calves that shared placental circulation in embryonic life were born with and retained for a long time red blood cells of each other. Based on Medawar's earlier study[5] calves with the same genetic difference were expected to reject the foreign erythrocytes. Thus the finding suggested that the exchange of blood cells between these calves in embryonal life must have led to a change in their immunological reactivity, so that they no longer reacted to the foreign cells encountered as embryos.

Burnet and Fenner[6] are credited for being the first to recognize in 1949 the biological impact of Owen's finding. The salient point here was that the immune system of dizygotic twins considered antigens not encoded in their own genome as self. Burnet and Fenner have thus concluded that self is a property that must be 'learned' somatically during embryonal life.

The idea of immunological tolerance acquired in embryonal life was then followed up and proven experimentally by Peter Medawar and his group. The results were published in a three-page *Nature* paper[1] by Billingham, Brent and Medawar in 1953, which could serve as a classic example for meticulous precision and lucidity, the two major virtues of experimental scientists. Their data, besides demonstrating tolerance to foreign tissues in embryos of two different species, have established a number of additional points. First, the animals injected with foreign cells as embryos were shown to accept in adult age skin grafts from the same donor. Second, the acquired tolerance was immunologically specific: animals tolerant to cells of one donor retained their capacity to reject grafts from a genetically different donor. Third, skin grafts from the tolerizing donor were accepted although skin cells were not used for tolerization, suggesting that the 'foreignness' recognized by the immune system was shared among different tissues. Fourth, tolerance was not due to a specific failure of the host's immune response or a modulation of antigenicity of the graft, because passively transferred immune cells could induce graft rejection. Thus tolerance appeared to affect only part of the immune system, notably the very part that would respond to the same antigen in adult age. Altogether, acquired tolerance has turned out to be the exact inverse of acquired immunity.

Simultaneously with the Medawar study, Milan Hasek and his group in Prague performed experiments using parabiotic chicken and duck embryos, and were able to demonstrate tolerance in these models.[7] But Hasek's studies remained largely unknown for a while, because he published all his work before 1955 in the Czech language.

Although tolerance as a natural and experimental fact became well established by the early 1950s, attempts to propose a feasible mechanism that would account for it had remained unsuccessful until Burnet[8] came up with the clonal selection theory in 1959 (see Section 1.1 for details). The central thesis of this theory, namely, that each lymphocyte should express receptors of one single antigen specificity, permitted to postulate a simple mechanism for tolerance: the elimination of self-reactive lymphocytes during embryonal life, a process termed clonal deletion.

'Burnet presumably arrived at the one-cell–one-receptor solution intuitively, primarily because this arrangement would provide the clearest explanation for known features of antibody production', adds Dr. G. 'For example, monoclonality would allow to run several immune responses parallel, it would explain the increase of antibody titers with time by the proliferation of the relevant clone, and the continued presence of antibody after elimination of antigen by the persistence of the clone. But the prime merit of the theory was that it suggested a clear-cut way of separating reactivities against self from those against non-self. Indeed, from the evolutionary point of view, the defensive capacity of the immune system does not stringently require monoclonality, whereas self–non-self discrimination does, and thus it is reasonable to assume that the need for self–non-self discrimination has been the evolutionary driver of monoclonality.'[9]

For the experimental demonstration and conceptualization of tolerance, Medawar and Burnet were awarded with the Nobel Prize in 1960. The relatively early decision of the Nobel Committee after the discovery is explained by the importance of the topic, and in part also by the perspicuous state of biomedical sciences in the 1950s.

In the subsequent decade, a number of additional features of the tolerant state were uncovered. First, it was shown that repeated injections of the same antigen were required to maintain tolerance, otherwise the animals recovered from the unresponsive state.[10] Second, the dose of antigen was found to be critical in the induction of response versus tolerance: very low and very high doses preferentially induced tolerance ('low-zone', and 'high-zone' tolerance), whereas medium-sized doses resulted in antibody response.[11] And finally, it was shown that the state of tolerance could be broken by the administration of a cross-reactive antigen, e.g., animals tolerant of bovine serum albumin (BSA) could produce anti-BSA antibody after challenge with horse serum albumin.[12,13] These features have been considered ever since to make up the 'classical phenomenology' of acquired tolerance.

The first fruitful period of tolerance research ended at this point. Although immunologists were aware that the next step should be to investigate whether clonal deletion would occur in reality, they also knew that the frequency of lymphocyte clones reacting to a single antigen (1 in 10 000 to 1 in 100 000) was far below the detection limit of the methods available to them, which rendered an experimental approach impossible. Therefore tolerance has remained a 'black box' for a long time that could only be lit by the torchlight of thought and fantasy. This set the stage for the era of theories.

9.2 THE ERA OF THEORIES

9.2.1 The Concept of Self–Non-Self Discrimination

It is not exaggerated to state that self–non-self (S–NS) discrimination is the most fundamental question of immunobiology, and therefore the way one thinks about it determines one's view about all other aspects of immunology. Unfortunately, many immunologists refuse to think about this problem, for them S–NS discrimination is nothing more than a slogan, and there is also a group of colleagues that denies its necessity. It seems therefore adequate to define S–NS discrimination more closely at this place. The following description will largely reflect Mel Cohn's thinking about this subject, most clearly stated in an essay of his[14] published in 2001. But care was taken to reproduce here only those statements which appeared self-evident, and thus hopefully would not constitute subjects of conflict between competing views.

Biological defense systems have one property in common: they are biodestructive, and as such dangerous for both intruder and host, similarly to the firearm by which one can kill the enemy as well as oneself. Therefore they must be equipped with a targeting device that directs the destructive power of effector mechanisms to the intruder. This is the basis of the concept that we refer to as S–NS discrimination. The evolutionary selection is on the precision of targeting: if it is not precise enough, pathogens are not eliminated efficiently, and significant damage to the host's own tissues occurs. It follows from this argument that *all* biological defense systems must make S–NS discrimination.

Defense systems are of two different kinds: germ-line-encoded and somatically generated. Current terminology refers to the former as 'innate' and the latter as 'adaptive' immune systems. All living creatures possess the innate system, but only vertebrates have, in addition, an adaptive immune system. The innate system of defense exists in different forms, e.g., bacteriocidal activities such as oxygen and nitrous oxide intermediates, lytic enzymes, toxic peptides, certain cytokines, etc. Common to all of them is that their targeting strategy is based on the recognition of *chemical features* common to many pathogens (bacterial lipopolysaccharides, mannans, glycans, double-stranded RNA, etc.) and absent from the host. Thus they distinguish between *self-of-the-species* and non-self. Most importantly, the recognitive components of the innate system are germline encoded. Thus if, for example, the targeting device mutates to recognize self, the individual will be eliminated.

The innate system provides the host with adequate protection as long as the pathogenic load is limited. For example, invertebrates that live in small ecologic niches can cope with the small number of pathogens they encounter by means of the innate system. In this case a steady state can develop between the hosts and pathogens. On the one hand, there is no selective advantage for the host species to increase the recognitive potential of its defense, because the pathogens no longer limit the survival and reproduction of most of its members. On the other hand, pathogens have no advantage in killing all hosts, because this would lead to self-termination.

In contrast to invertebrates, vertebrates populate vast areas of land and water, and migrate long distances and are thus likely to encounter a much larger variety of pathogens, many of which may evade the innate system. This situation must have set up the selective pressure for the evolution of the adaptive immune system. The targeting strategy of the adaptive system is qualitatively different, in that it is based on the recognition of epitopes, i.e., shape-patches on molecular surfaces, instead of chemical differences. Because the number of possible epitopes is enormous, the recognitive repertoire is correspondingly large, indeed it is large enough to cover even future changes of pathogens. This recognitive repertoire is generated somatically by random rearrangement of gene segments plus somatic mutations, and is then coupled to a limited number of effector mechanisms, the latter often being shared with the innate system.[15] Inherent to the new targeting strategy, the adaptive repertoire cannot make S–NS discrimination on a chemical basis, it must be made epitope-by-epitope. The distinction here is made between *self-of-the-individual* versus non-self, because self epitopes of one individual may be non-self for another. Furthermore, because the recognitive repertoire is generated somatically, S–NS discrimination must also result from somatic selection, which should eliminate cells instead of individuals.

If we wish, we could regard the somatic generation of immune receptor repertoire and its sorting into anti-S and anti-NS as processes of *somatic evolution* that is centered on providing advantage for the individual, in contrast to genetic evolution that confers advantage to the species (to the cost of some individuals).

'At this point it may be appropriate to emphasize that S–NS discrimination is not just a concept, it can also be regarded as the evolutionary driving force for fundamental mechanisms of the adaptive immune system', adds Dr. G. 'The one-cell-one-receptor arrangement ("clonality") is driven by S–NS discrimination, and so are the underlying mechanisms that enable clonality, e.g., allele- and isotype-exclusion of receptor genes, and perhaps also the fact that somatic rearrangement occurs at the DNA and not the RNA level. Natural selection probably acts via bi-specific lymphocytes where one specificity is anti-S and the other anti-NS. Some of these double-specific cells escape self tolerance and can be activated via anti-NS to produce anti-S that in turn causes autoimmunity. The specificity of antigen receptors (Ig, TCR) is probably also shaped by S–NS discrimination. While the increasing pathogenic load and its escape mutants are likely to drive the size of the recognitive repertoire, S–NS discrimination may affect the size of the antigen-combining site[16] the latter must be large enough to permit unambiguous (i.e., non-cross-reactive) distinction between S and NS.'

9.2.2 What is Immunological Self?

The term S–NS discrimination introduced by Burnet and Fenner[17] in 1948 is undoubtedly a very elegant and intellectually appealing one with a philosophical touch, but it is at the same time a notorious source of misunderstanding, in particular as far as the meaning of self is concerned.

Obviously, the general definition of self given in the *Concise Oxford Dictionary* as 'person's or thing's own individuality or essence' assumes different meanings when used in philosophy, psychology or immunology. Since immunology is an experimental science, the definition of immunological self has not been constant, it has been molded by new data as they came along. Perhaps this is why some colleagues felt even as late as the end of the twentieth century that immunological self was a mystic entity.[18]

The initial, purely intuitive definition of immunological self was 'everything in and under the skin', or in more scientific terms 'everything encoded in the genome of an individual'. But this had to be revised as it has turned out that normal unimmunized individuals possess 'natural' antibodies that can react with a variety of self constituents.[19] For many immunologists this finding has suggested that the immune system cannot distinguish between S and NS, and thus immunological self is just a metaphor.[20] Interestingly, only a few colleagues (e.g., Matzinger[21] and Langman and Cohn[22]) realized that something was wrong with the original definition, namely that immunological self must be defined by the immune system itself and not by the brains of immunologists. Natural antibodies also taught us something more important: their specificities for intracellular constituents, membrane components, senescent erythrocytes, etc., have revealed that they may be involved in the clearance of catabolic substances from the body.[23] The roles of the immune system thus seemed to include a previously unsuspected 'housekeeping' function, in addition to its known protective function against pathogens. Whether the debris of the body's own substances is S or NS has been the subject of heated semantic debates. But from the immune system's point of view it appears to be NS that has to be cleared. The case of natural antibodies raised the possibility for the first time that it may be more important for the immune system to 'know' what is to be saved or eliminated than what is S or NS. Another set of immunogenic self substances was identified at 'sequestered' sites of the body, such as the brain, testes and cornea; they also qualify as NS, because the immune system has no access to these sites and thus cannot develop tolerance to them. All these examples led to a change in the definition of immunological self: it has been proposed that S undoubtedly comprises autogenous substances, however, not every autogenous substance is S.

At this point it has become clear that S–NS discrimination, interesting as it might have appeared at the beginning, does not correctly describe the functional selectivity of the immune system, which is to preserve certain substances and eliminate others. That the former correspond to constituents of the body has remained self-evident. Recognizing the need for a change in terminology, Cohn and Langman[24] have proposed to replace S and NS with 'not-to-be ridded' (NTBR) and 'to-be-ridded' (TBR). But the new terms were long and cumbersome, and therefore the community has decided to continue using S and NS with the proviso that their correct meaning is 'to be preserved' and 'to be attacked', respectively. This wrangle about semantics was, however, just an interlude. The real question that kept both theoreticians and experimenters busy was how the immune system sorts its recognitive repertoire so that it can make the 'preserve or attack' distinction.

9.2.3 Early Theories of Self–Non-Self Discrimination

The idea of S–NS discrimination has its origin in the 'horror autotoxicus' theory put forward by Paul Ehrlich in 1901 (see in Silverstein[25]). Ehrlich studied the induction of hemolytic antibodies, and observed that these were readily formed against xenogeneic and allogeneic erythrocytes, but never against autologous red cells. To explain this result, Ehrlich argued that 'it would be exceedingly disteleologic, if in this situation self-poisons, autotoxins, were formed', and he proposed that 'the organism possesses certain contrivances by means of which the immunity reaction, so easily produced by all kinds of cells, is prevented from acting against the organism's own elements ... These contrivances are naturally of the highest importance for the individual'. The idea is so clearly formulated that all one has to do is to substitute 'contrivances' with self tolerance and 'horror autotoxicus' with S–NS discrimination to arrive at our understanding more than a century later.

'In my opinion, Paul Ehrlich was the greatest thinker ever in immunology', comments Dr. G. 'In his thinking he gave a clear priority to physiology, in contrast to the disease-centered thinking prevailing in medicine. I assume his sound basic principle could have been that health was the rule and disease the exception, and consequently mechanisms should exist to maintain health and their breakdown would cause disease. At that time, when darwinism had not yet found its way to medicine, Ehrlich invoked teleology in his arguments. But his reasoning was sound also from the evolutionary point of view, as evolution strives for functionality (health) by selecting against dysfunction (disease). Ehrlich also considered the immune response as a part of normal physiology, and not just as a reaction elicited by pathogens. This mental setting enabled him to make predictions about the immune system, which amaze us to date as being visionary. One of these predictions was "horror autotoxicus". Later generations of immunologists often misunderstood Ehrlich's theory as they thought that it would exclude the possibility of autoimmune disease for which there was increasing evidence.[25] Therefore they regarded "horror autotoxicus" as an obstacle to the progress in the research of autoimmune diseases. Now we know that Ehrlich was right. For self tolerance is the rule and autoimmune disease the exception. But they belong inseparably together: the former is the mechanism selected by evolution, and the latter represents the selective pressure for the development and maintenance of this mechanism.'

As already discussed (Section 9.1) Burnet and Fenner,[6] inspired by Owen's finding with dizygotic twin calves,[4] were the first to recognize the necessity of self tolerance in 1949. As they argued, the findings that foreign material or cells provoke an immune response while physically similar autologous material is inert demands the postulation of an active ability to distinguish between self and non-self. The merit of their thinking was that it directed the attention to a new, physiologically important mechanism (tolerance), and also offered a theoretical underpinning (S–NS discrimination) for it. Besides, they were the ones who introduced the terms 'self tolerance' and 'S–NS discrimination'. However, the mechanism they proposed – a 'self marker' that shuts down the immune response to all structures carrying it – was unsatisfactory, in fact, it did not even explain the Owen finding. Not surprisingly, it was soon refuted by scientists thinking about this problem, including Burnet himself.

The next intellectual incitement came with Jerne's natural selection theory of antibody formation[26] in 1955 (see also Section 1.1). This theory probably originated from Jerne's life-long fascination with natural antibodies (which culminated in his idiotype network theory 20 years later; see Section 5.4). Jerne envisaged the development of the immune system as a three-stage process (Fig. 9.1). At stage I, the generation of diversity (GOD) was proposed to occur by an undefined, possibly mutational process. (He elaborated on his view of GOD in his next theory in 1971; see Section 5.1.) The stage I repertoire was thought to be expressed as natural antibodies. Because at that time it became obligatory in every theory of immunity to provide an explanation for self tolerance, Jerne also had to deal with this question. His solution was to introduce stage II assumed to occur in embryonal life, at which the repertoire was exposed only to self antigens, and the antibodies which bound to (S) antigens were removed. Thus at

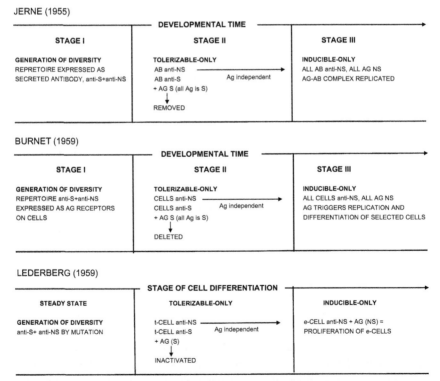

FIGURE 9.1 The three major early models of S–NS discrimination. AB: antibody, AG: antigen, NS: nonself, S: self. See text for further explanation. Based on References 8, 26, 31.

stage II the system was considered to be tolerizable-only. The remaining repertoire, by definition anti-NS, then entered stage III at which it was inducible-only.
Antibodies meeting their (NS) antigen at this stage were replicated.

This theory was a step forward regarding the explanation of tolerance, in that
it replaced the self marker of Burnet and Fenner by a selection step at stage II
for the elimination of anti-S. But the concept had also some obvious shortcomings. First of all, the antibodies binding antigen at stage III were considered to
direct their own replication, a view that was no longer tenable scientifically in
1955. Second, Jerne with all his admiration for the recognitive property of antibodies, disregarded their effector function. Thus stage II becomes unfeasible,
because antibodies binding to S would induce self-destruction. This thinking
error of Jerne turned out to be particularly instructive, because it helped realizing that the destructive effector arm of the immune system cannot be used for
S–NS discrimination. Third, the initial repertoire was expected to be vast, and
if it were expressed as secreted antibodies, no single antibody would attain sufficient concentration to function. But one cannot blame Jerne for this last error,
because most immunologists failed to appreciate this point until (and even after)
the appearance of the Protecton theory by Langman and Cohn[27] in 1987.

'Jerne's 1955 theory is usually praised as the first selectionist concept of immunology, but this is not quite correct for two reasons', add Dr. G. 'First, the theory had
instructionist elements, e.g., the self-replication of antigen-binding antibodies at
stage III. And second, if one defines a selectionist theory by the statement that the
antigen selects the appropriate specificity out of a pre-existing pool of antibodies,
then the first selectionist theory was in fact Ehrlich's side chain hypothesis in 1897
(see Section 1.1). Nevertheless, Jerne made one important step forward: whereas
Ehrlich could not conceive how the organism could be prepared in advance for
the virtually infinite range of antigens, Jerne pointed out that a great variety of
antibody specificities could be generated randomly at the beginning of the development of the immune system.'

One indisputable merit of Jerne's theory was that it served as an intellectual
stimulus, and thus seeded the next generation of concepts that strived for correcting its shortcomings. First in the row was Burnet, who published the initial version of his clonal selection theory in 1957 as 'A modification of Jerne's
theory...using the concept of clonal selection'.[28] A similar concept, also based
on the selection of cells instead of secreted antibodies was presented simultaneously by David Talmage.[29] By placing the antibody onto the surface of lymphocytes, and assuming that each lymphocyte has a single specificity, Burnet and
Talmage succeeded in correcting Jerne's first error (self-replicating antibodies)
as well as the second one (S–NS discrimination by absorption of antibodies to
self). The third error (a vast expressed antibody repertoire) was dealt with 2
years later by Talmage[30] and Lederberg.[31]

In the final version of the clonal selection theory[8] in 1959, Burnet proposed a hypothesis for S–NS discrimination (Fig. 9.1). He basically accepted

Jerne's three-stage scheme with the difference that at stage I the repertoire was expressed on cells, at stage II all cells reacting with S were deleted, and the remaining anti-NS cells then responded to antigen at stage III by proliferation and differentiation. Concerning the functional status of cells, at stage I they might have been inert (but this was unclear from the model), at stage II they were tolerizable-only, and the surviving (anti-NS) cells then differentiated in a presumably antigen-independent manner to stage III, inducible-only. In his model Burnet considered all stages to be dependent on the developmental time of the organism. Thus GOD as well as tolerance induction were thought to be once in a lifetime events. The problem with this view was that it considered tolerance induction as a static event, and thus could not account for the tolerization of anti-S cells that might arise later (by mutation) in the stage III population.

Lederberg,[31] who might have been dissatisfied with the static windows for GOD and tolerance, put forward a different model (Fig. 9.1). He proposed that GOD would operate throughout life (which makes good sense, as new lymphocytes also arise in a steady state), and he made the decision between tolerance or response dependent on the developmental stage of the cell, and not the organism. He assumed that lymphocytes were born as tolerizable-only ('t-cells'), and after a certain period when no antigen was encountered they would differentiate into effectors ('e-cells'), inducible-only. However, this model also had a problem of its own. As a consequence of the feature that t-cells cannot distinguish between S and NS, they become inactivated by both. Therefore S–NS discrimination in this model would only function properly in embryonal life when NS is practically absent. Later in life, in the presence of a pathogen load the precision of S–NS discrimination becomes the function of the time that t-cells need to differentiate into e-cells. If this time window is long, anti-NS cells become tolerized when NS (a pathogen) is present, and if the window is short anti-S cells will sneak through. Furthermore, the Lederberg model, similarly to the Burnet model, could not deal with unavoidable mutations to anti-S in the e-cell population.

This early upswing of S–NS discrimination theories was followed by a decade of fatigue for unknown reasons. Perhaps theoreticians realized that they could not clarify the problem any further without additional experimental input, or experimentalists became oversaturated with thoughts, which they were unable to translate into doable tests. Nevertheless, these early theories left long-lasting traces in the consciousness of immunologists so that the question of whether self tolerance would be established in the perinatal period (Burnet model) or throughout life (Lederberg model) was still a subject of debate four decades later.[32,33]

9.2.4 The Two-Signal or Associative-Recognition-of-Antigen Model

This model was first proposed by Bretscher and Cohn[34] in 1970, and has been updated and further refined over decades[14,35–39] so that now it stands alone as the most comprehensive theory of S–NS discrimination.

The seed of the two-signal idea came from Forsdyke,[40] who compared the activation of immune cells with the coincidence circuitry of a liquid scintillation counter, which reads one discharge in a single photo cell as noise, and only the simultaneous reading by both photocells is measured as a signal. Forsdyke[40] proposed that activation at one site might mean self for lymphocytes, and activation at both sites simultaneously might mean non-self.

The two-signal or associative-recognition-of-antigen (ARA) model, like its predecessors, was proposed in response to two kinds of need: first, there was a conceptual need to answer the questions left open by the previous models, and second, a practical need to account for new experimental findings.

Bretscher and Cohn recognized that the major common problem of earlier theories (Fig. 9.1) was the temporal separation of the 'tolerizable-only' and 'inducible-only' state of lymphocytes. Because cells in the 'inducible-only' state could no longer be tolerized, unavoidable mutations to anti-S in this cell population could not be controlled. In addition, the Burnet model could not account for the tolerization of newly arising cells produced throughout post-embryonal life, and the Lederberg model could only solve this problem at the cost of the precision of S–NS discrimination.

Of the new experimental facts, a series of hapten-carrier studies appeared to be most influential on the thinking of Bretscher and Cohn. In these experiments, antibody response to a small non-immunogenic molecule (hapten: H) coupled to an immunogenic carrier, e.g., poly-L-lysine (PLL), was measured.[41] In guinea pigs that could respond to PLL alone, H-PLL induced anti-H antibody, whereas animals genetically unresponsive to PLL failed to make antibody to the hapten. However, animals non-responders to PLL did produce anti-H antibody when immunized with the H-PLL conjugate complexed with a second immunogenic carrier, e.g., bovine serum albumin (BSA). But hapten-specific antibodies were not induced if the animals had previously been rendered unresponsive to BSA. In another set of experiments,[42] animals immunized with H-X (where X is a carrier protein) and another (non-cross-reacting) protein Y were shown to give a good secondary anti-H response when challenged with H-Y. This result has shown that the carrier-specific response must be induced, and this can happen independent of the anti-H response. Bretscher and Cohn interpreted these observations to indicate that:

1. For immunogenicity, at least two epitopes of an antigen (Ag) must be recognized
2. The recognition of the carrier (as well as hapten) epitope is specific
3. The carrier- (and possibly also the hapten-) specific cells are both inducible and tolerizable.

The initial version of the two-signal model[34] was based on the theoretical considerations and experimental facts above. Bretscher and Cohn proposed that all newly arising lymphocytes had two pathways open to them: inactivation (tolerance, paralysis, deletion, anergy) and activation. This was in contrast to previous models that considered lymphocytes to be born inactivatable-only. The decision between these pathways is brought about by two antigen-specific signals. Signal-1 follows the recognition of one epitope by the receptor of the cell to be induced, and Signal-2 the recognition of another epitope of the same Ag by a 'carrier antibody'. Signal-1 alone leads to paralysis, whereas signals-1+2 lead to activation. A unique feature of the model is that it 'delegates' S–NS discrimination to Signal-2. Signal-1 cannot discriminate, but if left alone it is interpreted by default as an interaction with S. At this point, the authors did not yet commit themselves to a particular cellular mechanism, but suggested that the 'carrier antibody' was likely to be T-cell-derived.

The stepwise amendments of the model (described in detail by Cohn[14,38]) will not be followed through here, only the matured version will be presented. The crucial postulates of this model are the following (Fig. 9.2A):

1. Stem cells give rise to monospecific ('clonal') lymphocytes that are in the 'initial' state (iB and iT), in which they can recognize Ag but cannot perform effector functions. Sorting of the repertoire into anti-S and anti-NS (i.e., S–NS discrimination) can only occur in the i-state, because this process entails the recognition of S which must remain without consequence (i.e., without destruction of S).

2. Interaction of the antigen-receptor of i-cells (iB, iT) results in Signal-1. This event drives the cells to the 'anticipatory' a-state, in which they become receptive to Signal-2. The proposal of an a-state was necessary to ensure that the signals are received in the correct order (Signal-1 followed by Signal-2).

3. The a-cell, in the absence of Signal-2, is put onto the inactivation (tolerance) pathway. Alternatively, the a-cell receives Signal-2 provided by an effector T helper (eTh) cell via associative (linked) recognition of the same Ag, and becomes activated. Because Signal-1 itself is non-discriminatory, the eTh cell must have previously undergone S–NS discrimination to be able to 'tell' the a-cell that the Ag is NS. Steps 2 and 3 complete S–NS discrimination (also referred to as Decision 1) under the ARA model.

4. An unseparable extension of the model deals with the fate of cells that have received both signals (activated cells). These cells become responsive to cytokines which promote their proliferation and differentiation into effector (e)-cells. The cytokine-driven step is necessary to ensure a sufficiently fast response to growing pathogens. At this stage S–NS is no longer monitored, but mutants to anti-S that may sneak through can be controlled by requiring e-cells to revert to the i-stage after the antigen was eliminated, or be short-lived and dead-end. Because the interplay of cytokines influences the effector response, step 4 is considered to be part of the 'determination of effector class', or Decision 2.

Several features of the ARA model require further explanation.

The importance of time in the model has to be emphasized. This applies, for example, to the length of the a-state. After receiving Signal-1, the a-cells will

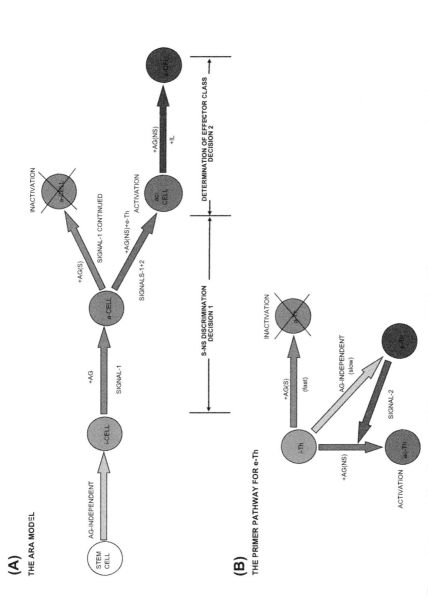

FIGURE 9.2   The associative-recognition-of-antigen (ARA) or two-signal model (A), and the proposed antigen-independent 'primer' pathway for e-Th cells (B). a: anticipatory, ac: activated, AG: antigen, e: effector, i: initial, IL: interleukin, NS: nonself, S: self, Th: T helper cell. Based on Reference 14.

be irreversibly inactivated with an estimated half life of about half a day[38] in the absence of Signal-2. To rescue the a-cell, Signal-2 must be delivered within this timeframe, which is a non-trivial requirement, because of the paucity of eTh cells recognizing the same Ag. Thus an appropriate steady-state frequency of eTh cells must be assured to be able to provide Signal-2 within the window of half a day. Another point where time is critical in the model is the generation of eTh cells as will be discussed below.

A critical question raised in connection with the ARA model was the following: if effector cells can only be generated by interaction with an eTh, how does the first eTh cell arise? Or in more general terms: how does the immune system get started? This was referred to as the 'primer problem' by the authors, and the 'chicken and egg problem' by their opponents. The solution to this problem proposed in 1983 and thereafter[3,35] was that there must be a third, *antigen-independent* pathway unique to helpers that provides the primer eTh (Fig. 9.2B). This pathway must also undergo S–NS discrimination, and therefore the time needed to differentiate into eTh in the absence of antigen must be longer than the time required for the inactivation of anti-S. If any Ag is encountered during this differentiation period, the iTh cell will be sent to the inactivation pathway. The pathway proposed for eTh cells thus works by a 'one signal versus no signal' mechanism, similarly to the Lederberg model (Section 9.2.3).

The way the immune system gets started was envisaged as follows. There is a period in ontogeny (embryonal life) when Ags defined as S are present ('prior'), those defined as NS are absent ('posterior'), and Ag-specific cells are absent. As i-cells start to emerge they will either meet Ag (by definition S) and be inactivated for lack of eTh to provide Signal-2, or do not find Ag and accumulate as anti-NS. At the same time, iTh anti-NS cells start their Ag-independent pathway to become eTh anti-NS. When a sufficient level of eTh is reached, the system becomes responsive, i.e., i-cells anti-NS can obtain Signal-2 and respond to Ags NS. Tolerance to S will be maintained as long as S is expressed ('persistent'), because of the lack of eTh anti-S. Thus under the ARA model self tolerance is established early in ontogeny, similarly to the Burnet model, but in contrast to the latter, the ARA model permits S–NS discrimination to continue life-long (as in the Lederberg model) under the control of eTh anti-NS.

One important limitation of the ARA model is that it permits lymphocyte activation by foreign Ags that share epitopes with S, which results in breaking of self tolerance and eventually autoimmune disease. Specifically, this situation arises when an i-cell recognizes a S epitope and the eTh a NS epitope of Ags S+NS. Since about 10% of NS Ags share epitopes with S, the ARA model would allow for an unacceptably high incidence of autoimmune diseases. To deal with this limitation, Langman and Cohn[43] proposed that there is competition between activation by S+NS and inactivation by S+S' at the level of the a-cell. Because S+S' Ags are persistent and usually available at larger amounts in the body than S+NS Ags, the competition is likely to be in favor of self antigens (= inactivation). It is therefore conceivable that such competition could keep the incidence of autoimmune diseases at the observed low (~1%) frequency.

Finally, a special feature of the ARA model, namely that it reaches beyond S–NS discrimination deserves mention here. As pointed out above, the Ag-receptor of each lymphocyte recognizes a single epitope, and this (Signal-1) leads to inactivation. Tolerance is thus epitope-by-epitope under this model (as well as in all previous models). However, an Ag is defined by the immune system as a set of linked epitopes, and thus a minimum of two linked epitopes must be recognized by a minimum of two different cells in order to identify an Ag. The ARA model, by requiring two associative recognition events for activation, implies that before the induction of an immune response epitopes are translated into an Ag, i.e., that induction occurs antigen-by-antigen (in contrast to previous models, in which both tolerance and induction were epitope-by-epitope). This feature is essential, as the immune system is selected upon to eliminate Ags and not epitopes, and to do this effectively the class of effector response ('Decision 2') to linked epitopes must be coordinated (e.g., for complement activation, antibodies to each epitope of the antigen should be complement binding; a mixture of complement binding and non-binding antibodies would be less effective or ineffective).

The description given here highlights the ARA model as an impressive intellectual edifice, and thus one would expect that the model should have gained wide acceptance in the immunological community. This has not been the case, however, for reasons that have to do mostly with mechanistic details rather than with the concept itself.

The origin of problems was that in 1970 when the model was first formulated nothing was known of either the antigen receptor of T cells or the nature of its ligand, and thus the cellular interactions required for the delivery of Signal-2 were assumed to take place through an 'antigen-bridge' (see in Fig. 8.3A). By 1975, however, it became clear that Th cells recognize antigen in a class II MHC-restricted fashion (Section 8.1.3), and this finding limited the possible interactions of Th cells to partners that constitutively express class II, i.e., B cells and dendritic cells. Because T cells usually fail to express class II, or the latter is only sporadically induced, the mechanism of postulated T–T-cell interactions has become obscure. The next problem came 10 years later with the discovery that T cells recognize peptide fragments of the antigen (Section 7.1.1), which rendered associative recognition through the antigen-bridge unfeasible. A 'surrogate' for linked recognition has, however, remained possible, provided that the peptides presented by an antigen-presenting cell (APC) all derive from one single antigen, i.e., that the APC is monospecific. This condition is met only in the case of Ig receptor-mediated antigen uptake by B cells (see Section 8.1.3 and Fig. 8.3B). Therefore, a strictly antigen-specific interaction as predicted by the model seems only possible in Th–B-cell collaboration.

MHC-restricted peptide recognition has thus become a serious challenge for the model as far as T–T-cell interactions are concerned. A number of studies addressed this problem experimentally. The first evidence for T–T-cell interactions came from experiments showing that the induction of cytotoxic T lymphocyte precursors (Tcp) required interaction with Th cells recognizing antigen on the same APC.[44–46] This implies that the Tcp must be in close physical proximity to the Th cell in order to receive help. More recent studies[47,48] have demonstrated that the actual help is delivered through a molecular interaction between CD40L expressed on the Th cell and CD40 on the APC. The preferred model for help thus envisages that the Th cell induces costimulatory activity of the APC, and the latter in turn activates Tcp. However, because some CD8 cells express CD40,[49] a direct Th–Tcp interaction is also possible.

The question of Th–Th-cell interaction has also been pursued experimentally, mostly by Peter Bretscher and his colleagues. Here the rules appear to be similar to those in Tcp–Th cooperation. Thus the epitopes recognized by the two Th cells must be physically linked[50–52] implying that they should be presented by the same APC. But some controversy has remained regarding the molecular interaction that mediates help. According to Bretscher and coworkers,[52,53] the OX40–OX40L interaction is responsible for this and the CD40–CD40L interaction is not involved, whereas Zanetti and colleagues[51] state that both interactions are required. Because OX40 and OX40L may be expressed on both Th cell and APC, it has remained unclear whether the delivery of help occurs through Th–APC or Th–Th interaction (or both).

Taken together, T–T-cell cooperations have been demonstrated beyond doubt, but the proposed three-cell-cluster arrangement (Tpc–Th–APC, or Th–Th–APC) cannot ensure Ag-specificity of the interaction, unless the APC only presented a single Ag at a time, which cannot be taken for granted. The specificity problem finally prompted Peter Bretscher to propose a modification of the model, in which Signal-2 would be delivered only when two interacting T cells recognized two epitopes presented by one and the same B cell.[39] This model would solve the problem, but has so far little experimental support.[54]

In summary, the ARA model appears mechanistically feasible in Th–B-cell interactions. The Achilles' heel of the model is T–T-cell cooperation, because Ag-specificity becomes fuzzy here, and thus this interaction cannot safely control S–NS discrimination.

'The ARA model had a rocky intellectual history.' adds Dr. G 'At first it was overshadowed for a decade by Jerne's idiotype network theory (see Section 5.4), which promised a solution for all aspects of immunoregulation. Particularly young scientists were enthusiastic about the network, because it represented a new way of thinking, and its acceptance thus permitted them a demarcation from the previous generation; a general ambition of the young. The "two-signal" concept appeared corny in comparison: it reminded them of some old ideas generated at a time when they were still in kindergarten. Of course, they ignored that all ideas in science have roots in the past (another privilege of the youth). After the network theory had faded away, the idea of a two-signal activation mode of lymphocytes became extremely popular, but there was disagreement about the nature of Signal-2 (see Section 9.2.5). Nevertheless, the core idea, i.e., that Signal-1 leads to inactivation and Signals-1+2 to activation, has gained general acceptance, and it is now considered to be the most important contribution to conceptual immunology since the clonal selection theory even by opponents of the ARA model.'[55]

9.2.5 Alternative Models

After 1970, most immunologists (except enthusiasts of the idiotype network) started to think in terms of a two-signal mechanism for lymphocyte activation, and thus the models to be described here all have this feature in common.

The first 'alternative' two-signal model to follow the Bretscher-Cohn theory was put forward by two outstanding thinkers at the John Curtin School, Kevin Lafferty and Alastair Cunningham,[56] in 1975. This model was based on Lafferty's previous work on allogeneic interactions, and was originally meant to explain alloreactivity. Over the course of his studies, Lafferty noted that alloantigen alone was not sufficient to trigger allograft rejection. In addition, a 'second signal' he called 'allogeneic stimulus' was required that was provided by a metabolically active allogeneic cell of hematopoietic origin.[57] In the absence of this 'stimulator cell' allogeneic organ grafts were accepted,[58] but adding small numbers of allogeneic spleen or peritoneal exudate cells induced rapid rejection of previously tolerated grafts.[59] Lafferty and Cunningham therefore proposed that the induction of alloresponses requires receptor-mediated interaction of lymphocytes with the antigen as a first signal, plus a second signal (later termed co-stimulator[60]) provided by a special stimulator cell. The authors also pointed out that the requirement for a stimulator (i.e., antigen-presenting cell; APC)-derived second signal may apply to all immune responses. Thus in this model, Signal-1 was identical with that of the Bretscher-Cohn scheme, although tolerogenicity of Signal-1 alone was not postulated. However, Signal-2 was entirely different: it was APC-derived (instead of Th-cell-derived) and was not antigen-specific. The precise nature of Signal-2 remained undefined.

The problem with this model is that the cell to be activated cannot 'know' whether the antigen (Signal-1) is S or NS, and the non-specific second signal cannot provide this information either, i.e., the model cannot account for S–NS discrimination. The proposed mode of activation would only work safely (i.e., without the risk of autoimmunity), if the repertoire were previously purged completely of anti-S reactivity. But mutations of anti-NS to anti-S as well as mutations of S itself after repertoire purging would remain a risk of uncontrolled autoimmunity. For fairness sake, one should point out, however, that the authors themselves did not regard their hypothesis as a model for S–NS discrimination. After the discovery of co-stimulatory molecules 10–15 years later (see Section 8.7.2), the Lafferty-Cunningham model transcended in all interpretations of the biological role of co-stimulation.

The next version of two-signal models, already with the aim of explaining S–NS discrimination, was proposed by Janeway.[15,61] In his model, Janeway acknowledged the necessity of clonal deletion for elimination of cells reacting to S antigens encountered early in lymphocyte development, as well as the requirement for a second signal to control the response versus tolerance decision later, upon encounter of antigen. The novel element of the model was the nature of the second signal. In his reasoning Janeway emphasized the role of the innate immune system. He pointed out that the innate system is uniquely equipped to recognize conserved microbial constituents absent from the host, referred to as pathogen-associated molecular patterns (PAMPs), by pattern recognition receptors (PRRs).[62] Because the effector mechanisms of the adaptive immune system are almost invariably 'borrowed' from the innate system, the PRRs of the latter could provide Signal-2 for lymphocyte activation. This way the adaptive system would only become activated against infectious NS, and would not react to innocuous (non-infectious) S. As to details of the mechanism, Janeway considered Signal-2 to be provided by co-stimulatory molecules. Expression of the latter is indeed induced by PAMPs in B cells and macrophages.[63] However, responses to pathogens that succeeded to evade recognition of their PAMPs remained to be explained. Janeway proposed that dendritic cells may represent the answer of evolution to this problem, because they express co-stimulatory molecules constitutively.

Although the infectious non-self concept is rather original, its usefulness in explaining S–NS discrimination is questionable. Instead of listing here the arguments supporting this statement, let us consider the complement system as an example of effector mechanisms used in both innate and adaptive immunity. Complement activation by the innate system (alternate pathway) is based on the recognition of PAMPs. However, the classical pathway is triggered alone by antibodies, and if the latter happen to be autoantibodies binding to a self molecule, complement would cause autoimmune damage. In this case the effector mechanism is decoupled from pattern recognition, and placed fully under the control of the adaptive system, consequently, only the latter can make S–NS discrimination. In general, because S–NS discrimination by the innate system is germ-line encoded, by definition, it cannot function in sorting a somatically generated random receptor repertoire into anti-S and anti-NS. However, this is not meant to underestimate the importance of PAMPs and PRRs in host defense. They are indispensable for the innate system, and may have another interface with the adaptive system in the regulation of effector response (discussed in Section 9.2.6).

'The essay presenting the infectious non-self model in *Immunology Today*[15] was probably Charlie's best brainchild', comments Dr. G. 'But not because of the parable of "infectious non-self versus non-infectious self" that was known by almost everybody including those who only read the title. Its real merit was that it represented the first serious effort to conceptualize the relationship between the innate and adaptive immune systems in terms of both function and evolution. This brilliant essay called the attention of immunologists to the previously neglected area of innate immunity, and it must have also provided the intellectual stimulus for the discovery of the immunological role of Toll-like receptors in Charlie's laboratory.'[64]

The most influential and popular version of two signal models was the 'danger hypothesis' proposed by Polly Matzinger. The model was first presented in an admirably lucid and insightful review article on T-cell tolerance.[21] Its leading thesis is that the immune system's task is to distinguish between dangerous and innocuous rather than NS and S. This idea is reminiscent of Janeway's infectious non-self versus non-infectious self[15] with the difference that 'danger' replaces infectious non-self.

'With all the merits of this essay I must add that it had also a generous dose of Matzingerian theatricality', interjects Dr. G. 'This applies particularly to the introduction where Polly made statements, such as: "This essay is about tolerance, but also about something deeper. about the belief that the immune system's primary driving force is the need to discriminate between self and non-self. I have abandoned this belief." This has almost the drama of a Shakespeare monologue (with the protagonist, Polly, standing alone, spotlit in the middle of the stage). Curiously, it has turned out from the subsequent detailing of the model that Polly could not get away entirely without S–NS discrimination either.'

Three types of argument were brought up for the need of a new paradigm to replace S–NS discrimination. First, it was the presence of autoantibodies and potentially autoreactive T cells. This aspect has already been discussed as the problem of how to define 'immunological self' (Section 9.2.2). Second, the existence of T-cell tolerance of peripheral self molecules not encountered in the thymus required explanation. Meanwhile this problem has largely been solved by the display of peripheral self in the thymus (discussed in Section 9.3.4). Third, the sheer number of self proteins to be tolerant of appeared too high. As we pointed out before (Section 8.4.4), by our calculation the deletion of TCR reacting to MHC-bound peptides derived from *all* self proteins is manageable without crippling the anti-NS repertoire. Another problem raised in this context was to induce tolerance to all distinct 'idiotypic' sequences of T- and B-cell receptors, the number of which was estimated to be 10^{12}! However, this number is clearly an overestimate, if for no other reason, because most vertebrates do not harbor so many lymphocytes. More recent data and theoretical considerations (Section 8.4.4) would limit the size of the functional T- plus B-cell repertoire to approximately 5×10^6. In principle, one receptor would produce ~2 hypervariable 'idiotypic' peptides (one per receptor chain), the overwhelming majority of which would be destroyed by antigen processing, and many of the remaining intact peptides would fail to bind to the MHC allotypes expressed in the host. Considering these limitations, the total 'idiotypic load' to self tolerance may be $\ll 10^6$ different peptides.

Taken together, the puzzling aspects of self tolerance that appeared to Matzinger 'intriguing, mystic and unsatisfactory' in 1994 have meanwhile found an explanation without the need for a new paradigm.

The actual danger model incorporated elements of all previous two-signal hypotheses. Its major postulates are the following.

1. Recognition of antigen, i.e., Signal-1, in the absence of Signal-2 leads to cell death. This should apply to both T and B cells (although it was not explicitly stated for the latter). Signal-1 is thus identical to that of the Bretscher-Cohn and Janeway models.

2. Signal-2 to B cells is provided by Th cells as in the Bretscher-Cohn model. Because B cells take up Ag specifically via their Ig receptor, they present under physiological conditions only one single Ag, and consequently the B–Th-cell interaction remains antigen-specific. The S–NS discrimination of B cells is thus placed under the control of Th cells.

3. Thymocytes cannot accept Signal-2, and thus recognition of (self) Ag in the thymus leads to deletion. Under this model only those thymocytes must be deleted, which recognize Ags normally found on APCs (i.e., those derived from the APCs' own proteins and from ubiquitous circulating proteins).

4. After leaving the thymus, naïve T cells purged of anti-S of APC are allowed to receive Signal-2 *only* from 'professional' APC (dendritic cells; DC). Signal-2 in this case is co-stimulation as in the Lafferty-Cunningham model. Recognition of Ag on any other cell type of the body would lead to deletion. This arrangement would allow tolerance of peripheral S Ags not encountered in the thymus, including those undergoing late somatic variation such as 'idiotypic' peptides presented on B cells. The proposed mechanism for peripheral tolerance is thus a mechanistic variant of the Bretscher-Cohn postulate that Signal-1 alone leads to inactivation.

'To my appreciation postulate 4 delegates too much responsibility to DCs', adds Dr. G 'which carries the risk of increased vulnerability. For example, assume that some activated T cells mutate to anti-S of APC, or that the APCs, due to some change in hormonal regulation or the like, alter their presented spectrum of self peptides. Both cases would result in generalized autoimmunity, or what may even be worse, in a complete depletion of APCs. Clearly, a DC-derived "generic" (not Ag-specific) second signal could only work in reality, if neither the T cell nor the APC changed, or if the frequency of changes were too low to provide a selective pressure against this mechanism.'

5. Effector cells (T and B) must ignore Signal-2. They should perform their function upon receiving Signal-1 (Ag recognition) regardless of any other signal. They should subsequently die or revert to the resting state in a short period of time (to restrict damage by effectors mutated to anti-S).

It is interesting to note that the eye-catcher 'danger' finds no application in this first formulation of the model. Only a short section at the end of the article deals with danger, defined as tissue destruction that activates APCs. It appears therefore that this is in fact a classical model of S–NS discrimination with a different label.

In later elaborations of the model[65,66] 'danger' was given a closer definition as a set of tissue-derived signals that inform about damage, for example, the exposure of hydrophobicity, nucleic acids, heat-shock proteins, interferon alpha, products of hyaluron, etc. By that time it has become increasingly clear that such danger signals may play an important role in the regulation of the effector response. But the new insights failed to provide any additional clue as to why these signals should also be involved in the *initiation* of immune response.

One common feature of the Janeway and Matzinger models is that they both 'borrow' the second signal from outside the adaptive immune system, signals that are more likely to be used in the regulation of effector response. What could have prompted the authors to postulate that signals such as pathogenicity and tissue damage should serve as the initiator of immune response?

'In addition to the arguments given by the authors, one reason could have been that it is extremely difficult to determine the point at which activation ends and effector differentiation begins', points out Dr. G. 'For example, certain pathogen-derived substances can "tune" DCs immediately after uptake of the pathogen toward the favored effector class.[67] In such a case activation and effector differentiation set out almost simultaneously. But this does not necessarily imply that these substances were used as Signal-2 for activation. It is more likely that the system utilizes ancient evolutionary experience as a "preliminary information" to shift the response toward the desired effector class as early as possible. By common sense (and under the ARA model), effector differentiation can only set forth *after* the cells became activated.'

'It is another question whether the initiation of immune response can rely solely on the activation of APCs by pathogen- or tissue-derived signals. I have some doubts about this. Firstly, because Charlie's PARPs are not associated with all antigens that must be eliminated. Secondly, the timepoint at which tissue destruction occurs to produce Polly's danger signals may be too late for starting an immune response against fast-growing pathogens. Thus the only conceivable way to use APC-derived co-stimulation as Signal-2 would be, if it were expressed irrespective of what antigen was taken up, or if its expression were constitutive. And, of course, this Signal-2 could never make S–NS discrimination, and thus it would only work in a T-cell repertoire that is *perfectly* free from anti-S.'

'Beside these considerations, there is recent evidence showing that a destructive immune response can develop in the complete absence of any pathogen- or host tissue-derived "danger" signal.'[68]

9.2.6 An Aside on the Regulation of Effector Response

As pointed out above, in the two most recent models of lymphocyte activation,[15,65] Signal-2 became intermingled inseparably with the regulation of effector response. In view of this, the question of how effector responses may be regulated merits a brief discussion at here. This discussion will also remain largely theoretical, because effector regulation is one of the least explored areas in immunology.

In principle, the goals of immune effector response are twofold: first, to deal with pathogens and other harmful substances as effectively as possible, and second, to do as little damage to self tissues as possible. Since the substances produced by the effector response can be equally harmful to both host and pathogen, these two goals are conflicting, and therefore the immune system can only control the response by monitoring progress toward these goals.

At least two aspects of the effector response are envisaged to require regulation. One is the choice of the appropriate effector class. Because not all classes are effective in eliminating a particular invader, the immune system must be able to decide about the type of effector response that deals with the attack most effectively, e.g., which antibody isotype, with or without complement, which cytokines, Th cell types, cytotoxic T cells, B cells, macrophages etc. The choice of effector response should comprise a selection for the more effective response types and suppression of the ineffective ones (because the latter would compete with the former). The second aspect is quantitative regulation, i.e., how much of the listed effector types is needed at any given stage of the response, including the termination of responses after the invader was eliminated.

How the immune system manages to exercise such a complex regulation is unclear, although some principles begin to emerge. The most important prerequisite for effector regulation is that the initial response should encompass a broad range of different effector types.[33,69,70] A broad initial response would allow the system to test each effector class and select the most efficient ones during the course of an infection. Although this statement is seemingly contradicted by findings showing that microbial products can influence effector differentiation very early after activation,[67,71–73] it should be emphasized that what these data demonstrate is a bias toward a given effector class and not a presetting of the response. It is generally agreed that a pre-determined, stereotyped response would be too rigid to be able to accomplish its goals.

As proposed by Segel and Bar-Or,[69] monitoring of the effector response should occur by feedback from the end results of the process. Feedback can be provided by different substances of the pathogen on the one hand, and by damaged self tissues on the other. For example, increased amounts of a pathogen-derived external or secreted molecule could indicate that the pathogen is growing, whereas an intracellular molecule would signal that the pathogen is being killed. Similarly, host tissue-derived 'danger' factors could serve as indicators of damage to self. The thoughtful analysis of Segel and Bar-Or thus places the Signal-2 candidates of Janeway[15] and Matzinger[21] in their proper context, for the use of 'pathogenicity' and 'danger' as success indicators of the effector response is much more likely than their presumed role in lymphocyte activation.

How the immune system senses and quantitates these signals is not quite clear. Presumably macrophages, the 'terminal station' of every effector response, play a major role here. Macrophages are 'professional eaters' like a restaurant tester, and are thus likely to be 'aware' of what they have ingested. And there is no reason to believe that they would retain this information rather than communicating it to other cells involved in the response. There is some evidence in the literature in support of this assumption. For example, it is known that *Leishmania major* and *Listeria monocytogenes*, when taken up by macrophages, establish intracellular infection. Infected macrophages then secrete IL-12 that drives the development of Th1 cells producing interferon-γ, the cytokine needed for the clearance of infection.[74] This example illustrates how a pathogen-derived signal is 'translated' into a cytokine signal, which in turn is used to communicate the 'event' with other cell types needed to participate in the response. In view of the known versatility of cytokines, it is reasonable to assume that they serve as the 'language' that permits communication between different effector cell types.

But cytokines are also major players as effector molecules, and this raises the question of how the optimal 'cocktail' of them is made up to suit the requirements of a given response. In this respect, the first useful insight was provided by the discovery of the effector subclasses Th1 and Th2 (Section 8.6.3). Meanwhile we also have Th3 and Th17, and thus the trend appears to be that effector Th cells will be divided into an increasing number of subsets that produce small, distinct arrays of cytokines. In this context a study by Paul Lehmann's group[75] deserves mention. These authors investigated cytokine co-expression by single cells using a two-color enzyme-linked immunospot assay. They demonstrated that the great majority (~95%) of 'committed' effector Th cells produced one single cytokine, a finding that has appeared enigmatic for more than a decade. But in the frame of this analysis, the expression of a single cytokine per cell represents the final resolution of functional subsets, which would permit the most precise composition of effector response by the recruitment of the desired numbers of cells producing certain cytokines.

The purpose of this brief mental exercise has been to illustrate how the immune system might use pathogen- and host-derived signals as feedback information for the regulation of its effector output aiming to achieve efficient elimination of pathogens with as little 'collateral damage' to the host as possible.

9.2.7 The Bottom Line

The question of how the immune system provides protection against invaders while in most cases avoids damage to host tissues has certainly been the most difficult one in immunology. Theoretical approaches to this problem have yielded a number of interesting insights, but could not completely solve the problem even after the conceptualization of recent data.

The most fruitful idea has been the two-signal hypothesis, whose postulates that Signal-1 alone should lead to inactivation (tolerance) could not be replaced by any better proposal until now. However, a number of problems have arisen with respect to Signal-2, which was postulated to be necessary for lymphocyte activation.

Under the associative-recognition-of-antigen (ARA) model (Section 9.2.4), Signal-2 is provided by an effector T helper (Th) cell upon simultaneous recognition of another epitope of the same antigen. The cell to be activated reads Signal-1 alone as self, and the 'GO' signal is the combined Signals1+2, of which Signal-2 should ensure that the antigen is foreign. Thus this model 'delegates' self–non-self (S–NS) discrimination to the effector Th cell. The model is mechanistically feasible in T–B-cell collaboration, because the B cell can only take up one single antigen by receptor-mediated endocytosis and present peptides thereof bound to its class II MHC molecules. Thus although antigen processing disrupts the continuity of epitopes, their origin from a single antigen is ensured. However, the application of the ARA model to T–T-cell interactions is problematic, because a direct interaction is unfeasible due to the incapability of T cells to process antigen and their failure to express class II MHC. Thus the interaction can only take place on the surface of a third cell, usually an antigen-presenting cell (APC) that is not monospecific, i.e., a dendritic cell or a macrophage. Because these APCs can present peptides of different antigens simultaneously, the two T cells may recognize peptides derived from different antigens, and thus the effector Th cell can no longer 'tell' its partner cell whether the antigen the latter recognizes is S or NS. The proposal that the APC would keep all peptides processed from a single antigen together on the cell surface[76] in a 'signalling patch' would solve the problem, but there is no mechanism for this known.

Other Signal-2 candidates such as 'pathogenicity' or 'danger' are not feasible as discussed before (Section 9.2.5). These signals are more likely to play a role in the regulation of effector response (Section 9.2.6).

The remaining option is to replace the antigen-specific Signal-2 of the ARA model with a non-specific co-stimulatory signal provided by the APC (Section 9.2.5). Indeed, most experimental support for the two-signal concept came from studies in which co-stimulation was considered to be Signal-2 (Section 8.7.2). The problem with this model is that it cannot account for 'peripheral' tolerance. Mutants anti-S of APC that may arise post-thymically in the mature T-cell population, or a change in the presentation of S antigens by APC would result in uncontrolled autoimmunity.

In conclusion, the hypothesis that came closest to an all-embracing explanation of S–NS discrimination was the ARA model. The weakness of this model lies in mechanistic problems of antigen-specific T–T-cell interactions. Alternative hypotheses that replace the antigen-specific second signal with a non-specific one fail to explain S–NS discrimination, and thus can only be regarded as models for lymphocyte activation.

9.3 THE ERA OF MECHANISTIC STUDIES

9.3.1 Clonal Deletion of T Cells

As discussed before (Section 9.1), the prediction of the clonal selection theory that self-reactive cell clones should be deleted during ontogeny has proven very difficult to approach experimentally for a long time (exactly for 28 years), because the frequency of individual clones is far below the detection limit of available methods. This technical limitation could never really be overcome. Fortunately, however, studies of T-cell receptor (TCR) expression toward the end of the 1980s opened up an unexpected novel approach. By this time serological studies of the TCR yielded a sizeable battery of monoclonal antibodies (mAbs), many of which proved to be specific for distinct V regions of the receptor. An obvious question to address with the aid of these antibodies was whether Jerne's prediction that TCR V regions are specific for allelic variants of the major histocompatibility complex (MHC) could be substantiated by experimental results.

To the disappointment of many immunologists, no clear correlation could be demonstrated between the expression of a particular TCR V segment and the MHC alleles present in the same mouse. But there were a couple of exceptions, the most notable being Vβ17a discovered by the Kappler-Marrack team in Denver.[2] Vβ17a is a rare allelic form of Vβ17 present only in four of the known inbred mouse strains, and detected specifically by the mAb KJ23a. The key finding was that the majority (up to 90%) of T-cell hybridomas prepared from Vβ17a$^+$ T cells reacted with the I-E class II MHC molecule, apparently irrespective of the other variable elements of TCR. Thus this germ-line-encoded V segment seemed to have per se an appreciable affinity for a particular MHC molecule. Three of the four *Vβ17a* mouse strains, SWR, SJL and C57L, also harbored a measurable frequency (~4–15%) of peripheral T cells expressing the corresponding V segment. These strains had one more property in common: they failed to express I-E molecules due to different genetic defects. In contrast, the fourth strain, C57BR, that expressed the I-E^k molecule had no Vβ17a$^+$ T cells despite the presence of the corresponding allele in the genome.[77] The KJ23a mAb was then used to demonstrate that the Vβ17a$^+$ T cells in this strain were eliminated before reaching maturation in the thymus. This was the very first demonstration of clonal deletion as a mechanism of tolerance to a self MHC molecule. It was enabled by the frequency of self-reactive Vβ17a$^+$ cells that was sufficiently high to be detected by flow cytometry.

Another, even more revealing set of studies utilized a non-MHC self antigen encoded by the *Mls* (minor lymphocyte stimulating) locus. The *Mls* locus discovered by Hilliard Festenstein in 1973 had been one of the long-standing enigmas in immunology.[78] It has at least two alleles, *Mls^a* and *Mls^b*, and the product of *Mls^a* stimulates a strong mixed lymphocyte reaction but no cytotoxic T-cell response in MHC-identical *Mls^b* strains. Thus the Mls antigen behaves as a class II MHC molecule but it is not encoded in the MHC. The use of TCR-specific mAbs helped to finally resolve the Mls puzzle in 1988, and at a stroke also provided the first evidence for clonal deletion as a mechanism of tolerance to non-MHC self antigens. These studies were conducted independently by two groups, one was again the Kappler-Marrack team in Denver, and the other the 'united Swiss immunology forces' including Rolf Zinkernagel's group in Zurich, and the Ludwig Institute for Cancer Research in Lausanne. Their results appeared side-by-side in *Nature*.[79,80] The Denver group used Vβ8-specific mAbs to demonstrate that one member of this V region family, Vβ8.1, was absent from the peripheral T cells of mice carrying the *Mls*[a] gene, whereas *Mls*[b] mice expressed Vβ8.1 in 4–8% of T cells. They then went on to demonstrate that immature cortical thymocytes expressed Vβ8.1 normally, but mature medullary thymocytes, similarly to peripheral T cells, were devoid of Vβ8.1^{+} cells. They concluded that these cells must have been eliminated at the stage of transition from immature to mature cells in the thymus. Analogous results were obtained by the Swiss group by the use of a newly produced Vβ6-specific mAb that detected 4–10% positive T cells in *Mls*[b] and practically none in *Mls*[a] mice. A year later a third Vβ segment, Vβ9, was reported[81] to react to and be deleted by Mls[a].

'At this place I would like to say a few words about Rob MacDonald, the senior author on the paper of the Swiss group', adds Dr. G. 'Rob was a quiet, superbly intelligent young (compared to me) Canadian immunologist, a permanent member of the Lausanne group. One of his specialities was his perfectly controlled precise language: when Rob gave a seminar, you could have written it down as said, and this would have made a publication without any further correction. Not surprisingly, he was extremely productive, publishing more than anyone else I've ever met. Furthermore, he was humble, without any trace of the almost epidemic egomania among immunologists, so that this quality alone would have sufficed to consider him unique.'

Taken together, the results above have made a strong case for clonal deletion as a mechanism by which self-reactivity is purged from the T-cell repertoire. Furthermore, they have explained the vigorous reactivity to Mls[a] by the participation in the response of T cells expressing three different Vβ segments, which can make up 10–20% of peripheral T cells. The Mls model also enabled the visualization of thymic deletion by immunohistology,[82] and the demonstration that the mechanism of deletion was apoptotic cell death.[83]

'But these results also had a disquieting aspect, when it came to the question whether the responses used in these studies could be regarded as representative of normal T-cell responses to peptide–MHC (pMHC) complexes', comments Dr. G. 'One difference was obvious: whereas the specificity of TCR to pMHC is usually dependent on the sum of its variable elements, in these particular responses a single V segment seemed to impose specificity on the TCR irrespective of the other variable elements. In the case of Vβ17a this was still conceivable, because the capability of TCR to dock on pMHC implies that the V segments may have a germ-line-selected specificity for MHC. However the finding that Mls[a], a single self molecule not involved in antigen presentation, can selectively react with three of the 20–30 germ-line-encoded Vβ segments was beyond any rationale. On the other hand, anti-Mls responses required class II MHC, usually I-E, one of the two expressed class II molecules in mice, and in this respect they resembled a normal T helper (Th) cell response. At this point the elucidation of the nature of anti-Mls response had to stop, because the stimulating molecule itself remained unknown.'

'As a way out of this deadlock, a search was started for known molecules with antigenic characteristics similar to those of Mls. This approach was a success, and soon a number of such molecules were identified including bacterial toxins[84–87] and endogenous retroviral proteins.[88–93] Indeed Mls itself was also likely to be the product of a retroviral gene.[87] All these molecules were collectively termed "superantigen", a designation that could have better served as a buzzword in a TV commercial than in science. But it was very effective in raising the interest of immunologists (who were, like everyone else, tamed to TV commercials). Binding studies with superantigens have revealed that they interact with conserved residues of class II MHC molecules that are distant from the peptide-binding site,[85,94–96] and with TCR Vβ residues that are also well away from the interaction site for pMHC.[97] Furthermore superantigens did not require antigen processing for their effect.[87] It has thus turned out that superantigens are indeed cross-linkers of class II MHC with TCR, and that they are not antigens in the physiological sense. So in the end, the term "superantigen" proved to be a misnomer in every respect.'

'Of course, much of the interest in superantigens was fuelled by the expectation that they would reveal a novel strategy of the immune system against pathogens. But studies demonstrating a purported usefulness of superantigens for the immune system were scarce and unconvincing[98] compared to their well-documented negative effect: the deletion of significant portions of the T-cell repertoire. Furthermore, there were data to demonstrate that exogeneous superantigens administered in vivo could also cause deletion and anergy.[84,99] Superantigens are therefore more likely to serve the agenda of pathogens in evading the immune system. The fact that phylogenetically distant pathogens such as viruses and bacteria use the very same strategy supports this assumption.'

Another approach to the demonstration of clonal deletion was to use TCR transgenic mice that tend to express the transgene in almost all T cells. The first study of this kind was undertaken by Harald von Boehmer and his colleagues in Basel.[100] They used a TCR transgene specific for the male minor histocompatibility (H-Y) antigen presented by the H-2D^b class I MHC molecule. In female mice the great majority of mature peripheral T cells expressed the transgene, and the proportion of CD4 and CD8 cells appeared normal. But the peripheral T cells from male mice revealed a number of abnormalities. Although they expressed the transgene at similar levels as female mice, the majority of cells lacked the CD4 and CD8 co-receptors. Of the remaining T cells the CD4$^-$8$^+$ subpopulation had very low levels of the co-receptor, and the CD4$^+$8$^-$ subset was represented at a very low proportion but with normal level of the co-receptor. Importantly, none of these populations responded to the H-Y antigen, indicating that the absence or low level of CD8 precluded the male-specific response. In the thymus most cells expressed the transgene in both female and male mice. But the total number of thymocytes was drastically (>10 fold) lower in male than in female mice. This difference could be accounted for by a severe depletion of CD4$^+$8$^+$ cells from the thymus of male mice.

Altogether, the TCR transgenic model, although rather artificial, has established a number of important features of T-cell tolerance. First, deletion of autoreactive cells in the thymus as a major mechanism has been confirmed. Second, a clear role of co-receptors in tolerance has been demonstrated, in that co-receptor-negative as well as CD8^{low} cells unable to respond to H-Y were shown to be spared from deletion despite the expression of the TCR transgene. The involvement of CD4 in tolerance has also been demonstrated by an independent approach: CD4-specific antibodies prevented intrathymic deletion.[101] Third, deletion has been shown to selectively affect immature thymocytes at the double-positive (CD4$^+$8$^+$) stage, a finding that has been confirmed by different laboratories.[102–105]

'The deletion of thymocytes at the double-positive stage led to some paradoxical results in these experimental models', adds Dr. G. 'Specifically, in the Mls model both CD4$^+$8$^-$ and CD4$^-$8$^+$ mature cells were depleted of Vβ8.1 and Vβ6 T cells, although only the CD4$^+$8$^-$ subset could react to Mls.[79,80,102] And in the transgenic model,[100] the CD4$^+$8$^-$ subset was also depleted, although only the CD4$^-$8$^+$ subset could respond to H-Y. Taken at face value, these results have suggested that the tolerance mechanism would delete a lot more T cells in the thymus than necessary.'

'A possible solution of the paradox emerges if we ascribe these results to the non-physiological nature of experimental models. In the Mls model deletion is caused by the cross-linking of a particular TCR Vβ segment with class II MHC. Because this Vβ segment is present in ~5% of all TCR, the deletion affects thousands of distinct T-cell clones that would have been distributed in both single positive (CD4$^+$8$^-$ and CD4$^-$8$^+$) subsets. It is therefore not surprising that deletion of the double-positive cells, the precursors of single-positive cells, caused a detectable depletion of the "innocent" subset, too. But this kind of deletion can only occur in a few unfortunate individuals carrying an endogenous viral superantigen. Normally, the specificity of TCR to a pMHC is determined by all of its variable elements, and thus the deletion affects individual clones whose frequency is 0.001 to 0.01%. The TCR transgenic model is even worse, because these mice are practically monoclonal, and if the transgene is anti-self the organism applies different compensatory mechanisms to circumvent the deletion of its entire T-cell compartment. One of these mechanisms appears to be the modulation of co-receptor expression.'

'In a physiological scenario, the question whether clonal deletion at the double-positive stage would cause unnecessary loss can be formulated as follows: Could the TCR of a CD8 T cell deleted by interaction with a class I pMHC have served as a functional receptor for a class II pMHC in a CD4 T cell (or vice versa)? In principle, the answer is "yes" implying that a single receptor, TCR1, can give rise to two different specificities: TCR1+CD4 and TCR1+CD8. The question really is how frequently such clones occur in a single individual. Although it is impossible to assign a concrete number of the frequency, I would argue that such clones are a rarity, and consequently their deletion would not cause appreciable loss in the "innocent" subset.'

9.3.2 Clonal Deletion of B Cells

The discovery that self-reactive B cells are also subject to clonal deletion followed immediately after the T-cell deletion studies, and went therefore almost unnoticed, receiving much less press coverage. For comparison, whereas clonal deletion of T cells was reported in four leading articles in *Nature* (the highest possible placement of a discovery, and every scientist's dream) as well as in about a dozen *Nature* letters (not to mention other journals), the report on clonal deletion of self-reactive B cells was a single short *Nature* letter.

'Of course, the extent of press coverage has never been a measure of importance, particularly because it happened all too often that a Nobel Prize-worth discovery was published as an inconspicuous short report', comments Dr. G. 'The actual reason why this was a hard time to study B cell tolerance was that in the euphoria of successful T-cell studies many immunologists started to believe that tolerance would be the exclusive domain of T cells. In other words, the failure to produce antibodies to self antigens would result from the deletion of self-reactive Th cells, i.e., the absence of T–B-cell collaboration required to turn on antibody production, rather than from any change in the B cells themselves. This was of course a misconception, because T–B-cell collaboration could also permit the activation of autoreactive B cells, for example, when the B cell recognizes a self epitope and the T cell a foreign epitope of the same antigen.'

The pioneering study of B-cell deletion was performed by David Nemazee, a profoundly thinking young B-cell immunologist, at that time at the Basel Institute, together with Kurt Bürki, a Swiss molecular biologist.[106] They produced transgenic mice using genes encoding an anti-class I MHC antibody (anti-H-2^k) of the IgM class. In H-2^d mice about 25–50% of splenic B cells were found to express the transgene, and high titers of IgM antibody of the same specificity were detected in the serum. In contrast H-2^{k}xH-2^d heterozygotes lacked B cells expressing the transgene, and no anti-H-2^k antibody was detectable in the serum. These results indicated that autoreactive B cells, even if present at very high numbers as in this model, could be eliminated by clonal deletion. The authors then went on to demonstrate that the bone marrow of H-2^k mice still contained B cells expressing low levels of the transgenic anti-H-2^k antibody, suggesting that clonal deletion might have occurred at the transitional stage from pre-B cell to mature B cell.[107]

These data would have firmly established clonal deletion as a major mechanism of B-cell tolerance, had other studies not been there with different results. The latter were performed by Christopher Goodnow and colleagues[108,109] in Sydney, using a double transgenic mouse that expressed genes for hen egg lysozyme (HEL) as a 'neo-self' antigen, and a high-affinity anti-HEL antibody. In this model, anti-HEL B cells did not undergo clonal deletion, but were unable to secrete anti-HEL antibody and expressed a markedly reduced level of surface IgM with unchanged level of surface IgD. Thus in this model self tolerance seemed to result from B-cell hyporesponsiveness[110] rather than clonal deletion. This finding was reminiscent of the phenomenon known as "anti-μ suppression" described more than a decade earlier.[111,112] The observation in these early studies was that the treatment of B cells with antibodies specific for the heavy chain of IgM caused a complete disappearance of cell surface IgM. Immature B cells were particularly sensitive to the treatment, in that low concentrations of anti-IgM for about 24 h caused a complete but reversible down-modulation of surface IgM, which became irreversible after 48 h, and an arrest of B-cell development occurred. Mature B cells were less sensitive to anti-IgM, they required higher antibody concentrations and the down-modulation was always reversible. The authors recognized that their finding might have implications for B-cell tolerance to self antigens. Taken together these results have raised the possibility that B-cell tolerance might be achieved by a non-deletional mechanism.

In a follow-up study, Goodnow and colleagues[113] sought for an explanation for the discrepancy between their data and those of Nemazee and Bürki. For these experiments they modified the HEL, anti-HEL double transgenic model so that HEL was expressed in membrane-bound form, and demonstrated that HEL in this form caused deletion of anti-HEL B cells. They have concluded that multivalent interaction with membrane-bound molecules induces deletion whereas monomeric or oligomeric soluble antigens cause non-deletional silencing (i.e., anergy; see Section 9.3.3) of B cells.

At this point the notion has emerged that T-cell and B-cell tolerance may be, at least in part, mechanistically different: whereas the prevailing mechanism of T-cell tolerance appeared to be clonal deletion, in B-cell tolerance non-deletional mechanisms might dominate. This difference has been explained by the different ways the specificity repertoires of T and B cells are generated.[114] In the case of T cells, the receptor repertoire is generated in the thymus upon TCR rearrangement, and it remains largely unchanged, except for low-frequency spontaneous mutations, after the cells left the thymus. It seems therefore appropriate that the bulk of tolerance is established by clonal deletion in the thymus. In contrast, the repertoire of B cells is generated in two stages, stage-1 being the expression of germ-line-encoded variable elements, which then undergo extensive somatic hypermutation after contacting antigen to form a more diverse stage-2 repertoire. Thus, clonal deletion at stage-1 would be counter-productive, because most of these cells are just substrates of mutations, which can result in either anti-self or anti-foreign specificities. The same argument applies to stage-2 B cells as long as their receptor further mutates. It is therefore not surprising that B cells preferentially use a non-deletional mechanism of self tolerance.

'Convincing as this argument may sound, I should mention that the evidence for both deletion and anergy of B cells was indirect, and as such open to different interpretations', points out Dr. G. 'For example, Gus Nossal,[115] Burnet's successor at the Walter and Eliza Hall Institute, who was a proponent of non-deletional mechanisms interpreted the Nemazee & Bürki data as "stripping" of surface Ig from the cells which rendered them undetectable, instead of being deleted. In contrast, Mel Cohn and Rod Langman[116] who did not believe in non-deletional tolerance argued that the existence of antigen-specific but unresponsive B cells has nothing to do with tolerance, it just reflects the presence of non-inducible surface Ig+ B cells that arise upon haplotype exclusion.'

'I must also add that the attempt to reconcile these two mechanisms[113] was not a very lucky one. The data taken at face value suggest namely that monomeric antigens presumably signaling the B cell by a conformational change can induce anergy, whereas a multivalent aggregational signal leads to deletion. In other words, the B cell can read an affinity-based signal as well as an aggregational signal that is based on the overall avidity of multiple interactions. This would be acceptable as long as the outcome of the signals is unresponsiveness. However, the widely accepted concept that tolerance results from Signal-1 (antigen recognition) alone entails that the same signal in the presence of Signal-2 leads to induction. And a multivalent Signal-1 becomes a problem for antibody response, because the same Igs would have too low affinity individually to be able to function in solution. Thus induction by aggregational signals would flood the body with useless antibodies that cannot mediate any effector function. Therefore I suspect that cell death induced by multivalent interactions may be a phenomenon unrelated to tolerance. Indeed, it has been reported that programmed cell death can be triggered by extensive cross-linking of different cell surface receptors, e.g., CD2, CD45, CD47, CD99, MHC class I and class II, etc., with antibodies.[117–122] The multivalent engagement of surface Ig may just be one more example for the same mechanism. On the other hand, there is evidence in the more recent literature for the involvement of different apoptotic pathways in B-cell development and tolerance.'[123]

'In view of all these considerations, I am afraid I cannot but conclude that the mechanism(s) of B-cell tolerance has remained a controversial issue.'

9.3.3 Clonal Anergy

Anergy is defined as a cellular state in which lymphocytes fail to give certain responses upon stimulation through the antigen receptor (as well as other receptors normally required for full activation). Because anergy is induced via the antigen receptor of lymphocytes and the resulting unresponsiveness is also antigen-specific, it has been considered to be akin to immunological tolerance from the very beginning.

The phenomenon was discovered and the term 'anergy' coined by Nossal and Pike[124] in 1980. These authors induced tolerance by injecting mice in the perinatal period with a soluble antigen (fluorescein coupled to human gamma globulin), and assayed the binding of fluorescein to B cells as well as antibody production to the tolerogen several weeks later. Surprisingly, tolerance induction caused only a modest decrease in the number of fluorescein-binding B cells. The remaining antigen-binding B cells showed binding profiles indistinguishable from those of non-tolerized B cells, suggesting that the expression of surface Ig was unaltered. Nevertheless, the fluorescein-specific B cells were incapable of responding to the antigen (or to mitogen) by antibody formation. This study has raised the possibility for the first time that B-cell tolerance may be largely achieved by functional silencing instead of clonal deletion. As discussed in the previous section, similar results were reported later, using a transgenic model of B-cell tolerance with the additional observation that tolerant B cells had reduced levels of surface IgM but continued to express high levels of surface IgD. However, the molecular mechanisms of B-cell anergy could not be pursued much further, because long-term culture and cloning of B cells was technically unfeasible.

T-cell anergy was discovered a few years later, somewhat fortuitously, by Lamb, and Feldmann and colleagues,[125] using human T helper cell clones specific for a peptide of influenza hemagglutinin. In this experimental system, preincubation of T cells with the antigenic peptide in the absence of antigen-presenting cells (APC) rendered the T cells incapable of mounting a proliferative response subsequently to the same antigen in the presence of APC. At face value, this result suggested that class II MHC-restricted T cells could be made unresponsive by the antigen alone, but a follow-up study clarified that for tolerance induction the peptide antigen was presented by class II MHC molecules of the T cells themselves.[126] Obviously, this experimental protocol would not have worked with murine T cells that usually do not express class II MHC.

Curiously, the first demonstration of anergy in murine T cells also resulted from a fortuity. As briefly alluded to before (Section 8.6.5), Jenkins and Schwartz[127] at the NIH set out to re-investigate an earlier claim, according to which antigens coupled to syngeneic spleen cells induced suppressor T cells. They found that peptide antigen coupled to syngeneic splenic APC by a chemical cross-linker failed to induce either proliferative T-cell response or suppression. What it did induce, however, was antigen-specific unresponsiveness of T cells in vivo as well as of T-cell clones in vitro, which appeared to be long-lasting (examined up to 24 days). The antigen and MHC specificity of the induction of unresponsiveness was identical to that required for T-cell activation. The authors have concluded that recognition of antigen/MHC by T cells under 'non-mitogenic' conditions results in functional inactivation. This rather general conclusion was supported by further data demonstrating induction of anergy by antigen presentation in planar lipid membranes containing only peptide plus MHC molecules,[128] and by stimulation of APC-free T-cell populations with mitogen[129] or anti-CD3 antibody[130] coated on a plastic surface. The implication of these results was that an APC-derived 'mitogenic' second signal would be required for T-cell activation in addition to antigen presentation, and this was also demonstrable experimentally.[131]

In vivo induction of anergy was observed in a number of additional experimental systems, for example, in Mls[b] mice injected with Mls[a]-expressing cells,[99] in mice injected with a high dose of soluble peptide antigen intravenously,[132] in Vβ8.1 transgenic mice[133] expressing Mls[a], and in double transgenic mice carrying an anti-H-2K[b] T-cell receptor and having H-2K[b] selectively expressed in pancreatic β cells.[134] These studies have raised the possibility that anergy may be a major mechanism of post-thymic ('peripheral') T-cell tolerance, in contrast to clonal deletion that usually takes place in the thymus.

The second signal that is assumed to decide between anergy and stimulation is referred to somewhat vaguely as co-stimulation. In most instances, co-stimulation denotes a bimolecular interaction between T cell and APC, through, for example, CD28 and B7, the well-known co-stimulatory receptor pair,[135,136] or via interaction between LFA-3 and CD2,[137] or LFA-1 and ICAM-1,[138] although the latter two interactions serve more cell adhesion, and the mechanisms by which they mediate co-stimulation are different from that of the CD28–B7 interaction. In some cases, co-stimulation can even be provided by soluble ligands, such as interleukin-1 (IL-1).[139]

As expected, the 'mitogenic' conditions required for T-cell activation have to do with the induction of IL-2, the major growth factor for T cells: anergic T cells are incapable of producing IL-2 upon restimulation.[140] The production of IL-3 is also diminished, as well as the reactivity of anergic cells to certain cytokines, but IL-4, interferon-γ, and cytotoxic activity are hardly affected. Thus T-cell anergy represents in fact partial responsiveness with a major defect in IL-2 production.

The feasibility of T-cell cloning and long-term culture enabled detailed investigations into the intracellular signalling pathways that operate during the induction of anergy. These studies will not be dealt with here, mostly because intracellular signaling is a complex science in its own right, and as such is beyond the scope of this book. Suffice it to say that a number of differences have been identified in the signaling pathways for anergy compared to activation, the common outcome of which is a transcriptional block of the IL-2 gene (see reviews by Ronald Schwartz[141,142] for more detail).

Finally an important and intriguing aspect of anergy remains to be mentioned, namely, that it can be reversed with high concentrations of IL-2 in murine,[143] and with IL-2 plus anti-CD2 antibody in human[144] experimental systems.

Altogether, anergy is a well-established experimental fact, and yet, no consensus has been reached in the immunological community about the role of this cellular state in self tolerance. Why?

'As always, the problem here, too, is insufficient understanding', answers Dr. G. 'As I have pointed out several times, satisfactory biological understanding can only be achieved by placing the phenomenon or mechanism in question into evolutionary context, and here is the rub with anergy. Since anergy is generally considered as a second "failsafe" mechanism to correct the shortcomings of clonal deletion, the following question arises; why should evolution have bothered to develop a second mechanism that is less perfect (cells remain alive, the state is reversible) than the first one? The usual answer of evolution to the weakness of a mechanism is to improve on it, instead of making a new one from scratch (which is worse in addition).'

'Evidently, this argument would only apply, if anergy were indeed a second mechanism, for which there is no evidence. However, as pointed out by Arthur Silverstein (personal communication), it may well be the first, more ancient mechanism that has remained, because it is physiologically neutral and thus could not be selected against.'

'Other views consider anergy as an intermediate stage toward apoptosis rather than a distinct mechanism. For example, Mel Cohn has argued that anergic cells may just represent the normal steady state of cells that have received Signal-1, and waiting for inactivation.[3] Polly Matzinger[21] expressed a similar thought in a more playful way: "If I were designing the immune system and wanted to ensure against reactions to self-tissues, I would not do it by pushing cells into a long-lived anergic state".'

'Another type of interpretation is that anergy represents a mechanism of "peripheral" tolerance, while the "central" mechanism is deletion by apoptosis. Although this is consistent with the majority of observations, there are also instances of central anergy and peripheral deletion. Furthermore, the two different outcomes remain unexplained, because there is no conceivable, selectable advantage arising from the anergic state.'

'Therefore, at the present state of affairs, it is safest to regard anergy as a potential or inherent property of the inactivation pathway initiated by Signal-1 (antigen alone). For example, certain "factors" may be required for the pathway to proceed to apoptosis, in the absence of which partially inactivated live cells would accumulate. Such cells would then be eliminated later by apoptosis due to senescence. Thus the physiological outcome would eventually be the same, and consequently, anergy would not be selected against.'

'Of course, in the absence of conclusive experimental evidence all interpretations remain speculative. The experimental question to be asked is whether the apoptotic deletion mechanism would fail, and to what extent, if anergy were absent.'

9.3.4 An Unexpected Turn: Display of Peripheral Self in the Thymus

By the end of the 1980s, the physical elimination of autoreactive T cells in the thymus (clonal deletion) asserted itself as a major mechanism of T-cell tolerance. However, it was also clear that this mechanism could only account for tolerance of self antigens expressed in the thymus, or carried to the thymus by the bloodstream. Tolerance of the remaining self proteins, for example those expressed selectively in particular organs, could obviously not be achieved by thymic deletion. For this reason most immunologists assumed that, in addition to the 'central' tolerance established in the thymus, there should be a second, 'peripheral' tolerance mechanism responsible for the inactivation of T cells that encountered autoantigens elsewhere in the body (i.e., after leaving the thymus). In the 1990s therefore significant experimental efforts were made to clarify the nature of this hypothetical peripheral tolerance.

The experimental systems for studies of peripheral tolerance usually involved a marker transgene placed under the control of an organ-specific promoter so that the transgene would be selectively expressed in that particular organ. For example, the approach taken by Hanahan and colleagues at the UCSF was to use the gene encoding the SV40 T antigen under the control of rat insulin promoter,[145] or by Flavell's group at Yale to use the same gene under the elastase I promoter,[146] in order to ensure a selective expression of the T antigen in the pancreas. Such studies served two interrelated purposes: first, they were expected to allow insight into the mechanism of peripheral tolerance, and second, they could have provided clues to the failure of tolerance in organ-specific autoimmune disease. However, the results coming out of these experiments defied the predictions of immunological common sense, indeed, they appeared rather esoteric. The reassuring aspect of the data was that the mice did establish tolerance to the transgene. But the unexpected turn was that the transgene was expressed, despite organ-specific promoters, also in the thymus.[145,146] Importantly, this thymic expression could not be regarded as a 'transgenic artefact', because insulin and elastase I were also expressed at low levels in the thymus, even in non-transgenic mice, along with other pancreatic proteins. The results thus raised the possibility that organ-specific genes could be expressed ectopically in the thymus. Similar results were obtained from other experimental models.[147,148] It was also demonstrated that the expression of organ-specific genes in the thymus occurred selectively in rare medullary epithelial cells, and that this spurious thymic expression was responsible for the establishment of tolerance rather than the 'proper' expression in the respective organ.[146–150]

'These results sounded almost like science fiction', comments Dr. G 'so that even old seasoned immunologists, well prepared for the tricks thymus can play, were taken aback. The reason for the consternation was that cell-, tissue- and organ-specific expression of certain genes was considered to be one of the most important biological mechanisms, the major instrument of ontogeny, without which embryonal development would be impossible. Violation of tissue-specific expression by the thymus appeared almost absurd, because no feasible mechanism could be envisaged that would allow this to happen.'

Another type of experimental question leading essentially to the same finding was asked by Bruno Kyewski and colleagues[151] in Heidelberg. These authors wondered how the immune system could manage to establish tolerance to inducible serum proteins whose concentrations could vary widely. They expected that non-induced, low levels of such proteins would cause a temporal limitation of antigen supply to the thymus, and thus prevent continuous tolerization of newly arising T cells. This was predicted to manifest in leaky tolerance to such proteins. The model they chose was the response to human C-reactive protein (hCRP), a major acute phase protein secreted by hepatocytes, whose concentration can increase up to 1000-fold during an acute-phase reaction. They introduced the hCRP gene into mice together with anti-hCRP T-cell receptor (TCR) genes, and found that tolerance was not leaky at all, and was mediated by intrathymic deletion of immature thymocytes, irrespective of widely differing serum concentrations of hCRP. The relevant antigen for deletion was not the circulating hCRP, but hCRP expressed by thymic medullary epithelial cells. This latter point was brought out even more clearly by another model, in which self tolerance to a disease-inducing autoantigen, proteolipid protein (PLP) of the myelin sheath, was shown to be limited to a particular splice variant of PLP expressed both in the thymus and in myelin.[152,153]

'Bruno Kyewski belongs to the faithful type of scientists, who has devoted his entire career to studying the thymus. He is one of the quietly thinking, non-aggressive, non-pushy characters, and I am all the more glad that he succeeded in making such an important contribution', adds Dr. G.

All these experiments have demonstrated that self tolerance of organ-specific antigens is established, contrary to expectations, in the thymus, with the aid of some mechanism that permits organ-restricted proteins to be expressed in thymic medullary epithelial cells. Furthermore, the results implied that much of self-tolerance that was believed to require an extra peripheral mechanism was indeed settled 'centrally' in the thymus, casting thereby doubts on the existence of peripheral tolerance as such. However, many immunologists remained skeptical about these results, for the lack of a plausible mechanism that could induce ectopic expression of diverse non-thymic proteins in the thymus.

The missing mechanism was then provided by the discovery of the 'autoimmune regulator' (AIRE). The *aire* gene was identified by two groups of human geneticists[154,155] studying a rare autoimmune disease called autoimmune poly-endocrinopathy-candidiasis-ectodermal dystrophy (APECED), also known as autoimmune polyendocrine syndrome type-1 (APS-1), a monogenic autosomal disease with recessive inheritance. Since this was the only known human auto-immune disease inherited in a Mendelian fashion, it provided a unique model to analyze the genetics of human autoimmunity. The single susceptibility gene termed *aire* was cloned and shown to be expressed prevalently in the thymus. It encodes a polypeptide with DNA-binding activity[156] and transcriptional trans-activating property.[157] In APS-1 patients the gene harbors a number of muta-tions that interfere with the transactivating function of the AIRE protein.[158,159] The results have thus demonstrated that defects in a single gene can cause auto-immune disease, and that the function of the unmutated gene has to do with activation of gene-transcription in the thymus.

The functional characterization of the AIRE protein was performed by the group of Diane Mathis and Christophe Benoist[160] (who moved meanwhile from France to Harvard). They 'knocked out' the murine homolog of *aire* gene by a deletion resulting in a frame shift and premature termination of transcrip-tion. The AIRE-deficient mice showing symptoms of APS-1 were then com-pared with normal mice in terms of a number of immunological parameters. The results have clearly shown that AIRE is responsible single-handedly for the ectopic expression of many tissue- and organ-restricted proteins in thymic medullary epithelial cells. The number of non-thymic proteins expressed in the thymus as a result of transcriptional activation by AIRE was estimated to be between 200 and 1200. The AIRE protein was shown to be expressed selec-

tively in thymic medullary epithelial cells,[161] and to be most active in the perinatal period, when the T-cell repertoire develops.[162] Thus AIRE has turned out
to be a major player in constructing a thymic replica of the self proteome for
the purpose of inducing T-cell tolerance. However, it may not be the only player
involved, as the thymic expression of many self proteins appears to occur independently of AIRE.[163] The complete scope of genes ectopically expressed in
the thymus has remained unknown. Estimates run up to ~3000, i.e., 10% of the
total genome,[163] but this may still be an underestimate due to limitations of the
methods used. It is reasonable to assume that ectopic expression should cover
the majority of potentially pathogenic self antigens, provided that the selective
pressure for this mechanism has been autoimmune disease.

'Thymic expression of diverse self molecules, or the "projection of an immunological self shadow within the thymus", as Diane Mathis used to put it[160], was a
key finding that has changed the way immunologists think about self tolerance',
explains Dr. G. 'Although the phenomenon appeared bizarre to most of us at the
beginning, the case of AIRE demonstrating that a specific molecular mechanism
has evolved for this purpose convinced almost everybody. So we had to reconcile
with the fact that in this case biological reality defied our imagination. The most
important conceptual change induced by this finding has been the realization that
the elimination of self reactivity from the T-cell repertoire was prioritized by evolution to occur predominantly, if not entirely, in the thymus. Whether this decision
was just a caprice of evolution or due to the lack of a viable alternative is difficult
to disentangle in retrospect. But the present status suggests that the selective pressure of autoimmune diseases must have acted primarily (or perhaps exclusively)
on the process of clonal deletion in the thymus, instead of driving a separate
peripheral tolerance mechanism as expected by most immunologists. A corollary
to this statement is that self–non-self discrimination for T cells begins and ends in
the thymus, i.e., cells that leave the thymus must be by definition anti-non-self.
I believe many colleagues would still vehemently object against this view, and
argue that this arrangement would leave the body unprotected from autoimmunity
caused by TCRs that mutate to anti-self after leaving the thymus. This argument
is of course correct. However, the frequency of such mutations may be too low
to provide sufficient selective pressure for an additional mechanism. Therefore,
unless a feasible mechanism for peripheral T-cell tolerance will be discovered,
we have to live with the somewhat disquieting alternative that the elimination
of self-reactivity from the T-cell repertoire may be settled once and for all during
ontogeny in the thymus.'

9.4 CAN SELF TOLERANCE BE UNDERSTOOD?

The answer of most immunologists to this question would be 'yes, partially'.
Only a small over-critical and insecure minority would reply with 'no', whereas
another handful of self-confident immunologists would say 'yes', although
they may not understand more than their insecure colleagues. It is therefore of
interest how Dr. G would relate to this question.

'My answer would be that of most immunologists', replies Dr. G 'but I believe this is not the point here. I would rather try to paint a picture of self tolerance, and point out what can be understood on the basis of presently available information, and what has remained controversial.'

9.4.1 Importance of the Perinatal Window

'It has been recognized since the very beginning that the time window in which the immune systems arises, i.e., the late embryonal to early postnatal life, is the most critical period for the establishment of self tolerance', continues Dr. G. 'The period before birth is particularly well suited for the development of tolerance, because the embryo lives in a practically sterile environment, and therefore every antigen recognized by the immune system is self. Indeed, there is a large body of evidence, although mostly indirect, that self tolerance is established by and large in this period. According to other views, the early postnatal life also belongs to this privileged time period, but the advantage of having only self antigens around does not apply any more, and thus the newborn's own immune system must get gradually started, in inverse ratio to decreasing maternal immunity. Because it is not quite clear when exactly the time window closes, this period is usually referred to as the "perinatal window".'

'Provided that evolution favored the late embryonic life for the establishment of self tolerance, one could also envisage that a specific tolerance mechanism should exist that is operating only in this period. The most likely candidate for such a mechanism would be that both T and B lymphocytes recognizing antigen in this period would be sent, irrespective of their developmental state and anatomical location, onto a death pathway. This idea is just a more up-to-date formulation of what Burnet[8] proposed in 1959, and was reiterated in subsequent concepts of tolerance,[15,21] so that by now it has gained almost universal acceptance. However, the proposition has remained hypothetical until now, because there is no experimental evidence either for or against it. The available data permit us only to extrapolate to the existence of a stereotype "death-on-recognition" reaction before birth. For example, immature thymocytes have been shown to undergo apoptosis after stimulation via their antigen receptor.[164–167] It is also known that the terminal phase of B-cell genesis in the bone marrow is associated with a considerable loss,[168] and that anti-IgM antibody treatment of neonatal mice deletes all developing B cells.[169,170] At face value, however, these data demonstrate that immature lymphocytes are more prone to death upon antigen recognition, i.e., they support the Lederberg model[171] according to which the differentiation state of the cell is what matters, and not the developmental state of the animal. Mel Cohn's two signal model (Section 9.2.4) explains the massive inactivation of cells during the perinatal window simply by stating that only Signal-1 exists at this early stage of lymphoid development, i.e., another mechanism is not necessary. Thus it may well be that there is nothing "special" about the perinatal window, except that the immune system arises at this time, and therefore all developmental processes including tolerance induction occur at a larger scale.'

'In conclusion, the idea that the perinatal window is a critical period for the establishment of self tolerance remains valid, but whether or not this entails a distinct mechanism of tolerance is unclear.'

9.4.2 What Happens After the Perinatal Window Closed?

'Whatever the operating principles in the perinatal window may be, the immune system must be ready for a protective mode with the appearance of the first, potentially pathogenic microbes. This should happen around birth.'

'According to all current concepts,[15,21,34] the postnatal principle would permit lymphocytes to go two different pathways: inactivation or activation. This is envisaged to operate by a two signal mechanism, whereby Signal-1, antigen recognition, alone would result in inactivation, and Signals-1+2 in activation. It appears that the inactivating first signal can be received by all lymphocytes as soon as they start to express antigen receptors, i.e., by mature cells as well as their precursors. However, probably only mature lymphocytes can accept the activating second signal.'

'Another characteristic although not exclusive feature of postnatal tolerance is that the inactivation after Signal-1 does not necessarily manifest in cell death. In some instances, an extended period of unresponsive state – anergy – develops. Anergy appears to be the preferred modus of postnatal tolerance of B cells (Section 9.3.2), but T cells can also become anergic after encounter with antigen presented by "non-professional" antigen-presenting cells (Section 9.3.3). However, the functional significance of anergy and the reasons for its frequent use in postnatal tolerance are unknown.'

'The core problem of postnatal and adult tolerance is that the lymphocyte repertoires developed in the perinatal window are constantly turned over, and replenished with newly arising cells. Consequently, mechanisms are required to ensure self tolerance throughout the entire lifetime. These mechanisms are partially different for B and T cells.'

9.4.3 Adult Tolerance in the B-Cell Compartment

'Studies of B-cell population dynamics suggest that the "first round" of B-cell tolerance induction occurs already at the precursor stage in the bone marrow. The data show that the number of mature B cells produced in the adult bone marrow is less than half of what would be expected from the number of their immediate precursors.[172] The remaining precursors undergo apoptosis at the pre-B to B-cell transition. Indirect evidence indicates that the reason for cell death is two-fold: first defective Ig-gene rearrangements,[173] and second, elimination of autoreactive cells.[169] Although the extent to which these two causes contribute to cell death is unknown, it is justified to assume that B cells with high affinity for ubiquitous self antigens are likely to be eliminated in the bone marrow by clonal deletion. This mechanism apparently does not make self–non-self (S–NS) discrimination, i.e. foreign antigens reaching the bone marrow will also delete the respective clones.'

'The young B cells traverse the wall of bone marrow sinusoids, and accumulate in the lumen awaiting release into the blood. The exact number of B cells entering the blood every day cannot be determined, because of the wide distribution of bone marrow. But observations are consistent with an estimated number of 2×10^7 B cells per day,[168] which corresponds to approximately 20% of the total peripheral B cell pool of an adult mouse.'

'B cells exported from the bone marrow are taken up, after a brief period of circulation, in the peripheral lymphoid organs (spleen and lymph nodes). Approximately half of the B cells in the periphery are renewed rapidly (in 3–4 days),[174,175] and the other half are long-lived (on average 4–6 weeks, up to several months).[176] Thus the daily output of new B cells from the bone marrow is mostly "spent" on replenishing the fast renewing population.'

'The short-lived B-cell population poses little danger of autoimmunity, because the life-span of the cells is insufficient to differentiate into antibody-forming cells after antigen encounter. In contrast, the long-lived population carries a high risk of autoimmunity, particularly because many of these cells are antigen-primed and undergo somatic hypermutation,[177–179] which can result in a sizable proportion of autoreactive B cells. (Iterative cycles of hypermutation and antigen selection account for affinity maturation,[179] which is a physiologically important process in antibody responses, as antibodies function in solution and should thus have high affinity.) It is therefore self-evident that the long-lived "immune repertoire" of B cells must be strictly patrolled for autoreactivity by an additional "peripheral" tolerance mechanism.'

'There are good reasons to believe that peripheral tolerance of immune B cells is ensured by a Bretscher-Cohn-type[34] two-signal mechanism, in which the S–NS decision is made by an antigen-specific T helper (Th) cell. As pointed out before (Section 9.2.7), because a B cell can take up only one single antigen by receptor-mediated endocytosis, the peptides recognized by Th cells on its surface are derived by definition from the same antigen. This way the Th–B-cell interaction remains antigen-specific despite the fragmentation of antigen into peptides by processing. Thus B-cell activation can rely on the Th cells, whose repertoire was pre-sorted to be anti-NS. If a particular B cell mutates to anti-S, it will not receive the activating second signal from Th cells, and will be inactivated by default. Under this mechanism it is still possible to break B-cell tolerance by cross-reactive antigens,[12,13] notably, if the B cell recognizes a S^B epitope and the Th cell a NS^T epitope of the same antigen.[180] As discussed before (Section 9.2.4), the frequency of such an event is limited by a competition between the $S^B + NS^T$ and $S^B + S^T$ (self) antigen for the same B cell.'

9.4.4 Adult Tolerance in the T-Cell Compartment

'Starting again with cell population dynamics, it is important to note that in young adult mice the thymic output of new T cells is ~1% of total thymocytes per day,[181] which corresponds to <1 million cells. In animals older than 6 months the relative output is only 0.1%, and considering thymic involution this corresponds to just a few thousands cells per day. Thus the renewal rate of the peripheral T-cell pool ($<10^6$ of $~10^8$ T cells/day) is much slower than that of the B-cell compartment (2×10^7 of 10^8 B cells renewed per day; see Section 9.4.3). In contrast, the thymus itself turns over its cell content every 5–7 days,[181] which indicates that 93–95% of all thymocytes die within the thymus.'

'These data suggest that in case of the T-cell repertoire dramatic changes occur only during development in the thymus (positive and negative selection; see Section 8.4.3), but once it is formed it remains by-and-large constant. Furthermore, T cells, in contrast to B cells, do not hypermutate after antigen encounter. Therefore we can conclude that the requirement for a peripheral toler-ance mechanism is much less stringent for T cells than for B cells.'

'The question then arises: does peripheral tolerance exist at all for T cells? And with this we have arrived at the most controversial chapter of self tolerance.'

'Mel Cohn would argue that self–non-self (S–NS) discrimination by T cells at the periphery would also occur by a two signal mechanism, i.e., the T cell must recognize the antigen and receive a second signal from a T helper (Th) in order to be activated (Section 9.2.4). However, this would demand an antigen-specific T–T-cell interaction, which has not been demonstrated experimentally thus far. Indeed, the interaction between precursors of cytotoxic T cells and Th cells or between two Th cells does not exhibit strict antigen specificity. The only limita-tion for these interactions appears to be that both T cells must recognize antigen on the same antigen-presenting cell (APC).[44–46,50–52] Since the uptake of antigens by APCs is not antigen-specific (except for B cells), interactions can take place between T cells seeing different antigens on the same APC, which renders S–NS discrimination leaky.'

'The only T-cell tolerance scenario consistent with the presently available data is the following. Elimination of autoreactive clones occurs in the thymus, by interaction with bone-marrow-derived APC for ubiquitous antigens, and with medullary thymic epithelial cells ectopically expressing tissue-restricted antigens (Section 9.3.4). In the thymus, interaction with any antigen should lead to clonal deletion including foreign antigens that may enter the thymus. Thus the central tolerance mechanism, as also in the case of B-cell tolerance in the bone marrow, does not seem to care about losses caused by the deletion of some anti-NS clones. All T cells leaving the thymus are operationally anti-NS.'

'In the periphery a "surrogate" two signal mechanism seems to operate, which controls T-cell activation but does not make S–NS discrimination. This mecha-nism determines the site where T-cell activation is permitted to occur: this is the professional APC in lymphoid organs.[21] The second signal is provided by co-stimulatory molecules expressed on the APC, i.e., it is not antigen-specific. The likely biological need for such a mechanism is that T cells activated elsewhere would cause tissue destruction. Accordingly, antigen recognition on cells other than professional APC leads to unresponsiveness (anergy). In this model T–T-cell interactions (see above) just serve to optimize the activation of resting cells.'

'The model as outlined cannot control anti-S reactivity that may arise due to mutation of a T-cell receptor, or due to change in the pattern of self peptide pre-sentation by professional APC. However, such changes may be too infrequent to serve as a selective pressure. Alternatively, as I suspect, this model is not yet the "final truth".'

9.4.5 Final Plea

'The foregoing represents a sincere effort on my part to assemble the available information into a coherent picture of self tolerance. But all I have achieved by the end is a sketch. Moreover, I am afraid many colleagues will not agree with it. This is because our present understanding of tolerance is based to a large extent on conjectures and inferences, which are subject to personal taste and allow a number of different scenarios. Therefore I would like to plead here "not guilty".'

'Self tolerance is doubtless the most difficult subject in immunology both conceptually and experimentally, so it is not really surprising that we have not got much further during the past half a century that has passed since its discovery. But the slow pace of progress has cost a loss of image. Interested outsiders often consider the field "an obscure, utopian research backwater", as worded in an online magazine of the biotechnology industry (www.singalsmag.com accessed 07.11.2001). This is, of course, the opinion of business people, who are thought to be superior to anyone of us in grasping reality, because they are dealing with money: the ultimate reality. This prejudice can be straightened easily by defining money as a rectangular piece of colored paper without intrinsic value, or as a number in the computer of a bank. Yet, such opinions will not remain without consequence, when it comes to the funding of tolerance research.'

'Therefore the future of the tolerance field, in my opinion, lies primarily in the research of autoimmune diseases. Namely, autoimmunity has to do with the breakdown of self tolerance, and thus mechanisms of the former can provide new insights into the latter, as exemplified beautifully by the discovery of AIRE (Section 9.3.4). But for the time being we must be content with the sketchy picture we have', concludes Dr. G.

REFERENCES

1. Billingham RE, Brent L, Medawar PB. *Nature* 1953;**172**:603.
2. Kappler JW, Wade T, White J, Kushnir E, Blackman M, Bill J, et al. *Cell* 1987;**49**:263.
3. Cohn M. *Res.mmunol.* 1992;**143**:323.
4. Owen RD. *Science* 1945;**102**:400.
5. Medawar PB. *J.Anat.* 1944;**78**:176.
6. Burnet FM, Fenner F. *The Production of Antibodies*. Melbourne: MacMillan; 1949.
7. Hasek M, Hraba T. *Nature* 1955;**175**:764.
8. Burnet FM. *The Clonal Selection Theory of Acquired Immunity*. London: Cambridge Univ. Press; 1959.
9. Cohn M, Langman RE. *Immunol.Rev.* 1990;**115**:1.
10. Smith RT, Bridges RA. *J.Exp.Med.* 1958;**108**:227.
11. Mitchison NA. *Proc.Roy.Soc.Ser.Biol.Sci.* 1964;**161**:275 6.
12. Weigle WO. *J.Immunol.* 1964;**92**:791.
13. Humphrey JH. *Immunol.* 1964;**7**:449.
14. Cohn M. In: Moulin AM, Cambrosio A, editors. *Singular Selves. Historical Issues and Contemporary Debates in Immunology*. France: Elsevier; 2001. p. 53.
15. Janeway Jr CA. *Immunol.Today* 1992;**13**:11.
16. Percus JK, Percus OE, Perelson AS. *Proc.Natl.Acad.Sci.USA*. 1993;**90**:1691.
17. Burnet FM, Fenner F. *Heredity* 1948;**2**:289.
18. Silverstein AM, Rose NR. *Immunol.Rev.* 1997;**159**:197.
19. Avrameas S. *Immunol.Today* 1991;**12**:154.
20. Tauber AI. *The immune self: theory or metaphor?* Cambridge: Cambridge University Press; 1994.
21. Matzinger P. *Annu.Rev.Immunol.* 1994;**12**:991.
22. Langman RE, Cohn M. *Scand.J.Immunol.* 1996;**44**:544.
23. Grabar P. *Immunol.Today* 1983;**4**:337.
24. Cohn M, Langman RE. *Cell.Immunol.* 2002;**216**:15.
25. Silverstein AM. *A History of Immunology*. San Diego: Acad. Press; 1989, 162.

26. Jerne NK. *Proc.Natl.Acad.Sci.USA.* 1955;**41**:849.
27. Langman RE, Cohn M. *Mol.Immunol.* 1987;**24**:675.
28. Burnet FM. *Aust.J.Sci.* 1957;**20**:67.
29. Talmage DW. *Ann.Rev.Med.* 1957;**8**:239.
30. Talmage DW. *Science* 1959;**129**:1643.
31. Lederberg J. *Science* 1959;**129**:1649.
32. Miller JFAP, Basten A. *Curr.Op.Immunol.* 1996;**8**:815.
33. Silverstein A, Rose N. *Immunol.Rev.* 1997;**159**:197.
34. Bretscher P, Cohn M. *Science* 1970;**169**:1042.
35. Cohn M. Progress in Immunology. In: Yamamura VY, Tada T, editors. Orlando: Academic Press; 1983. p. 839.
36. Langman RE. *The Immune System.* San Diego: Academic Press; 1989.
37. Bretscher P. *Immunol.Today* 1992;**13**:74.
38. Cohn M. *Annu.Rev.Immunol.* 1994;**12**:1.
39. Bretscher P. *Proc.Natl.Acad.Sci.USA.* 1999;**96**:185.
40. Forsdyke DR. *Lancet* 1968;**291**:281.
41. McDevitt HO, Benacerraf B. *Adv.Immunol.* 1969;**11**:31.
42. Rajewsky K, Schirrmacher V, Nase S, Jerne NK. *J.Exp.Med.* 1969;**129**:1131.
43. Langman RE, Cohn M. *Mol.Immunol.* 1987;**24**:675.
44. Pilarski LM. *J.Exp.Med.* 1977;**145**:709.
45. Keene J, Forman J. *J.Exp.Med.* 1982;**155**:768.
46. Mitchison NA, O'Malley C. *Eur.J.Immunol.* 1987;**17**:1579.
47. Bennett SRM, Carbone FR, Karamalis F, Flawell RA, Miller JFAP, Heath WR. *Nature* 1998;**393**:478.
48. Schoenberger SP, Toes REM, Voort EIH van der, Offringa R, Melief CJM. *Nature* 1998;**393**:480.
49. Armitage RJ, Tough TW, Macduff BM, Fanslow WC, Spriggs MK, Ramsdell F, et al. *Eur.J.Immunol.* 1993;**23**:2326.
50. Tucker MJ, Bretscher PA. *J.Exp.Med.* 1982;**155**:1037.
51. Gerloni M, Xiong S, Mukerjee S, Schoenberger SP, Croft M, Zanetti M. *Proc.Natl.Acad.Sci. USA.* 2000;**97**:13269.
52. Peters NC, Kroeger DR, Mickelwright S, Bretscher PA. *Int.Immunol.* 2009;**21**:1213.
53. Kroeger DR, Rudulier CD, Peters NC, Bretscher PA. *Int.Immunol.* 2012;**24**:519.
54. Strutt TM, Uzonna J, McKinstry KK, Bretscher PA. *Int.Immunol.* 2006;**18**:719.
55. Fuchs E. *Immunol.Today* 1993;**14**:236.
56. Lafferty KJ, Cunningham AJ. *Aust.J.Exp.Biol.Med.Sci.* 1975;**53**:27.
57. Lafferty KJ, Misko IS, Cooley MA. *Nature* 1974;**249**:275.
58. Lafferty KJ, Cooley MA, Woolnough JA, Walker KZ. *Science* 1975;**188**:259.
59. Talmage DW, Dart G, Radovich J, Lafferty KJ. *Science* 1976;**191**:385.
60. Lafferty KJ, Warren HS, Woolnough JA, Talmage DW. *Blood Cells* 1978;**4**:395.
61. Janeway Jr CA. *Cold Spring Harbor Symp.Quant.Biol.* 1989;**54**:1.
62. Medzhitov R, Janeway Jr CA. *Science* 2002;**296**:298.
63. Liu Y, Janeway Jr CA. *Int.Immunol.* 1991;**3**:323.
64. Medzhitov R, Preton-Hurlburt P, Janeway CA. *Nature* 1997;**388**:394.
65. Matzinger P. *Science* 2002;**296**:301.
66. Matzinger P. *Nature Immunol.* 2007;**8**:11.
67. de Jong EC, Vieira PL, Kalinski P, Schuitemaker JHN, Tanaka Y, Wierenga EA, et al. *J.Immunol.* 2002;**168**:1704.

68. Gray DH, Gavanescu I, Benoist C, Mathis D. *Proc.Natl.Acad.Sci.USA.* 2007;**104**:18193.
69. Segel LA, Lev Bar-Or R. *J.Immunol.* 1999;**163**:1432.
70. Cohn M. *Immunol.Res.* 2005;**31**:133.
71. Hsieh CS, Macatonia SE, Tripp CS, Wolf SF, O'Garra A, Murphy KM. *Science* 1993;**260**:547.
72. Mezhitov R, Preston-Hurlburt P, Janeway Jr CA. *Nature* 1997;**388**:394.
73. Urban JJ, Katona I, Paul WE, Finkelman FD. *Proc.Natl.Acad.Sci.USA.* 1991;**88**:5513.
74. Liew FY, Millott S, Lelchuk R, Chan WL, Ziltener H. *Eur.J.Immunol.* 1989;**19**:1227.
75. Karulin AY, Hesse MD, Tary-Lehmann M, Lehmann PV. *J.Immunol.* 2000;**164**:1862.
76. Cohn M. *Springer Semin.Immunopathol.* 2005;**27**:3.
77. Kappler JW, Roehm N, Marrack P. *Cell* 1987;**49**:273.
78. Festenstein H. *Transplant.Rev.* 1973;**15**:62.
79. Kappler JW, Staerz U, White J, Marrack PC. *Nature* 1988;**332**:35.
80. MacDonald HR, Schneider R, Lees RK, Howe RC, Acha-Orbea H, Festenstein H, et al. *Nature* 1988;**332**:40.
81. Happ MP, Woodland DL, Palmer E. *Proc.Natl.Acad.Sci.USA.* 1989;**86**:6293.
82. Hengartner H, Odermatt B, Schneider R, Schreyer M, Wälle G, MacDonald HR, et al. *Nature* 1988;**336**:388.
83. MacDonald HR, Lees RK. *Nature* 1990;**343**:642.
84. White J, Herman A, Pullen AM, Kubo R, Kappler JW, Marrack P. *Cell* 1989;**56**:27.
85. Karp DR, Teletski CL, Scholl P, Geha R, Long EO. *Nature* 1990;**346**:474.
86. Rust CJJ, Verreck F, Vietor H, Koning F. *Nature* 1990;**346**:572.
87. Bowness P, Moss PAH, Tranter H, Bell JI, McMichael AJ. *J.Exp.Med.* 1992;**176**:893.
88. Marrack P, Kushnir E, Kappler J. *Nature* 1991;**349**:524.
89. Frankel WN, Rudy C, Coffin JM, Huber BT. *Nature* 1991;**349**:526.
90. Woodland DL, Happ MP, Gollob KJ, Palmer E. *Nature* 1991;**349**:529.
91. Dyson PJ, Knight AM, Fairchild S, Simpson E, Tomonari K. *Nature* 1991;**349**:531.
92. Choi Y, Kappler JW, Marrack P. *Nature* 1991;**350**:203.
93. Acha-Orbea H, Shakhov AH, Scarpellino L, Kolb E, Müller V, Vessaz-Shaw A, et al. *Nature* 1991;**350**:207.
94. Fraser JD. *Nature* 1989;**339**:221.
95. Herman A, Labrecque N, Thibodeau J, Marrack P, Kappler JW, Sekaly RP. *Proc.Natl.Acad. Sci.USA.* 1991;**88**:9954.
96. Karp DR, Long EO. *J.Exp.Med.* 1992;**175**:415.
97. Pullen AM, Bill J, Kubo RT, Marrack P, Kappler JW. *J.Exp.Med.* 1991;**173**:1183.
98. Scherer MT, Ignatowitz L, Pullen A, Kappler J, Marrack P. *J.Exp.Med.* 1995;**182**:1493.
99. Rammensee HG, Kroschewski R, Frangoulis B. *Nature* 1989;**339**:541.
100. Kisielow P, Blüthmann H, Staerz UD, Steinmetz M, von Boehmer H. *Nature* 1988;**333**:742.
101. MacDonald HR, Hengartner H, Pedrazzini T. *Nature* 1988;**335**:174.
102. Fowlkes BJ, Schwartz RH, Pardoll DM. *Nature* 1988;**334**:620.
103. Sha WC, Nelson CA, Newberry RD, Kranz DM, Russell JH, Loh DY. *Nature* 1988;**336**:73.
104. Swat W, Ignatowicz L, von Boehmer H, Kisielow P. *Nature* 1991;**351**:150.
105. Vasquez NJ, Kaye J, Hedrick SM. *J.Exp.Med.* 1992;**175**:1307.
106. Nemazee DA, Bürki K. *Nature* 1989;**337**:562 122.
107. Nemazee D, Buerki K. *Proc.Natl.Acad.Sci.USA.* 1989;**86**:8039.
108. Goodnow CC, Crosbie J, Adelstein S, Lavoie TB, Smith-Gill SJ, Brink RA, et al. *Nature* 1988;**334**:576.
109. Goodnow CC, Crosbie J, Jorgensen H, Brink RA, Basten A. *Nature* 1989;**342**:385.
110. Adams E, Basten A, Goodnow CC. *Proc.Natl.Acad.Sci.USA.* 1990;**87**:5687.

111. Sidman CL, Unanue ER. *Nature* 1975;**257**:149.

112. Raff MC, Owen JJ, Cooper MD, Lawton 3rd AR, Megson M, Gathings WE. *J.Exp.Med.* 1975;**142**:1052.

113. Hartley SB, Crosbie J, Brink R, Kantor AB, Basten A, Goodnow CC. *Nature* 1991;**353**:765.

114. Goodnow CC, Adelstein S, Basten A. *Science* 1990;**248**:1373.

115. Nossal GJV. *Science* 1989;**245**:147.

116. Cohn M, Langman RE. *Immunol.Rev.* 1990;**115**:11.

117. Deas O, Dumont C, MacFarlane M, Rouleau M, Hebib C, Harper F, et al. *J.Immunol.* 1998;**161**:3375.

118. Lesage S, Steff AM, Philipoussis F, Page M, Trop S, Mateo V, et al. *J.Immunol.* 1997;**159**:4762.

119. Pettersen RD, Hestdal K, Olafsen MK, Lie SO, Lindberg FP. *J.Immunol.* 1999;**162**:7031.

120. Pettersen RD, Bernard G, Olafsen MK, Pourtein M, Lie SO. *J.Immunol.* 2001;**166**:4931.

121. Skov S, Klausen P, Claesson MH. *J.Cell.Biol.* 1997;**139**:1523.

122. Drenou B, Blancheteau V, Burgess DH, Fauchet R, Charron DJ, Mooney NA. *J.Immunol.* 1999;**163**:4115.

123. Defrance T, Casamayor-Palleja M, Krammer PH. *Adv.Cancer Res.* 2002;**86**:195.

124. Nossal GJ, Pike BL. *Proc.Natl.Acad.Sci.USA.* 1980;**77**:1602.

125. Lamb JR, Skidmore BJ, Green N, Chiller JM, Feldmann M. *J.Exp.Med.* 1983;**157**:1434.

126. Lamb JR, Feldmann M. *Nature* 1984;**308**:72.

127. Jenkins MK, Schwartz RH. *J.Exp.Med.* 1987;**165**:302.

128. Quill H, Schwartz RH. *J.Immunol.* 1987;**138**:3704.

129. Mueller DL, Jenkins MK, Schwartz RH. *J.Immunol.* 1989;**142**:2617.

130. Jenkins MK, Chen C, Jung G, Mueller DL, Schwartz RH. *J.Immunol.* 1990;**144**:16.

131. Jenkins MK, Ashwell JD, Schwartz RH. *J.Immunol.* 1988;**140**:3324.

132. Kearney ER, Pape KA, Loh DY, Jenkins MK. *Immunity* 1994;**1**:327.

133. Blackman MA, Gerhard-Burgert H, Woodland DL, Palmer E, Kappler JA, Marrack P. *Nature* 1990;**345**:540.

134. Morahan G, Hoffmann MW, JFAP Miller Proc. *Natl.Acad.Sci.USA.* 1991;**88**:11421.

135. Linsley PS, Brady W, Grosmarie L, Aruffo A, Damle NK, Ledbetter JA. *J.Exp.Med.* 1991;**173**:721.

136. Freeman GJ, Gribben JG, Boussiotis VA, Ng JW, Restivo VAJ, Lombard LA, et al. *Science* 1993;**262**:909.

137. Bierer BE, Peterson A, Gorga JC, Hermann SH, Burakoff SJ. *J.Exp.Med.* 1988;**168**:1145.

138. Springer TA, Dustin ML, Kishimoto TK, Marlin SD. *Annu.Rev.Immunol.* 1987;**5**:223.

139. Durum SK, Schmidt JA, Oppenheim JJ. *Annu.Rev.Immunol.* 1985;**3**:263.

140. Jenkins MK, Pardoll DM, Mizuguchi J, Chused TM, Schwartz RH. *Proc.Natl.Acad.Sci.USA.* 1987;**84**:5409.

141. Schwartz RH. *Science* 1990;**248**:1349.

142. Schwartz RH. *J.Exp.Med.* 1996;**184**:1

143. Beverly B, Kang SM, Leonardo MJ, Schwartz RH. *Int.Immunol.* 1992;**4**:661.

144. Boussiotis VA, Freeman GJ, Griffen JD, Gray GS, Gribben JG, Nadler LM. *J.Exp.Med.* 1994;**180**:1665.

145. Joliceur C, Hanahan D, Smith KM. *Proc.Natl.Acad.Sci.USA.* 1994;**91**:6707.

146. Antonia SJ, Geiger T, Miller J, Flavell RA. *Int.Immunol.* 1995;**7**:715.

147. Oukka M, Colucci-Guyon E, Tran PL, Cohen-Tannoudji M, Babinet C, Lotteau V, et al. *Immunity* 1996;**4**:545.

148. Oukka M, Cohen-Tannoudji M, Tanaka Y, Babinet C, Kosmatopoulos K. *J.Immunol.* 1996;**156**:968.

149. Smith KM, Olson DC, Hirose R, Hanahan D. *Int.Immunol.* 1997;**9**:1355.

150. Derbinski J, Schulte A, Kyewski B, Klein L. *Nat.Immunol.* 2001;**2**:1032.

151. Klein L, Klein T, Rüther U, Kyewski B. *J.Exp.Med.* 1998;**188**:5.

152. Klein L, Klugmann M, Nave KA, Tuohy VK, Kyewski B. *Nat.Med.* 2000;**6**:56.

153. Anderson AC, Nicholson LB, Legge KL, Turchin V, Zaghouani H, Kuchroo VK. *J.Exp.Med.* 2000;**191**:761.

154. Nagamine K, Peterson P, Scott HS, Kudoh J, Minoshima S, Heino M, et al. *Nat.Genet.* 1997;**17**:393.

155. Finnish-German APECED Consortium. *Nat.Genet.* 1997;**17**:399.

156. Kumar PG, Laloraya M, Wang CY, Ruan QG, Davoodi-Semiromi A, JX She KJ Kao. *J.Biol. Chem.* 2001;**276**:41357.

157. Pitkänen J, Doucas V, Sternsdorf T, Nakajima T, Aratani S, Jensen K, et al. *J.Biol.Chem.* 2000;**275**:16802.

158. Rosatelli MC, Meloni A, Meloni A, Devoto M, Cao A, Scott HS, et al. *Hum.Genet.* 1998;**103**:428.

159. Björses P, Halonen M, Palvimo JJ, Kolmer M, Aaltonen J, Ellonen P, et al. *Am.J.Hum.Genet.* 2000;**66**:378.

160. Anderson MS, Venanzi ES, Klein L, Chen Z, Berzins SP, Turley SJ, et al. *Science* 2002;**298**:1395.

161. Hubert FX, Kinkel SA, Webster KE, Cannon P, Crewther PE, Proeitto AI, et al. *J.Immunol.* 2008;**180**:3824.

162. Guerau-de-Arellano M, Martinic M, Benoist C, Mathis D. *J.Exp.Med.* 2009;**206**:1245.

163. Derbinski J, Gäbler J, Brors B, Tierling S, Jonnakuty S, Hergenhahn M, et al. *J.Exp.Med.* 2005;**202**:33.

164. Smith CA, Williams GT, Kingston R, Owen JJ. *Nature* 1989;**337**:181.

165. McConkey DJ, Hartzell P, Amador-Perez JF, Orrenius S, Jondal M. *J.Immunol.* 1989;**143**:1801.

166. Murphy KM, Heimberger AB, Loh DY. *Science* 1990;**250**:1720.

167. Nakayama T, Samelson LE, Nakayama Y, Munitz TI, Sheard M, June CH, et al. *Proc.Natl. Acad.Sci.USA.* 1991;**88**:9949.

168. Osmond DG. *Immunol.Today* 1993;**14**:34.

169. Fulop GM, Gordon J, Osmond DG. *J.Immunol.* 1983;**130**:644.

170. Opstelten D, Osmond DG. *Eur.J.Immunol.* 1985;**15**:599.

171. Lederberg J. *Science* 1959;**129**:1649.

172. Opselten D, Osmond DG. *J.Immunol.* 1983;**131**:2635.

173. Osmond DG, Kim N, Manoukian R, Phillips RA, Rico-Vargas SA, Jacobsen K. *Blood* 1695:79.

174. Everett NB, Tyler RW. *Int.Rev.Cytol.* 1967;**22**:205.

175. Press OW, Rosse C, Clagett J. *Cell.Immunol.* 1977;**33**:114.

176. Förster I, Rajewsky K. *Proc.Natl.Acad.Sci.USA.* 1990;**87**:4781.

177. Weigert MG, Cesari IM, Yonkovich SS, Cohn M. *Nature* 1970;**228**:1045.

178. Bernard O, Hozumi N, Tonegawa S. *Cell* 1978;**15**:1133.

179. Rajewsky K, Förster I, Cumano A. *Science* 1987;**238**:1088.

180. Mamula MJ, Lin RH, Janeway Jr CA, Hardin JA. *J.Immunol.* 1992;**149**:789.

181. Scollay RG, Butcher EC, Weissman IL. *Eur.J.Immunol.* 1980;**10**:210.

Chapter 10

Autoimmunity

Autoimmunity can be broadly defined as a specific immune *effector* response against self components that inflicts harm on the host. The self-damaging response is often of inflammatory nature, but other effector mechanisms, e.g., complement activation by autoantibodies bound to self structures, can also be the major cause of pathology. Autoimmunity should be distinguished from autoreactivity, the latter denoting the presence of self-specific antigen receptors and antibodies in the body that remain without harmful consequences. The manifestations of autoimmunity are called autoimmune diseases (AIDs), which represent a rather large assemblage of different illnesses with distinct symptoms, locations and pathomechanisms. The only commonality of AIDs on which most participants of the field agree is that the pathology is the consequence of a failure in one or another mechanism of self tolerance. Therefore, autoimmunity can be regarded as the down-side of self tolerance, as well as the most likely selective pressure that has driven self–non-self discrimination. In this context, the frequency of AIDs in the population (up to 5%) may reflect the limit of natural selection, i.e., that the latter cannot operate to perfection, only to adequacy defined as the level of harm that no longer threatens the procreation of the species.

Naturally, many of the diseases now known or assumed to be of autoimmune origin, particularly the more frequent ones, have been known since ancient times, and a large body of information has been gathered on their symptoms and pathology. But that an immune response against self components can be the cause of disease was first recognized at the beginning of the twentieth century.[1] The advent of immunobiology ('the immunological revolution') was an important impetus also for autoimmunity research, and thus a large number of diseases have been added to the list of AIDs from the 1950s on.

The history of the early period of autoimmunity research[2] as well as the individual diseases[3,4] were abundantly covered earlier. The focus of this chapter will be on how new insights into specific areas of immunology, such as the mechanisms of self tolerance, the biological role of the major histocompatibility complex, and the nature of antigen recognition by T cells, have led to a deeper and more precise understanding of autoimmunity.

A History of Modern Immunology. http://dx.doi.org/10.1016/B978-0-12-416974-6.00010-7

10.1 GENETIC FACTORS PREDISPOSING TO AUTOIMMUNE DISEASE

Autoimmune diseases (AIDs) clearly have heritable components, and this fact is easiest to appreciate through the increased prevalence of a particular disease within the same family.

For example, insulin-dependent diabetes mellitus (IDDM) has a prevalence of ~0.1% in the general population, whereas monozygotic twins are ~50% concordant, and HLA identical siblings ~20% concordant for the disease.[5] These numbers indicate that about half of the susceptibility factors are genetically determined, and that almost half of the genetic predisposition is contributed by the major histocompatibility complex (HLA). Or to put it differently, every second individual with full genetic susceptibility may get the disease, and the same applies to one in five individuals with a susceptible HLA allele. The remaining ~50% of predisposition is not heritable, usually referred to as 'environmental', which may include factors as diverse as infections, nutrition, environmental pollution, etc.

The genetic component of susceptibility tends to vary depending on the disease. For example, in rheumatoid arthritis (RA), it is smaller than in IDDM. Here the monozygotic twin concordance rate is ~20%, and the sibling occurrence risk is ~7%, at a population prevalence of ~1%.[6]

As these examples illustrate, most AIDs are multifactorial, with complex etiology and pathogenesis that comprise varying numbers of genetic and environmental factors. The identification of every single factor is therefore a significant challenge and still an ongoing effort.

10.1.1 Genetic Association with the Major Histocompatibility Complex

Among the numerous gene loci that may affect autoimmune diseases (AIDs) the major histocompatibility complex (MHC) stands out as the strongest predisposing factor. The association of AIDs with the MHC is observed as an increased frequency of particular alleles at a certain class I or class II MHC locus in patients compared to the healthy population. For example, the class II allele DRB1*0401 is present in >50% of Caucasian rheumatoid arthritis (RA) patients,[7] whereas its frequency in the healthy population is 14%. This finding indicates that the DRB1*0401 allele confers increased risk of RA to the individuals carrying it, the relative risk being about 3.6 times (50:14) higher than for DRB1*0401-negative individuals.

MHC association was first demonstrated in the early 1970s for ankylosing spondylitis, a chronic inflammatory joint disease, which was found to occur preferentially in individuals carrying the HLA-B27 class I allele.[8,9] The number of HLA-associated diseases then increased rapidly, so that a comprehensive listing in 1985 already encompassed more than 70 diseases.[10]

The precision with which MHC-linkage of a given AID could be determined was primarily contingent upon the technological stand of HLA typing. The earliest typing method was serology utilizing alloantisera (later also monoclonal antibodies), which defined major HLA types, for example HLA-DR1, DR2, DR3, etc. In retrospect, it has turned out that most of these antibodies detected epitopes shared among a number of related HLA allele products, and thus serological typing provided neither gene-specific not haplotype-specific information. Serology was then supplemented with cellular typing using T cells activated in mixed lymphocyte cultures against allogeneic cells. The resolution of cellular typing was higher than that of serology, so that the typing cells could distinguish a number of subtypes, designated Dw, within the broad serological specificities. For example, DR4 was subdivided by cellular typing into Dw4, Dw10, Dw13, Dw14, Dw15, and Dw'KT2'. The final resolution of HLA alleles was brought about by the advance of molecular biology, namely the polymerase chain reaction (PCR) permitted the rapid amplification and sequencing of the polymorphic regions of all previously unknown alleles. Taking again DR4 as an example, the molecular biology approach resulted in the identification of 19 distinct allelic variants of the polymorphic DRβ chain within this single serological specificity.

The new and possibly final state of knowledge about HLA polymorphism necessitated a new nomenclature, which was introduced by the WHO Nomenclature Committee in 1994.[11] By the new terminology the loci are designated by capital letters, e.g., HLA-A, HLA-B, HLA-C for class I, and DRA, DRB, DQA, DQB, DPA, DPB for the genes coding for class II α and β chains. Because DRβ chains are encoded in more than one locus, these loci are designated DRB1, DRB2 etc. The gene designations are followed by an asterisk and a number for the actual allele. For example, the allele previously known as DR4Dw4 becomes DRB1*0401 by the new nomenclature (the DRA gene encoding the α chain is monomorphic and thus can be omitted from the allele designation). The new nomenclature has been used for quite a while in parallel with the old one, and therefore readers of MHC–disease associations should be aware of both. The good news is that the terminology has not changed since 1994.

Technology was not the only limiting factor in determining precisely an MHC-associated susceptibility gene. Another type of complication arose from the feature of MHC genes referred to as linkage disequilibrium. As known, the rate of recombination between two genetic loci is usually proportional to their distance from each other: the further they are apart the higher the recombination rate and vice versa. But this rule does not apply to some MHC loci. Here the recombination rate is often lower than expected on the basis of distance, probably due to co-selection of the two loci by evolution. This results in a situation that a particular allele at one locus occurs almost always in combination with a defined allele at the second locus. Consequently it is not easy to distinguish whether the detected gene itself is responsible for the disease association, or a linked gene on the same haplotype. This applies particularly to DR and DQ genes, and examples to follow will illustrate the difficulties this linkage disequilibrium caused in the definition of MHC association for certain diseases.

Obviously it is neither possible nor necessary at this place to deal with the discovery of all MHC–AID associations. Instead, we will attempt to follow-up how the general principles and technological progress as outlined above have contributed to the definitive mapping of susceptibility genes in the case of a few selected diseases. Readers interested in more detail are referred to the work of Barbara and Gerry Nepom at the Virginia Mason Research Center in Seattle, who belonged to the most dedicated investigators of HLA–disease associations.

Rheumatoid arthritis represents the most thoroughly studied and best-documented example of an HLA-associated AID. The first reports[12,13] date back to the time when only serological and cellular typing were available, and thus these studies demonstrated association with the broad serological specificity DR4, and the most prevalent T-cell-defined subtype Dw4 (DRB1*0401). Subsequent investigations identified a second DR4 subtype, Dw14 (DRB1*0404) to be associated with RA.[14,15] Haplotype segregation in families with multiple cases of RA confirmed these results. But the genetic association still remained incomplete, first, because not all DR4 subtypes were found to be associated with RA, and second, a substantial proportion (20–35%) of RA patients was DR4-negative.

The complexity of HLA–RA associations was partially resolved by introducing more stringent criteria to define RA and exclude other joint diseases.[16] But the final clarification came from studies using genetic typing with allele-specific oligonucleotide probes, and involving patient populations of different ethnic origins. The picture that arose from these studies was still very complex. In Caucasian populations DRB1*0401 and 0404 were shown to account for approximately 70% of RA patients, while the majority of non-DR4 patients turned out to carry the DR1 (DRB1*0101) allele. The DR4Dw10 (DRB1*0402) allele was shown definitively not to be associated with RA. In Japanese, however, where the 0401 and 0404 alleles are extremely rare in the normal population, RA was found to be highly associated with another DR4 allele Dw15 (DRB1*0405).[17] In Israelis the situation was again different: the most commonly found DR4 allele here was 0402 in the healthy population, which is not associated with RA, and the most frequent allele in RA patients was DR1 (DRB1*0101).[18] Another interesting case was that of the Yakima Native American tribe with a highly increased prevalence of RA. Here the disease was most strongly associated with the allele Dw16 (DRB1*1402),[19] which is completely unrelated to DR4 and DR1.

Thus altogether five DRB1 alleles, 0101, 0401, 0404, 0405, and 1402, some of them seemingly unrelated, were found to be associated with RA, whereas the related allele 0402 was not associated. This finding posed a perfect puzzle. One possible explanation would have been that the identified DR associations just masked the 'real' association of the disease with a closely linked DQ allele, but this assumption was not supported unequivocally by typing data. The solution to the enigma finally came from sequencing of all these genes. Comparison of the deduced amino acid sequences of the DRβ chains encoded by the RA-associated alleles has namely revealed a short stretch from codon 67 to 74 that is shared by all these alleles (Table 10.1). A prominent feature of this sequence is a positively charged polymorphic residue, Arg or Lys, at position 71. In contrast, the RA-unlinked 0402 allele has a negative residue, Glu at this position (plus an adjacent negative residue, Asp70). Thus, the opposing charges at position 71 correlate with susceptibility versus resistance to RA. The remaining conservative exchange, Leu to Ile at position 67 may be of little functional consequence. Two important conclusions follow from this sequence comparison: first, it seems to be the DRB1 gene itself that is associated with RA (not some linked gene), and second, the positive charge of residue 71 appears to determine disease association by an unknown mechanism.

'The 67–74 sequence of RA-associated DRβ chains was widely referred to in the literature as the "shared epitope"[20], adds Dr. G. 'This term probably has its origin in the fact that these allelic DR variants were originally defined by serological and cellular typing, i.e., through epitopes recognized by antibodies or alloreactive T cells. That this sequence influences allorecognition has also been demonstrated directly.[21] Nevertheless the term remains somewhat confusing, because it implies that direct recognition of the 67–74 sequence by T cells should be a disease mechanism in RA. Clearly, speculations about a possible role of the shared epitope in RA[20] were premature at that time. This question could only be reasonably addressed some years later, after the discovery of HLA-DR structure and the rules of peptide binding to these molecules.'

TABLE 10.1 Amino Acid Sequences of DRβ Chains at Positions 67 to 74

DRB1* Allele	Association with RA[a]	Amino Acid at Position							
		67	68	69	70	71	72	73	74
0101	yes	L[b]	L	E	Q	R	R	A	A
0401	yes	–[c]	–	–	–	K	–	–	–
0404	yes	–	–	–	–	–	–	–	–
0405	yes	–	–	–	–	–	–	–	–
1402	yes	–	–	–	–	–	–	–	–
0402	no	I	–	–	D	E	–	–	–

[a] Rheumatoid arthritis.
[b] Single letter code for amino acids.
[c] Residue identical with that of 0101.

Insulin-dependent diabetes mellitus (IDDM) was recognized by the mid-1980s to be the result of an autoimmune response against insulin-producing beta cells in the Langerhans islets of pancreas.[22] In population studies,[23] IDDM was found to be strongly associated with the serological specificities HLA-DR3 and DR4, weakly associated with DR1 and DR8, and negatively associated with DR2.[24] This associations needed, of course, further precision, which was provided by the discovery of the molecular diversity underlying each serological type.

The clearest case of disease association could be established for haplotypes within the DR4 serological group. As shown in Table 10.2, the DR4 serotype is subdivided by genetic and cellular typing into several alleles, each of which is in linkage disequilibrium with a particular DQ allele. Interestingly, it has turned out that IDDM segregates more clearly with one of the linked DQ alleles, DQB1*0302, than with any of the DRB1 alleles. This is particularly revealing in the case of DRB1*0401, which is linked to DQB1*0302 only in a subset of individuals, and this subset is susceptible to IDDM, whereas the majority of the population carrying the DRB1*0401-DQB1*0301 haplotype is not.[25] Altogether, DQB1*0302 has been found in ~95% of Caucasian IDDM patients who carry a DR4-positive haplotype (and in ~70% of all Caucasian IDDM patients), and is thus the gene most highly associated with diabetes.[26]

Another remarkable finding was the dominant protective effect of the DR2-linked DQB1*0602 allele.[26] Heterozygotes carrying this allele together with a susceptibility allele on the other parental haplotype were shown to have a relative risk significantly below one becoming diabetic.

TABLE 10.2 Association of IDDM with Haplotypes in the DR4 Serological Group

Association with IDDM[a]	Haplotype		
	DQB1	DQA1	DRB1
no	0301	0301	0401[b] (Dw4)[c]
yes	0302	0301	0401 (Dw4)
yes	0302	0301	0402 (Dw10)
no	0301	0301	0403 ((Dw13)
yes	0302	0301	0404 (Dw14)
no	0401	0301	0405 (Dw15)

[a] Insulin-dependent diabetes mellitus.
[b] Allele defined by genetic typing.
[c] Allele defined by cellular typing.
Based on Reference 25.

The remaining HLA associations of IDDM were weak, complex, and difficult to rationalize. In general, the disease appeared to be more closely associated with DQ alleles than with DR alleles, but exceptions to this rule were also found.[5] Furthermore, in most cases both parental HLA haplotypes seemed to influence disease susceptibility,[5] so that a weaker DQ susceptibility allele in combination with other alleles often behaved as neutral, suggesting recessive inheritance of susceptibility. Even the strongest susceptibility allele, DQB1*0302, was found to confer different degrees of susceptibility depending on the second parental DQ allele.[26]

'The complex and partially confused HLA associations of diabetes made frustrat-ingly little sense for the conceptualizing mind', comments Dr. G. 'Nevertheless, they are justifiable from the evolutionary point of view. Consider that before the discovery of insulin, IDDM killed all affected individuals at a young age, and was thus a very rigorous selective pressure. Consequently, even if there had been dominant susceptibility alleles at earlier points in time, they would have been rapidly eliminated by natural selection, and so we would not see them. That we still can detect at least one strong susceptibility allele (DQB1*0302) is solely due to the existence of a dominant protective allele (DQB1*0602), which renders the susceptibility allele recessive, and thereby permits its escape from the iron grip of natural selection. A similar trend can be seen in the case of weaker susceptibility alleles that tend to be neutralized in heterozygosity with other alleles. Altogether, the recessive or recessive-like inheritance of diabetes susceptibility can perfectly account for the present state of HLA associations. Of course, with the introduc-tion of insulin therapy, IDDM was taken out of the hands of natural selection, and so in the long run, the frequency of susceptibility alleles will probably increase.'

In the search for the structural basis of HLA–IDDM associations, Hugh McDevitt's group[27] at Stanford University took a direct, Occam's razor kind of approach. Using a new method for the rapid cloning and sequencing of enzy-matically amplified DNA segments,[28] they sequenced the DRB, DQA and DQB genes from IDDM patients and from healthy controls. Sequence comparisons led to a number of interesting observations. First, all sequences found in patients were also found in healthy controls, indicating that the autoimmune process was not due to a mutant HLA allele unique to the disease (indeed, this applies to all MHC–disease associations). Second, the DQβ chain amino acid sequence was directly correlated with predisposition to IDDM. Third, the DQ-determined susceptibility was largely dependent on the amino acid at position 57 of the β chain: all DQB alleles positively associated with IDDM encoded Ala, Val, or Ser, whereas all neutral or negatively associated alleles Asp at position 57. This correlation was further supported by the sequence of the Aβ chain (the murine homologue of DQβ) expressed in non-obese diabetic (NOD) mice[29] that develop a spontaneous autoimmune diabetes similar to IDDM. The Aβ sequence of NOD mice is unique in that it has Ser at position 57, in contrast to all other known Aβ allelic forms with Asp at this position. According to these findings the complex HLA associations of IDDM can be reduced to the effect of a single amino acid at position 57 of the respective class II β chain: Asp57 confers resistance and non-Asp57 susceptibility to diabetes.

'The discovery of the Stanford group brought a significant degree of clarity into the confusing field of IDDM genetics. Similar results were reported later by the pioneer of PCR, Henry Erlich and his colleagues,[30] and the validity of the "position-57 story" was also confirmed in large populations[26] and family studies[31], adds Dr. G. 'Nonetheless, the concept failed to enjoy unanimous acceptance, in fact, it caused some fury particularly in circles of HLA-typers. The major objection of the latter was that the "rule-57" was not generally applicable. For example, IDDM in Japan is associated with Asp57 alleles of DQB,[32] and even Caucasian IDDM patients often carry one Asp57 allele.[26] They argued therefore that codon 57 itself could not account for the genetic association with IDDM. However, the finding that >99% of Caucasian diabetics carries at least one non-Asp allele[26] could not be explained away, at most, the dominant protective role of Asp57 could be questioned[33] that was not explicitly stated in the original study[27] anyway. So the 57-opponents finally offered as a compromise to treat position 57 as a "linked marker",[5] whatever this might mean.'

'The debate about position 57 may be regarded, on the one hand, as another example of the usual conflict between "reductionists" and "complicators". On the other hand, it reflects fundamental differences in the way experts of distinct fields were thinking about the MHC. Geneticists, of course, preferred to take a genetic locus at face value, whereas immunologists, who were by that time well aware of the role of MHC in antigen presentation and T-cell recognition, preferred to view MHC–AID associations as being indirect, brought about by immunological mechanisms.'

Pemphigus vulgaris (PV) is a life-threatening blistering disease of the skin and mucosa caused by autoantibodies against desmoglein 3, a keratinocyte cell adhesion molecule.[34] Population studies revealed strong association of PV with two distinct class II alleles, DRB1*0402 (DR4Dw10) and DRB1*1401 (DR6Dw9). These two associations appeared to be independent, without synergy. The first association could be ascribed to the DRB1*0402 allele itself, as practically all DR4 PV patients carried this allele, in contrast to a much lower frequency in healthy DR4 controls. However, the DRB1*1401 association turned out to be virtual, the real susceptibility allele being DQB1*0503, which is in linkage disequilibrium with the DR allele above.[35]

Sequence comparisons of the susceptibility genes with related alleles revealed two interesting points. First, the DRB1*0402 association correlated closely with the amino acid at position 71 of the DRβ chain as also found in RA. In fact the PV and RA associations were mirror images: a positively charged residue at position 71 translated into susceptibility to RA and resistance to PV, and a negative residue had the opposite effect. Second, the DQB1*0503-

associated susceptibility to PV correlated with Asp at position 57 of the DQβ chain, i.e., the exact opposite to IDDM susceptibility.

A common denominator of all these studies was that a single amino acid at position 71 of the DRβ and position 57 of the DQβ chain, respectively, seemed to be instrumental in determining susceptibility to different AIDs. It was therefore very likely that these amino acid positions would affect the structure and/or function of the respective molecule in a fundamental way.

10.1.2 Selective Antigen Presentation: A Possible Mechanism for MHC–Disease Association

As the autoimmune disease (AID)-linked major histocompatibility complex (MHC) alleles were found to be perfectly normal (i.e., not mutants), it was reasonable to speculate that the disease associations had to do with the physiological function of MHC: antigen presentation to T cells. According to this notion, certain allelic forms of MHC molecules can present particular autoantigens selectively, and the T cells thus activated are responsible for the pathology either directly or through their help to autoreactive B cells resulting in autoantibody formation. The question was only how the selectivity of antigen presentation could be accomplished.

'Actually the idea of selective antigen presentation was not new', points out Dr. G. 'It was proposed two decades earlier to explain the effect of MHC-linked immune response (Ir) genes (see Section 6.2.6). So for those of us who have ever worked on Ir genes, the analogy of the latter with MHC-linked autoimmunity was immediately obvious. Namely, Ir genes are manifested in MHC allele-dependent responses to foreign antigens, and AIDs may be induced by MHC allele-dependent responses to self antigens. Therefore it made sense to test out the mechanisms of Ir-gene control in autoimmune models. This explains also why so many colleagues who had formerly worked on Ir genes, including Hugh McDevitt himself the discoverer of these genes, ended up later studying MHC–AID associations.'

The experimental approach to selective antigen presentation was to compare disease-associated and non-associated MHC molecules for peptide binding, and to establish differences in binding specificity that would correlate with disease association. Such experiments were feasible for HLA-DR molecules, the only class II proteins whose peptide-binding specificity was reasonably well characterized at that time.[36,37] Based on the findings of previous genetic studies (Section 10.1.1), the question to be addressed was whether sequence 67–74 and more specifically position 71 of the DRβ chain implicated in disease associations would influence peptide binding.

The first study of this kind reported by Hammer et al.[38] utilized peptide libraries[39] to compare the binding specificity of DR4 molecules, two of which (DRB1*0401 and 0404) were associated and the third (0402) not associated with rheumatoid arthritis (RA). As shown in Table 10.1, these molecules differ in the 67–74 region, the prominent difference being at position 71, where RA-associated molecules carry a positively charged residue (Arg or Lys), and the non-associated variant a negative residue (Glu). The rationale of the study received strong support from the crystal structure of HLA-DR complexed with a single peptide published just the year before.[40] In the three-dimensional structure, position 71 turned out to be located in the centre of the α-helical region of DRβ (see Fig. 7.2), and was shown to form part of a pocket that accepts position 4 (relative to anchor position 1) of the bound peptide.

The peptide-binding data[38] showed a clear preference at relative positions 4, 5 and 7 for residues whose electrostatic charge was complementary to that of the DRβ-71 residue. Thus a negative charge at these positions of the peptide enabled binding to the RA-associated DR4 types, and abolished binding to the non-associated molecule, and positive charge had the opposite effect. Substitution of position 71 to an oppositely charged residue reversed these binding preferences. It was thus clear that charge attraction vs. repulsion between DRβ-71 and the middle portion of the peptide accounted for the selective binding. This new information combined with the known HLA-DR binding motifs (see in Table 7.2) permitted the authors a search for selectively binding peptides of self proteins implicated in RA, in the expectation of identifying the unknown autoantigen(s) responsible for the disease. Although this hope was not fulfilled, a number of peptides binding to RA-associated DR4 molecules were identified, about one third of which were selective.[38] One of the selective peptides, type II collagen 1168–1180, was later co-crystallized with DRB1*0401, and the Lys residue at DRβ-71 was shown to form salt-bridged hydrogen bonds with the Asp side chain at relative position 4, and interacted also with position 5 of the peptide.[41] Importantly, the dominant arthritogenic epitope of human type II collagen (sequence 261–273)[42] was also found to carry a negative residue (Glu) at relative position 4.

An interesting, somewhat related case was presented in treatment-resistant Lyme arthritis, an autoimmune-like condition associated with DRB1*0401, as is RA. The disease is triggered by a dominant T-cell epitope in the outer surface protein-A of *Borrelia burgdorferi* and maintained by a homologous self epitope in the leukocyte function-associated antigen-1 (LFA-1).[44] Noteworthy in this context is that both the triggering and the cross-reactive epitope had the negatively charged residue Glu at relative position 4.

The chronologically second study reported by Wucherpfennig et al.[43] approached the problem from the opposite side. They used pemphigus vulgaris (PV) as a model, which is associated with a negative charge at position 71 of DRB1*0402. Since the disease-inducing autoantigen, desmoglein 3, was known, they searched the sequence of this protein for peptides with the known DR4 binding motif, plus a positively charged residue at relative position 4. Seven such peptides could be identified, four of which were able to recall T-cell responses from PV patients (the remaining three may not have been produced by processing of the autoantigen in vivo). As expected, these peptides were selectively presented by 0402 and not by the closely related RA-associated molecules 0401 and 0404.

But charge preference is not the only mechanism, by which position 71 of the DRβ chain can impose selectivity on peptide binding. For example, multiple sclerosis is assumed to be initiated by T cells recognizing a dominant epitope (residues 84–102) of myelin basic protein (MBP) presented by DR2Dw2 (DRB1*1501) molecules.[45] An unusual feature of DR2 is the presence of Ala at β71; all other known DRB1 alleles encode Lys, Arg, or Glu at this position. Crystal structure of the DR2 protein together with the dominant core peptide (MBP 85–99) revealed a large hydrophobic position-4 (P4) pocket, which arose due to the presence of the small Ala residue at β71 (instead of the large residues of other DR types).[46] The P4 pocket was occupied by a Phe residue of the MBP peptide, which represented the major anchor for binding. Other DR types with large residues at β71 could not accommodate a Phe residue at position 4, and would therefore be unable to bind this peptide. Thus, in this case, size limitations of the P4 pocket account for the selectivity of peptide binding.

'Since the "position-71 story" was clear and simple enough, Kai Wucherpfennig and Jack Strominger[47] at Harvard University felt encouraged to propose that selective binding of autoantigenic peptides by disease-associated MHC molecules would be the mechanism underlying the genetic linkage of AID with MHC', adds Dr. G. 'As alluded to before, this concept was analogous to the "determinant selection" hypothesis put forward by Shevach and Rosenthal two decades earlier to explain the action of MHC-linked Ir genes (see Section 6.2.6 and Fig. 6.2). Because the selective presentation concept was well-founded many colleagues considered the puzzle of MHC–disease association solved, and stopped thinking about it. However, this was premature, because selective presentation did not solve the problem, just shifted it to a different level. To appreciate this point, it should be recalled that HLA-DR molecules can bind peptides without any charged residue in the middle perfectly well.[37] This binding is, of course, not selective, i.e., it cannot account for disease association. So if we wish to keep the hypothesis, we must make the additional assumption that the autoimmune process is *always* initiated by T cells responding to a single peptide (or a small set of homologous peptides) bound selectively. Why?'

'As there is no clear answer to this question, all I can do is to employ the Sherlock Holmes strategy, i.e., exclude all possibilities except one, and hope that the remaining one will be the truth. First, I must point out that in vitro binding studies with random peptide libraries did *not* identify any charged residue as a position 4 anchor.[36,37] In contrast, the majority of naturally presented abundant self peptides eluted from DR4 (DRB1*0401) molecules had a negative residue, Asp or Glu, in the middle.[48] Thus it is not the binding itself, but something else in the physiology of antigen presentation that leads to the dominance of peptides with a charged position 4. For "something else" three possibilities can be envisaged: antigen processing, peptide loading onto MHC, and the stability of peptide–MHC complexes. It is highly unlikely that antigen processing would preferentially yield peptides with charged residues, as the latter do not stabilize against proteases, but do rather the opposite by serving as protease recognition sites. Peptide loading onto MHC class II is controlled by the HLA-DM molecule, which removes peptides with insufficient anchors from the class II binding site (see Section 7.3.3). Although HLA-DM appears to act on the P1 and not on the P4 pocket of the binding groove,[49] it is still possible that a strong interaction with the P4 pocket improves the chance of peptides to survive the "editing" action of HLA-DM, and become dominant. Thus a possible effect of position 4 on peptide loading is difficult to exclude. Finally, a strong interaction of the peptide with the P4 pocket may induce a more compact conformation of the peptide–MHC complex, leading to higher stability and longer in vivo half-life of the latter. Single residue differences are known to have tremendous impact on these parameters.[50] This would be my favored mechanism for the establishment of epitope dominance, while peptide loading appears to me somewhat less likely. Perhaps Mr. Holmes would be unsatisfied with this outcome, but I cannot offer anything better.'

'If we now make one more ad hoc assumption, namely that autoimmunity can *only* be triggered by dominant (i.e., abundantly presented) self peptides, we have managed to save the idea of selective presentation, except that it has become selective epitope dominance. Because P4 is the most polymorphic pocket in the HLA-DR binding site (see in Fig. 7.2), it is not surprising that its effect on epitope dominance exhibits allele-specific features and can thus be read out as a genetic association of AIDs with particular DR alleles. Of course, the next question is: why are these dominant self peptides not under self tolerance? This aspect will be discussed later.'

Translation of the position-57 effect into mechanisms followed a similar path, except that it was investigated in somewhat less detail than position 71. As pointed out before (Section 10.1.1), the amino acid at position 57 of the DQβ chain appeared to determine single-handedly the susceptibility vs resistance to at least two different AIDs, insulin-dependent diabetes mellitus (IDDM) and pemphigus vulgaris (PV). Alleles with DQβ57 residue Ala, Ser, or Val conferred susceptibility, whereas those with Asp resistance to IDDM, and the reverse association applied to PV. The question was therefore addressed, whether the Asp57 vs non-Asp57 difference would affect the peptide-binding specificity of the respective molecule. And the answer was a clear yes[51] for a tight binding to non-Asp57 molecules, peptides required a negatively charged residue at relative position 9. On the contrary, negative charge at position 9 inhibited peptide binding to molecules with Asp57. Thus here again, similarly to the case of position 71, electrostatic attraction or repulsion caused selectivity of peptide binding.

The underlying molecular mechanism was, however, different from that of the position-71 effect. In class II molecules with Asp57 an interdomain salt bridge was detectable between Asp57 of the β and Arg76 of the α chain. This interaction is conserved in most DR, DQ, and DP molecules, and is assumed to stabilize the right-hand end of the peptide-binding groove.[52,40] In the IDDM-associated DQB1*0302 chain, Asp57 is replaced by Ala, and thus the interchain salt bridge cannot form. But a negative residue of the bound peptide, e.g.,

Glu, occupying the P9 pocket forms salt bridged hydrogen bonds with $Arg76\alpha$, thus replacing the interchain interaction.[53] In the $I\text{-}A^{g7}$ molecule of non-obese diabetic (NOD) mice, Asp57 is replaced by Ser, which participates in a triplet hydrogen-bonding interaction with $Arg76\alpha$ and the position 9 Glu of the bound peptide.[54] It seems therefore that a negative residue at peptide position 9 is favorable to achieve a compact structure of non-Asp57 molecules, and thereby a higher stability of peptide–MHC complexes.

Concerning the link between peptide binding and susceptibility to IDDM, it is probably relevant that the autoantigen implicated in the disease, glutamic acid decarboxylase 65[55,56] forms dominant epitopes with the NOD class II molecule,[54,57] and these epitopes have a negative charge at position 9. It is therefore possible that the genetic association of disease with position 57 is exerted through selective epitope dominance, as in the case of position 71.

For completeness' sake it should also be mentioned that the effect of position 57 is not limited to DQ, and of position 71 to DR molecules. Indeed, the position 57 of $DR\beta$[51] as well as 71 of $DQ\beta$[58] can also affect the peptide-binding specificity and disease association of the respective molecule.

Based on all these studies it appears safe to conclude that the curious association of certain AIDs with single polymorphic residues in class II β chains is the consequence of a key role these residues play in peptide–MHC interactions. Although this alone would suffice to explain disease associations, additional ways by which MHC molecules could influence autoimmunity are not ruled out.

10.1.3 Other Possible Mechanisms for MHC–Disease Association

MHC molecules interact not only with peptides but also with the antigen receptor of T cells (TCR), and thus they can be expected to control disease susceptibility through influencing T-cell recognition, instead of or in addition to peptide presentation. The effect of MHC alleles on the selection of the normal TCR repertoire was known from studies of MHC restriction (Section 8.4.3). It seemed therefore reasonable to seek for MHC allele-dependent TCR-repertoire differences that would be relevant for disease mechanisms. The goal of this type of experiments was to establish a tripartite correlation between a disease-associated MHC allele, the TCR repertoire selected by this allele, and the pathogenic T cells from this repertoire that are causative of the respective disease.

A number of studies in this vein were performed, some using animal models, others investigating directly the TCR repertoire of patients suffering from autoimmune disease (AID). Of course, these studies had to deal per force with both processes, i.e., positive and negative thymic selection, that shape the TCR repertoire. A few of the relevant reports will be discussed here for illustrative purposes.

The favorite animal model for these investigations was the non-obese diabetic (NOD) mouse. For example, Ridgway et al.[59] demonstrated a very labile state of self tolerance in these mice that could have been the result of a defect in tolerance induction, but whether the defect was in repertoire selection or elsewhere was not identified. Another approach was to graft the thymic epithelium of NOD mice into newborn athymic non-autoimmune C57BL/6 mice.[60] The resulting chimeras regularly showed autoimmunity to pancreatic beta cells and salivary glands. Although the conclusion that repertoire selection by NOD thymic epithelium being sufficient to induce autoimmunity was justified, it remained unclear whether the NOD class II molecule, or other non-MHC genes expressed in the graft were responsible for the effect. Furthermore, how the T cells selected on NOD MHC interacted at the periphery with allogeneic MHC molecules of the recipient was not clarified, and thus the pathogenesis of the observed autoimmunity was obscure. Another series of experiments addressed the puzzling question of why a second class II molecule not associated with diabetes prevented the NOD class II-driven disease. The results demonstrated that the protective effect was due to negative selection,[61] or not due to negative selection,[62] or due to positive selection,[63] in other words no unequivocal solution was offered.

Aberrations of the TCR repertoire in AID was most extensively studied in rheumatoid arthritis (RA) by Conny Weyand and Jörg Goronczy and their colleagues at Mayo Clinic. Of course, in these experiments thymic selection could not be studied directly, only the status of the peripheral T-cell repertoire permitted inferences to repertoire selection. Their major findings were the following. Clonal expansion of CD4 T cells was characteristic in RA patients, not found in healthy controls or other joint diseases.[64] The expanded clonotypes were present both in blood and synovia, and were found in both naive and memory T-cell populations.[65] The expanded clones caused an approximately ten-fold contraction of the peripheral repertoire.[66] The expanded clones were autoreactive and often of aberrant phenotype.[67] The authors argued[68] that these aberrations might largely result from a defect in thymic selection. This argument was based on the presence of expanded clones among naive peripheral T cells. However, the absence of expanded clones from MHC-matched healthy controls suggests that normal thymic selection cannot result in selective clonal expansion, i.e., these clones might have arisen upon priming at the periphery, and reversed later to the naive phenotype. Alternatively, there might have been a disease-specific defect in thymic selection. In any case, the expanded clonotypes correlated with the disease but not with the MHC type.

The merit of all these studies was that they uncovered a number of aberrations in the T-cell repertoire that may be relevant for the pathogenesis of certain AIDs. However, these data failed to establish the tripartite correlation between MHC allele, TCR repertoire and pathogenic T cells, and therefore did not really constitute evidence for repertoire selection as an underlying mechanism of MHC–AID association.

A rather straight-forward mechanism for MHC–AID association would be, if the implicated MHC molecule itself served as the target of autoimmune attack. Indeed, there is some experimental evidence suggesting that this mechanism may operate in certain AIDs. One of the diseases investigated was reactive arthritis that was known to be induced by specific pathogens, e.g., *Shigella, Salmonella, Chlamidia* and *Yersinia*, and associated with HLA-B27.[69] The experimental approach taken was to investigate anti-HLA-B27 and anti-*Yersinia* antibodies for possible cross-reactivity.[70] Cross-reactivities in both directions (anti-HLA to *Yersinia* and anti-*Yersinia* to HLA) could be demonstrated, of which most informative was the reaction of an antibody raised against the polymorphic part of HLA-B27 with a *Yersinia* component. It was inferred from the data that antibodies to a pathogen could react to self MHC molecules and thus cause an MHC-associated autoimmune-like condition. A similar approach was taken to demonstrate cross-reactivity between a heat shock protein (HSP) of *E. coli* and the RA-associated DRβ chain 67–74 sequence, known as the 'shared epitope'.[71] The cross-reactive anti-HSP antibodies recognized the RA-associated shared epitope selectively and this fact established a perfect correlation between genetic association and possible disease mechanism. The pathomechanism suggested by both studies was, of course, contingent on the assumption that the effector response to an ubiquitous self antigen (HLA) could have local manifestation in the joints, for which there was some precedence.[72] But the question of whether the cross-reactive antibody-based mechanism operates also in the actual diseases has remained open.

Another candidate mechanism for MHC–AID association would be if the disease were not associated with MHC proper, but with a closely linked non-MHC gene that participates directly in the pathogenesis. A mechanism of this kind may be operating in systemic lupus erythematosus (SLE), a complex AID with a wide spectrum of manifestations, including attacks to the joints, kidney, central nervous system, blood vessels, and myocardium. Although SLE was shown to be associated with class II MHC alleles, it was unclear whether the class II gene itself, or another closely linked gene was responsible for the predisposition. Because the genes encoding tumor necrosis factor (TNF) α and β are located within the MHC close to class II genes in both mouse[73] and human,[74] it was reasonable to assume that some abnormality of one or the other TNF gene might be involved in disease development. The first support for this hypothesis came from studies of (NZBxNZW)F_1 mice that develop a spontaneous lupus-like AID. The data reported by Jacob and McDevitt[75] demonstrated a restriction fragment length polymorphism in the TNF-α gene, the NZW variant of which was associated with lupus nephritis and correlated with reduced production of TNF-α. Replacement therapy with TNF-α caused a delay in the development of nephritis suggesting a protective role of this cytokine against the disease. In a follow-up study McDevitt's group investigated TNF-α production by normal human lymphocytes and monocytes from HLA-typed donors.[76] The results demonstrated a class II-associated quantitative dimorphism of TNF-α, in that DR2 and DQw1 donors exhibited low, whereas DR3 and DR4 subjects high production of TNF-α. In SLE patients carrying DR2 or DQw1, the low TNF-α levels were associated with an increased incidence of nephritis. In contrast, DR3 patients with high TNF-α production were not predisposed to nephritis, and in DR4 patients the high inducibility of TNF-α correlated negatively with lupus nephritis. Taken together, these studies indicated that the class II MHC association of lupus nephritis could be explained by quantitative differences in the expression of the TNF-α gene that is located within the MHC, in the neighborhood of class II genes.

A rather surprising aspect of the studies discussed in this and the previous section is that the analysis of only half a dozen AIDs has revealed at least three completely different mechanisms that can account for the MHC association of disease. Taken the large number of AIDs, it is possible that additional mechanisms may also be discovered in the future.

10.1.4 Non-MHC Genes Predisposing to Autoimmunity

Although the major histocompatibility complex (MHC) accounts for a large proportion of the genetic susceptibility to autoimmune diseases (AIDs), most of the predisposing genetic factors are not related to the MHC. Since single non-MHC genes with major impact on the disease usually could not be identified, it has been assumed that this part of genetic predisposition represents the cumulative effect of a number of genes. Indeed, genetic studies have revealed a polygenic control for at least some AIDs.[77–79] The consequence of polygenic inheritance is that the contribution of each single gene is minor, and thus the identification of such genes requires uncommon efforts.

The search for susceptibility (or resistance) genes in multifactorial diseases is usually performed by applying two different strategies: the candidate gene approach, and the genome-wide linkage analysis, as well as combinations of both.

The candidate gene approach presupposes some knowledge about the pathomechanisms of a particular disease, which would permit making educated guesses about the involvement of certain genes. For example, taken the well-known fact that many AIDs are caused by an inflammatory T helper (Th)-cell response, one can suspect associations with genes encoding or regulating inflammatory cytokines and their receptors,[80,81] or with genes for different immune receptors on lymphocytes.[81–83] Perhaps the most well-known example for the candidate gene approach was the identification of the insulin gene, or more exactly the promoter region of the insulin gene, as a susceptibility factor in diabetes.[84,85] Once a hypothesis is formed the procedure is then to search for common alleles of the candidate gene, and test them for disease association, similarly to the way it was done for the MHC, with the difference that the association would be weaker, and therefore much larger test samples are required to achieve significance of the results. In animal models the procedure may be different: here one can use transgenic or knockout technology to introduce or inactivate the candidate gene, respectively, and monitor the resulting phenotype for symptoms of autoimmunity.

The genome-wide linkage analysis is a more recent approach of great importance, because it permits, in principle, the identification of all loci where disease association could be demonstrated. Technically, this is done by polymerase chain reaction amplification of DNA using a number of primers specific for microsatellite markers spanning all autosomes. The markers used for screening can be selected from available genome databases. By this method one can identify chromosomal regions associated with a disease, and then find candidate genes in these regions. The genome-wide analysis is usually performed on affected sib-pairs, plus their parents and/or unaffected sibs for comparison. In animal models involving inbred strains, the analysis is done on hybrids between susceptible and resistant strains and backcrosses or F_2 segregants thereof. The genome-wide approach was first taken to analyze insulin-dependent diabetes mellitus, the 'golden standard' for dissection of polygenic diseases, in both human[86,87] and mice.[88,89]

'The genetic analysis of multifactorial diseases has retained, despite all technological progress, a never-ending, Sisyphean character', comments Dr. G. 'This is because even the genome-wide analysis is unable to detect small individual risk contributions, and it is often difficult to assign a role for the products of linked genes in the pathomechanism of disease. Taking the most extensively studied disease, diabetes in NOD mice, as an example, almost a decade of genetic studies have identified 11 susceptibility loci on nine chromosomes in addition to the MHC, but the total number of susceptibility loci is likely to be higher, and a mechanistic explanation for the pathogenetic role of only two or three genes of the 11 could be provided.[90] I believe, new ways of analysis will be mandatory in order to accelerate this kind of studies.'

This short section was only meant to give a foretaste of the investigations required for the genetic dissection of AIDs. Because the work itself commenced in the 1990s, and is far from being completed, this field is obviously premature for a historical account.

10.2 HOW IS AUTOIMMUNITY INITIATED?

The most mysterious facet of autoimmune diseases (AIDs) is the way they are initiated. This process apparently requires a number of genetic factors, many of which are poorly understood, and a strong contribution of external events or environmental factors that are even less well known. In addition, the initiating factors involved in one disease may be different from the ones needed for another, and it is even possible that a single disease is triggered in many different ways. Due to this situation it is virtually impossible to make a generally valid statement as to how AIDs get started.

In an attempt to provide a meaningful frame for this topic, we will restrict ourselves to the discussion of AIDs that are known to commence with the activation of autoreactive T cells, and are caused either by the effector response of T cells or autoantibodies (resulting from T–B-cell collaboration). We then define the sine qua non conditions, without which such diseases could not arise, and discuss evidence for each of these 'essential ingredients'.

10.2.1 Escape from Central Tolerance

It is obvious that self epitopes causing deletion of the T cells recognizing them in the thymus cannot serve as targets for autoimmune attack at the periphery. Even more obvious is the corollary to this, i.e., that escape of T cells from central (thymic) tolerance is a prerequisite for autoimmune diseases (AIDs), or plainly stated AIDs cannot arise without autoreactive T cells.

The prohibitive role of central tolerance in autoimmunity was best illustrated by the case of the 'autoimmune regulator' (AIRE) discussed in detail before (Section 9.3.4). The AIRE protein is a transcriptional transactivator that causes ectopic expression of extrathymic organ-specific proteins in medullary thymic epithelial cells (mTECs). Mutations in the *aire* gene that inactivate the protein lead to a spontaneous autoimmune disease termed autoimmune polyendocrinopathy-candidiasis-ectodermal dystrophy (APECED), also known as autoimmune polyendocrine syndrome type-1 (APS-1), in both human[91,92] and animal models.[93] In addition to AIRE, other mechanisms were also implicated in the expression of organ-restricted self molecules in the thymus, and as a result the total spectrum of 'thymically expressed-peripheral-self' might represent all tissues of the body.[94] The obvious purpose of ectopic protein expression in the thymus is the induction of central tolerance to these molecules, and thereby prevention from autoimmunity.[95] Indeed, a clear link between the expression of a single peripheral self antigen in the thymus and a defined autoimmune phenotype has been established.[96]

Common sense would therefore suggest that self proteins ectopically expressed in the thymus should not be involved in AIDs. Curiously, however, this is not the case: many pathogenic self antigens, among others glutamic acid decarboxylase 65 (GAD65) implicated in diabetes as well as myelin basic protein (MBP) and proteolipid protein (PLP) implicated in multiple sclerosis were shown to be expressed ectopically in the thymus.[95] It thus appears that tolerance induction to ectopically expressed proteins in the thymus is a 'leaky' process. In some instances, the causes for this leakiness have been elucidated. For example, GAD65 was shown to be expressed at very low levels in mTECs compared to pancreatic β cells.[97] Thus in this case quantitative differences in gene expression between these two cell types explain deficient tolerance to GAD65, as well as the pathogenic capacity of the latter at the periphery. The pathogenicity of PLP was found to result from differential mRNA splicing in mTECs versus oligodendrocytes: because mTECs skip one exon, this portion of the protein remains exempt from thymic tolerance and can readily induce autoimmunity.[98,99] In addition to the mentioned quantitative and qualitative differences in gene transcription, differences in post-translational modifications, and in antigen processing and presentation could all contribute to a somewhat different display of self epitopes on mTECs compared to peripheral antigen-presenting cells. Thus some discrepancy between central tolerance and peripheral self appears to be unavoidable, simply because it is a sheer impossibility that the mTECs could faithfully emulate the expression and presentation mechanisms in various tissue- and organ-specific ways.

'The discovery of ectopic gene expression in the thymus has profoundly changed immunologists' view on the role of central tolerance in autoimmunity', comments Dr. G. 'Previously it was widely assumed that central tolerance could only be established to peripheral antigens that accessed the thymus via blood circulation, and so the control of most T-cell reactivity to organ-specific antigens was left to mechanisms of peripheral tolerance. In the light of the new knowledge the scope of central tolerance seems much wider than anticipated. Indeed thymic tolerance appears to be so comprehensive that only its mechanistic imperfections permit some autoreactive T cells to sneak through to the periphery. It is therefore not far-fetched to conclude that central tolerance must have been the major instrument chosen by evolution in order to keep the frequency of AIDs acceptably low.'

10.2.2 Escape from or Breaking of Peripheral Tolerance

As pointed out in Section 10.2.1, central tolerance can be leaky, permitting T cells specific for certain autoantigens or epitopes thereof to reach the periphery in a functional state. These cells, upon encounter of the respective autoantigen, respond to it, as if it were a foreign antigen.

Such non-tolerant T cells may be responsible for the initiation of certain autoimmune diseases (AIDs). For example, the lack of tolerance to certain epitopes of myelin basic protein and proteolipid protein[95] could be the cause of multiple sclerosis, and deficient tolerance to glutamic acid decarboxylase[97] may be involved in the induction of autoimmune diabetes.

This assumption is substantiated by results obtained using transgenic models. For example, a recurrent finding in studies with T-cell receptor (TCR) transgenic mice was that TCR transgenes specific for organ-restricted antigens were not deleted in the thymus, and in these cases spontaneous AID developed sooner or later, depending on the presence of genetic susceptibility factors.[89,100,101] Thus a number of AIDs may be induced by autoantigens that are foreign from the immune system's point of view. Under physiological conditions such antigens are usually inaccessible for lymphocytes, and thus peripheral tolerance cannot develop to them.

Autoimmunity could also arise when the tolerant state of peripheral lymphocytes is broken. This assumption is based on the classical finding[102,103] that animals tolerized with a particular antigen can respond to a cross-reactive antigen, and the antibodies formed not only recognize epitopes unique to the immunogen, but also those shared between tolerogen and immunogen. The mechanistic explanation for tolerance-breaking needs three components: first, a *live* (undeleted) tolerant cell recognizing an epitope shared between self and cross-reacting antigen, second, another cell activated by a foreign epitope on the cross-reacting antigen, and third, a cooperation between these two cells that enables induction of the tolerant cell.

Although there is no direct evidence for the involvement of tolerance-breaking in AIDs, this can be reasonably assumed to be the case in a number of instances. This mechanism operates most likely in AIDs induced by *ubiquitous* self antigens that should normally be under self tolerance. Perhaps the most illustrative example is provided by diseases associated with HLA-B27, i.e., reactive arthritis, and ankylosing spondylitis. Pathology in these diseases is caused by autoantibodies specific for the self major histocompatibility complex (MHC) class I molecule HLA-B27. Because tolerance of both B and T cells to self MHC is one of the most firmly established facts in immunology, HLA-B27-specific autoantibodies could only arise after breaking of B-cell tolerance. The latter seems to happen as a result of molecular mimicry[104,70] between certain microbial proteins of *Klebsiella* and *Yersinia*, and a 'private' epitope of HLA-B27. The most likely scenario here is that the surface Ig receptors of tolerant B cells bind the microbial protein via the self-mimicking epitope, then internalize, process and present it to T helper (Th) cells activated by foreign epitopes of the same molecule. The Th cells, by providing 'help', rescue the B cells from the tolerance pathway and facilitate their differentiation into antibody-forming cells. Implicit in this mechanism is that the disease should spontaneously remit after clearance of the pathogen for lack of foreign helper epitopes, which seems to be the case in reactive arthritis. However, when the disease takes a chronic course after elimination of the pathogen as in ankylosing spondylitis, one has to assume that Th-cell tolerance to HLA-B27 was also broken, probably via interaction between anti-self and anti-foreign Th cells.

Presumably a similar mechanism operates during the induction of AID in animal models, the widely used protocol for which prescribes the use of heterologous protein antigens. For example, bovine or human type II collagen readily induces arthritis in mice, which is accompanied with antibodies and T-cell response to the related autologous protein.[105] The role of breaking self tolerance during disease induction was addressed in collagen arthritis models by Holmdahl and colleagues.[106–109] In mice, arthritis could only be induced by heterologous (rat) type II collagen (CII), and unimmunized mice harbored T cells tolerant to autologous CII.[106] Tolerance was also induced to rat CII epitopes introduced into the mouse protein.[107,108] In contrast, in certain rat strains arthritis could be induced by autologous CII, and self CII-specific T and B cells were demonstrated in unimmunized animals.[109] Thus, these two species seem to differ in terms of self tolerance to CII. Therefore it appears that the induction of certain AID models, such as collagen arthritis in mice, is contingent on breaking of self tolerance, but this may or may not be the case in other species or other disease models.

'For sake of historical fidelity I must mention, although it may sound unfair, that the original reason for choosing heterologous proteins for autoimmune models had nothing to do with breaking of self tolerance', adds Dr. G. 'Before the biotechnology era, immunologists actually had no other choice, because most proteins of laboratory rodents were either commercially unavailable or offered at exorbitant prices. Obviously the isolation of a protein from a single ox was an easy undertaking, compared to obtaining the same yield from 25 000 mice. Thus the rationale of breaking tolerance was attached to most of these experiments a posteriori, which of course does not decrease its validity.'

10.2.3 Availability of Autoantigen

The requirement for autoantigen is so self-evident that its statement qualifies for a platitude. However, this topic has some internal complexity, which makes its discussion indispensable.

Autoantigens can be expressed at two different locations: in the respective tissue and in the thymus. Lack of thymic expression tends to result in autoimmune disease (AID), for which the best illustration is the repeatedly cited AIRE deficiency.[93] Conversely, thymic expression should induce tolerance to the great majority of potentially immunogenic self proteins. Quantitative aspects of expression also deserve mention here, for both tolerance induction and T-cell activation operate with a lower threshold, i.e., both events happen preferentially when the antigenic epitope is abundantly expressed. This phenomenon is known as epitope dominance. Under constant rate of protein turnover, epitope dominance is determined solely by the interaction of peptides with major histocompatibility complex (MHC) molecules (Section 10.1.2) which is independent of the anatomic site, and thus epitopes dominant at the periphery should also be dominant in the thymus. Since the initiation of AID usually requires a dominant self epitope, the preferential tolerization of T cells specific for dominant epitopes effectively prevents AID in most cases. There are, however, exceptions to this rule: a number of proteins expressed in the thymus can still induce autoimmunity at the periphery, suggesting deficient tolerance induction even to dominant epitopes. Most of the known autoantigens implicated in disease belong to this category.[95] The full scope of peripheral self representation in the thymus is estimated to be at least 3000 proteins,[94] while the number of known autoantigens that fail to induce central tolerance despite thymic expression is ~30. Thus the efficiency of thymic tolerance in preventing autoimmunity appears to be surprisingly high.

The fact that only a small fraction (<1%) of proteins expressed in the thymus fails to induce tolerance implies that the number of autoantigens at the periphery that can initiate one given AID is unlikely to be >1. After antigen processing each protein usually yields a single dominant epitope (and 2–3 'subdominant' ones), and thus most AIDs are likely to be induced by T-cell response to a single dominant epitope. The narrow range of the initiating response explains why a stable and high presentation of the triggering epitope is mandatory in the affected organ. During the course of disease tissue destruction occurs, which increases the available amount of autoantigen, and thus the response can 'spread' to previously unseen epitopes and eventually to other autoantigens.[110,111]

The availability of autoantigen can also depend on the anatomical location, as there are sites in the body that are not accessible for the immune system. In such cases immunologists speak about 'sequestered antigen'. The classical example for this situation is lens proteins that can only become immunogenic after a penetrating injury to the eye.[112] A more modern and AID-relevant example is provided by myelin basic protein (MBP) that is expressed exclusively in the central nervous system (CNS), and involved in the induction of multiple sclerosis (MS) and its animal model, experimental autoimmune encephalomyelitis (EAE). The sequestered state of MBP results from the blood–brain barrier that prevents access of resting MBP-specific T cells to the CNS,[113] although they are present in the normal peripheral T-cell repertoire.[114] Invasion of CNS thus requires MBP-specific T cells to be activated outside the CNS,[113] which is achieved by intentional immunization in the case of EAE, and probably via cross-reactive antigens in the case of MS (discussed in Section 10.2.4).

In conclusion, the initiation of autoimmunity is a rare event depending on the coincidence of a number of different factors. The sustained presence and abundance of the initiating autoantigen appear to be important in providing an extended timeframe and sufficient stimulus for this event to happen.

10.2.4 Environmental Triggers

As discussed above (Section 10.2.3) organ-specific autoantigens are in some instances sequestered by barriers from the immune system and thus cannot induce autoimmunity. There are also indications that many autoantigens are inaccessible to T cells even in the absence of a physical barrier, and that this indeed may be the rule rather than the exception. The cause of inaccessibility is that resting T cells do not migrate into tissues,[115] and thus cannot meet the autoantigen. Consequently the activation of autoreactive T cells must occur in the peripheral lymphoid system *in the absence of the autoantigen*. This could conceivably happen when an environmental antigen entering the body happens to carry an epitope that is identical or at least similar to the dominant epitope of an organ-specific autoantigen. The presence of identical or equivalent epitopes in unrelated antigens is referred to as 'molecular mimicry'. The major protagonist for the role of mimicry in autoimmunity has been Michael Oldstone at the Scripps Research Institute.

The most likely source of environmental antigens that could enter the body is pathogenic microbes. It is thus not surprising that the majority of data is on pathogen-derived epitopes mimicking self.

Initial experiments conducted in the early 1980s dealt exclusively with epitopes for antibodies, as the nature of T-cell epitopes was still unknown at that time. A popular approach was to generate monoclonal antibodies (mAbs) against viruses and test them for reactivity with host tissues. Examples are mAbs to simian virus T antigen reacting with different cellular proteins,[116] anti-reovirus mAbs recognizing a number of normal tissues,[117] anti-human T-cell leukemia virus mAbs reacting with HLA-B histocompatibility molecules,[118] anti-measles virus mAbs recognizing host heat shock proteins,[119] and mAbs specific for vaccinia[120] or measles[121] virus binding to intermediate filaments. By these early experiments molecular mimicry established itself as a rather frequent, fortuitous phenomenon.

The next generation of studies aimed more specifically at linking mimicry to a disease. In these experiments virus infections were chosen that were associated with autoimmune disease (AID), for example, reovirus type 1 infection of mice known to result in an autoimmune polyendocrine disease. Mabs isolated from these mice were shown to react with the islets of Langerhans, the pituitary, and a number of hormones.[122] Even more conclusive were experiments in which sequence homologies were searched for between viral proteins and autoantigens, for example, a protein of adenovirus type 12 and A-gliadin, the antigen involved in celiac disease,[123] and between myelin basic protein involved in multiple sclerosis (MS) and hepatitis B virus polymerase.[124] The homologous sequences were then used as peptides to raise antibodies that indeed reacted with both virus and autoantigen. A similar approach was taken to show mimicry between HLA-B27 associated with ankylosing spondylitis and Reiter's syndrome, and bacteria such as *Yersinia paratuberculosis*[70] and *Klebsiella* pneumonia,[104] and to demonstrate antibodies in patients' sera reacting with the shared peptides. Taken together these data have satisfactorily established the role of molecular mimicry in the induction of pathogenic autoantibodies.

Searching for mimicry at the level of T-cell epitopes was a pursuit in the 1990s. Because T-cell epitopes are short linear peptides, the identification of mimicking epitopes was expected to be easy on the basis of sequence homology. Surprisingly, however, this was not the case: whereas mimicry of B-cell epitopes was often based on clear sequence homology,[125] mimicking T-cell epitopes could not be identified in many instances by simple sequence alignment. This was most convincingly shown in a study by Wucherpfennig and Strominger.[126] These authors searched for mimicry peptides capable of activating human T-cell clones specific for an immunodominant T-cell epitope (residues 84–102) of myelin basic protein (MBP), an autoantigen implicated in MS. The search criteria included anchor residues required for binding to major histocompatibility complex class II molecules, key residues contacting the T-cell antigen receptor, as well as additional parameters, such as viruses known to cause human pathology and prevalent in the northern hemisphere (where MS occurs frequently), and bacterial sequences associated with inflammatory diseases of the central nervous system. A fraction (70) of the peptides thus identified was then synthesized and tested on the MBP-specific T-cell clones. The most striking finding was that only one of the seven active mimicry peptides had visible sequence homology with the MBP peptide, consequently, the other six would not have been predicted by sequence alignments. The observation that a single TCR could interact with a number of peptides with unrelated sequences was quite intriguing at that time. Meanwhile this has been recognized as a normal feature of T-cell recognition known as 'polyspecificity' (see Section 8.4.4). Another interesting finding was that each mimicry peptide derived from a distinct pathogen (six different viruses and one bacterium), implying that any of these agents could serve as an environmental trigger of MS.

Nevertheless, sequence homology between autoantigenic and mimicking T-cell epitopes could also be demonstrated in a number of cases, usually in diseases or disease models where a clear causal link existed between infection by a particular pathogen and a subsequent autoimmune condition. For example, in a model of herpes stromal keratitis seven of eight amino acids were identical in the inducing autoantigenic peptide and an epitope in a coat protein of herpes simplex virus type-1.[127] Similarly, in treatment-resistant Lyme arthritis a six-residue-long stretch of the OspA 165–173 peptide of *Borrelia burgdorferi* was found to be homologous to a peptide of leukocyte function-associated antigen-1 acting as autoantigen in this disease.[44] A more modest sequence motif of four contiguous residues was found to be shared by the heart muscle-specific α myosin and an outer membrane protein of *Chlamydia*, the latter known to be linked to human heart disease. Peptides with this motif from both myosin and *Chlamydia* were shown to induce heart disease in a murine model.[128] Finally, in a study with human T cells from prediabetic and recent diabetic patients, a significant homology could be demonstrated between glutamic acid decarboxylase, a β-cell autoantigen, and the P2-C protein of Coxsackie B virus.[129]

Altogether, molecular mimicry of T-cell epitopes has turned out to be a complex phenomenon that is either based on sequence homology, or reflects the polyspecificity of T cells. In the latter case mimicry can only be detected at the level of the responding T cell.

That antigenic mimicry can indeed trigger AID has been demonstrated most elegantly in a transgenic model developed independently in Rolf Zinkernagel's[130] and Michael Oldstone's[131] laboratories. The authors introduced a transgene encoding a viral protein under the insulin promoter into mice, which resulted in selective expression of the protein in β cells of Langerhans islets. Interestingly, these mice were neither tolerant to the transgenic protein, nor did they develop diabetes. However, after infection of mice with the respective virus, β-cell destruction and diabetes ensued. These data have clearly shown that an inaccessible, organ-specific antigen cannot induce T-cell response, unless priming to the antigen occurs in the peripheral lymphoid system.

For completeness' sake it should be pointed out that molecular mimicry is not the only mechanism by which pathogens may induce autoimmunity. For example, tissue injury caused by the pathogen could lead to autoantigen release and subsequent sensitization.[132] In certain diseases, it has indeed remained a point of debate whether the trigger is mimicry or pathogen-induced damage.[133,134] Microbial superantigens[135] or inherent adjuvant properties of the pathogen[128] may also be able to trigger the autoimmune response, although the role of the latter is questioned.[136]

Conclusive data to demonstrate a role for non-infectious environmental triggers in AID are rather scarce. One example to be mentioned here is the role of cow milk as a possible environmental factor in insulin-dependent diabetes mellitus (IDDM). Animal studies identified a 17-amino-acid-long peptide of bovine serum albumin (BSA) that might contain a mimicking epitope.[137] All diabetic patients tested had elevated serum concentrations of anti-BSA antibodies, most of which were directed against the peptide, but no antibodies against other milk proteins. In contrast, only 2.5% of a large panel of healthy controls had such antibodies. The antibodies against the BSA peptide reacted with a β-cell specific surface protein, and could thus contribute to the development of IDDM.

The body of data discussed in this section provides in its entirety convincing although mostly indirect evidence for the role of environmental factors in the initiation of autoimmunity. Much remains to be done, however, until a full understanding is reached of how and to what extent these factors influence AIDs.

'I am afraid this section wouldn't be complete without discussing a widespread misunderstanding among immunologists about mimicry', adds Dr. G. 'This is the notion that the mimicking epitopes themselves break self tolerance, which attests a vague distinction between mimicry and cross-reactivity. Mimicking epitopes are ligands that are functionally recognized by a single receptor,[138] i.e., they are equivalent in activating cells carrying that particular receptor.[126] Consequently, if one member of the mimicking set is under self tolerance, all others will also be subject to tolerance. Therefore, immunization with a mimicking epitope, e.g., synthesized as a peptide, could never activate any T cell, if another member of the mimicry set were under tolerance. Conversely, if activation occurred, this would mean normal priming of non-tolerant cells.'

'Breaking of self tolerance is only possible with a *cross-reactive* antigen, which carries self/mimicry epitopes as well as foreign epitopes. In this case a cell recognizing a foreign epitope would help the self-specific cell "wake up" from its tolerant state. Of course, in natural cases, the infecting pathogen carries both mimicking and foreign epitopes, and therefore no distinction can be made between mimicry and cross-reactivity. Those who are interested in finding out whether or not tolerance was broken during disease induction have to investigate healthy susceptible individuals for the presence (or absence) of response to the mimicking epitope *alone*.'

10.3 SOME ASPECTS OF PATHOGENESIS

Generally speaking, the very same effector mechanisms cause pathology in autoimmune disease (AID), and eliminate pathogens during a useful immune response. Perhaps this is the reason why the pathogenesis of AIDs attracted less attention of immunologists than the initiation and genetics of these illnesses. Of course, there are also unique aspects in the pathogenesis of each AID, which are, however, topics of pathophysiology rather than immunology. Here we will recapitulate a few selected features of pathogenesis that directly pertain to immunology and were elaborated mostly by immunologists.

As pointed out earlier (Section 10.2), many AIDs commence with a T-cell response to an autoantigen. But the effector response causing pathology is not necessarily T-cell-mediated. For example, in myasthenia gravis (MG), the initial T-cell response against the acetylcholine receptor[139] helps B cells to produce autoantibodies, which in turn block signal transmission in the neuromuscular junctions,[140] and reduce the number of acetylcholine receptors by down-regulation and complement-mediated destruction.[141] Thus the typical symptoms of MG, muscle weakness and fatigability result from autoantibodies. In fact, the neuromuscular abnormalities of the disease can be passively transferred with antibodies to mice.[142]

In contrast to MG, in a number of AIDs, for example in multiple sclerosis (MS) and insulin-dependent diabetes mellitus (IDDM), pathology is largely if not entirely T-cell-mediated.

In the mouse model of MS, experimental autoimmune encephalitis (EAE), the full array of symptoms and pathology could be induced by injecting small numbers of cloned myelin basic protein (MBP)-specific T helper (Th) cells, as shown first by Larry Steinman and his colleagues[143] at Stanford University. However, in addition to Th (CD4) also CD8 cells seem to play a role in the pathogenesis, as illustrated by CD8 knockout mice that have milder acute EAE but more relapses,[144] suggesting that CD8 cells may participate as both effectors and regulators in this disease model. But the precise function of CD8 T cells in the disease has not been clarified in detail.

The cellular requirements for diabetes were investigated in the non-obese diabetic (NOD) mice, the animal model of IDDM. Diabetes occurs in this model spontaneously at the age of 12–30 weeks. As shown first by Linda Wicker and her colleagues,[145] diabetes could be induced in young, irradiated NOD mice by adoptive transfer of lymphocytes from diabetic mice. Disease induction was dependent on both CD4 and CD8 cells, and both subsets had to come from diabetic donors. Here again, the involvement of CD4 T cells in the pathogenesis was confirmed,[146] whereas the role of CD8 cells has remained unclear.

A special case of AIDs is represented by rheumatoid arthritis (RA). Th cells are implicated in the disease by linkage to major histocompatibility complex class II (Section 10.1.1) and other evidence (Section 10.1.2). However, the most severe pathological changes are not caused directly by either lymphocytes or antibodies. During joint inflammation synovial fibroblasts undergo profound hypertrophic-proliferative changes (probably triggered by lymphocytes), resulting in the formation of synovial pannus. The pannus then invades the periarticular tissue and causes severe cartilage and bone destruction via constitutive production of enzymes and cytokines.[147]

Immunologists have often striven to find common features in the pathogenesis of AIDs, which was difficult in view of the extreme diversity of these conditions. In the 1990s, a popular question in this vein was concerning the role of inflammatory Th1 and non-inflammatory Th2 cells in the pathogenesis of AIDs.[148] Because many AIDs were shown to be of an inflammatory nature, it was reasonable to assume that they were driven by autoreactive Th1 cells. The Th1 and Th2 cell subsets were known to cross-regulate each other via cytokines (Section 8.6.3, Fig. 8.9): thus interferon γ (IFNγ) inhibited Th2, whereas interleukin (IL)-4 and IL-10 blocked Th1 development. The lead idea was therefore to 'divert' autoreactive Th1 cells toward Th2 development and thereby prevent or possibly even cure disease.

Most experiments addressing this hypothesis were done in two AID models, EAE and the NOD mice. In the EAE model, several lines of evidence supported Th1 cell dependence of the disease: first, the disease was induced by MBP-specific Th1 but not Th2 cells,[149] second, infiltrating cells in the central nervous system produced IFNγ and IL-2 but much less IL-4,[150] third, IFNγ, tumor necrosis factor (TNF) and IL-2 dominated in the brain at the height of the disease,[151,152] whereas the recovery phase was associated with increased levels of IL-4, IL-10 and transforming growth factor (TGF)-β6.[13] Much less clear was, however, the role of Th2 cells in the disease. Although MBP-specific Th2 cells were shown to inhibit proliferation of Th1 cells of the same specificity, in vitro,[153] Th2 cells in immunodeficient mice induced EAE rather than protecting from the disease.[154] Finally, a number of papers[155–157] reported on CD4 suppressor or regulatory T (Treg) cells with Th2 phenotype that inhibited EAE, but the lack of a distinguishing marker at that time prevented the authors from determining whether these cells were Th2 or Treg. Similar results were obtained in the NOD model. The role of Th1 cells in the disease was conclusively demonstrated,[111,158–160] but a protective effect of Th2 cells was not seen.[160]

The conclusion from these experiments was that Th1 cells were indeed causative of certain T-cell-mediated AIDs and Th2 cells were not, but the question of whether 'immune deviation' from Th1 to Th2 would be doable, and if so this would favorably influence the disease, has remained open. Of course, the hope that the 'Th1–Th2 paradigm' would apply to most AIDs turned out to be unrealistic.

More recent approaches have turned away from the commonalities of AIDs, and treat each disease as a separate entity with the hope that this would lead to the discovery of novel relevant details of pathogenesis.

10.4 APPROACHES TO IMMUNOTHERAPY

In principle, therapy is a topic that would be more appropriately dealt with in the frames of pharmacology or medicine than immunology. However, autoimmune diseases (AIDs) represent an exception, because most of their mechanistic details have been discovered by immunologists, and thus it was natural that the same researchers continued their studies to provide proofs of principle for therapy.

Because AIDs are initiated by the same machinery as useful immune responses, it has been reasonable to assume that targeting any part of this machinery would have an effect on disease. However, this strategy is a double-edged sword: its result is beneficial as long as it affects a pathological response, but potentially dangerous if it compromises host defense against pathogens. Therefore the selectivity of immunotherapy has been a major consideration (and concern) from the very beginning.

In general, immune intervention can be directed to three different types of event, namely, antigen recognition, intracellular signaling and effector mechanisms. Because of the breakthrough discovery in the 1980s that a 'trimolecular complex' between major histocompatibility complex molecule, antigenic peptide, and T-cell antigen receptor initiates both immune response and AID, the initial approaches to therapy were strongly biased toward the antigen recognition process, including the trimolecular complex as well as other 'accessory' interactions taking place between T cells and antigen-presenting cells upon T-cell activation.[161] Subsequent efforts tried to exploit immune effector mechanisms, mostly cytokines and their receptors.[162] Some of the popular therapeutic approaches will be discussed in detail below according to the targeted molecules/mechanisms.

10.4.1 Targeting Antigen Presentation by MHC Molecules

Of the two classes of MHC molecules, class II was the primary target for immune intervention for the following reasons: first, class II molecules activate T helper (Th) cells that are central to immunoregulation, second, many autoimmune diseases are genetically associated with certain class II alleles (Section 10.1.1), and third, class II molecules are expressed only on cells of the immune system, which provides a margin of selectivity. Class II-targeted approaches were aimed at interrupting either the interaction of TCR with MHC molecule plus antigenic peptide, or the interaction between the MHC molecule and the antigenic peptide.

The drug candidates for interrupting TCR–MHC interactions were anti-class II monoclonal antibodies (mAbs), many of which were known to inhibit Th cell activation, and also efficient in different models of AIDs.[163–166] The potential advantage of this approach was that one could use class II allele-specific mAbs for selectively inhibiting responses channeled through an AID-associated MHC molecule provided that the basis for MHC association was selective autoantigen presentation (see Section 10.1.2). Such antibodies would be quite selective, as they would only affect ~10% of T cells. However, a number of mAbs showed significant toxicity for largely unknown reasons,[165,167,168] which substantially damped enthusiasm for this approach.

The second type of approach was to replace autoantigenic peptides in the class II binding site with tightly binding, non-antigenic ligands. This was based on known crystal structures of peptide–class II complexes (Section 7.2.2), and on binding motifs for the class II peptide binding cleft (Section 7.1.3). The rationale was to construct peptide ligands with all required MHC anchor residues, but without the TCR contact residues that drive the disease, and use them as competitive antagonists of antigen presentation. The selectivity of this approach was comparable to that of allele-specific anti-class II mAbs. The principle was proven in vivo, in T-cell responses[169] and autoimmune models.[170–173] However, the peptide-based program failed due to poor pharmacokinetics and proteolytic instability.[174] These shortcomings were then largely corrected by designing unnatural peptidomimetic ligands.[175,176] Yet, the compounds have not reached the clinic: the project was de-prioritized in favor of more promising approaches.

10.4.2 Targeting the Antigenic Ligand

Tolerance induction by the relevant autoantigen(s) represents a possible way of 'silencing' T cells that initiate and drive a certain autoimmune disease (AID). Indeed, tolerance has been regarded as the 'holy grail' of immunotherapy, because it affects only those T cell clones involved in the disease (far below 1% of total) and leaves the rest of the immune repertoire intact.

One limitation of tolerance therapy was that it required precise knowledge of the relevant autoantigen and its potentially pathogenic epitopes, which was not available for many AIDs. Another problem was that a safe and uniformly applicable method for tolerance induction was not known.

Experimental tolerance could be induced in a variety of ways, e.g., by injection of the antigen in soluble form,[177,178] antigen with incomplete Freund's adjuvant,[179–181] soluble MHC molecules complexed with antigenic peptide,[182] or by administering antigen through mucous membranes, i.e., orally[183] or by inhalation.[184] Many of these approaches[179–184] showed efficacy in AID models. However, some of these protocols could not be used in humans, and others were ineffective and/or unsafe.[185]

Thus, antigen-specific tolerance, attractive as it might have been, has not found therapeutic application in AID.

Another interesting, although somewhat mysterious, antigen-based approach involved the use of what was referred to as 'altered peptide ligand'. This was based on the observation that a myelin basic protein (MBP) peptide (MBP Ac1-11) that induced experimental autoimmune encephalitis (EAE) in mice could be turned by a single amino acid exchange into a ligand of different biological activity. The altered ligand, Ac1-11[4A], bound to the restricting class II molecule better than the antigenic peptide, and it stimulated encephalitogenic T-cell clones better in vitro, but in vivo it was not immunogenic and prevented EAE.[170,186,187] The mechanism of action of altered peptide ligands has remained unclear: tolerance induction and Th1 to Th2 cytokine shift were implicated.[187,188]

The therapeutic utility of altered peptide ligands was limited by the same factors as those of tolerance induction, and it also shared the fate of the tolerance approach.

10.4.3 Targeting the T-Cell Antigen Receptor

Monoclonal antibodies (mAbs) specific for the T-cell antigen receptor (TCR) can prevent the interaction of TCR with its ligand (peptide+MHC), and thereby interfere with T-cell activation. The mAbs depending on their specificity can be pan-TCR, chain-specific, variable (V)-region specific, or clonotypic. Many of these antibodies were available in the 1990s for diagnostic purposes.[189]

The use of mAbs with broad specificity was mostly considered in transplantation, although some of them were also reported to be efficient in autoimmune disease (AID) models.[190–192]

The more selective anti-TCR mAbs were considered in certain AIDs, in which a preferential use of a limited set of receptors was demonstrated. Evidence for a limited TCR usage came from autoimmune models, notably from studies of experimental autoimmune encephalomyelitis (EAE).[193] The attractiveness of this approach was that mAbs specific, for example, for a single V region would allow an immunosuppressive therapy with a degree of selectivity, affecting 1 to 30% of T cells (depending on the expression-frequency of the particular V region). Preferential use of particular TCRs was also demonstrated in pathogenic T cells isolated from multiple sclerosis patients.[194,195] However, the possibility that elimination of these T cells would enrich for minor pathogenic T-cell clones carrying a different receptor[196] could not be excluded, and this fact represented a serious limitation to the clinical use of this approach.

Another approach targeting the TCR was referred to as 'receptor vaccination'. This was based on the finding that short synthetic peptides corresponding to a V region or joining region sequence of the TCR caused functional inactivation of T cells expressing this sequence. Thus, provided that T cells involved in autoimmune pathology preferentially expressed a particular TCR sequence, vaccination with the corresponding synthetic peptide might have a therapeutic effect.[197,198] The mechanism by which such peptides would cause immunosuppression has remained unclear. The therapeutic utility of this approach was again limited by the potential heterogeneity of TCR usage in pathogenic T cells.

The CD3 complex, the signaling machinery of TCR, was also targeted for the purpose of immunosuppression. Anti-CD3 mAbs were usually found to cause total immunosuppression, and for this reason one of them (OKT3) has been used successfully in clinical transplantation. But the lack of selectivity of this therapy made its use prohibitive for AID indications.

10.4.4 Targeting Co-Receptors, Co-Stimulation, and Cell Adhesion Molecules

During T-cell activation, T cells and antigen-presenting cells (APCs) are kept together by a number of interactions between receptors collectively referred to as 'accessory molecules'. The accessory molecules, depending on their function, can serve as co-receptors (CD4 and CD8), others regulate the magnitude of T-cell response (co-stimulatory molecules), and the remaining ones facilitate cell-to-cell adhesion. Interference with any of these molecular interactions is expected to influence T-cell activation, and thus also the development of autoimmune diseases (AIDs).

Of the two co-receptors usually only CD4 has been considered as a pharmacological target, because it is selectively expressed on the AID-relevant Th cell class, and co-ligates class II major histocompatibility complex (MHC) molecules together with the T-cell antigen receptor (TCR). Anti-CD4 monoclonal antibodies (mAbs) were extensively used in animal models of AIDs,[199] providing sufficient proof for CD4-blockade as a therapeutic principle. However, in human trials CD4-specific mAbs showed only moderate effect[200] and caused long-lasting total Th-cell depletion by induction of apoptosis upon ligation.[201] Thus these mAbs were not indicated for AIDs, but the discovery of Herman Waldman and colleagues[202] that such mAbs induced long lasting tolerance suggested that they might be useful in transplantation. More recently, non-depleting anti-CD4 mAbs have been produced that hold promise of entering AID therapy. Meanwhile a novel although not unexpected indication has opened up for non-depleting anti-CD4 mAbs. At least one of these mAbs (Ibalizumab) was found to inhibit human immunodeficiency virus-1 in entering Th cells and thus significantly decrease virus load.[203]

There were numerous attempts to target co-stimulatory molecules for immunotherapy, one of which deserves discussion here, because it has become a true success story. This approach targeted the CTLA-4 molecule expressed on the surface of T cells and serving as a negative regulator of T-cell proliferation (see Section 8.7.2). This molecule was known to bind to B7 molecules on APC with up to 50 fold higher affinity than the positive regulator CD28. Researchers constructed a soluble fusion protein of CTLA-4 with the Fc portion of IgG_1 (CTLA4Ig), and showed that this construct interfered with T-cell activation and also induced tolerance to the antigens encountered by T cells during the treatment.[204,205] Up to this point, the finding was just a successful proof of principle, as done for many other targets of immunotherapy before. Miraculously, however, CTLA4Ig easily passed all subsequent steps of drug development. It is now approved under the trade-mark 'Abatacept' for the treatment of rheumatoid arthritis, and other indications will probably follow.

Cell adhesion molecules, in view of their importance for the function of the immune system, were also considered as therapeutic targets in AIDs. One of the successful approaches aimed at interrupting the adhesive interaction between leukocyte function-associated antigen (LFA)-3, and CD2 (LFA-2). This pair of molecules facilitates adhesion between cells of the immune system, including the T cell–antigen-presenting cell (APC) interaction. The construct produced for this purpose was LFA3TIP,[206] a fusion protein between the first domain of LFA-3 and the Fc portion of IgG_1. The construct was shown to bind to CD2 molecules on T cells and inhibit T cell activation. Moreover LFA3TIP induced T-cell unresponsiveness, suggesting that its function was not restricted to cell adhesion, but it also influenced T-cell signaling. This fusion protein is now approved for the treatment of psoriasis (trade-mark 'Alefacept'), although it is effective in only about 50% of patients for unknown reasons, and its mode of action has also remained unclear.

Another successfully targeted adhesion molecule was VLA-4, a receptor with multiple functions including the migration of activated T cells into tissues, adhesion and signalling in T cell-APC interaction, differentiation of T cells to effector cells, and activation of myeloid cells.[207] A humanized anti-VLA-4 mAb ('Natalizumab') that managed to reach the clinic was found effective in relapsing-remitting multiple sclerosis,[208,209] and was approved for this indication. The most likely mode of action is inhibition of crossing the blood–brain barrier by activated T cells and dendritic cells.[210]

10.4.5 Targeting the Effector Response

Most of these approaches were directed to cytokines or their receptors. Efforts to develop such therapies met initially some skepticism, because of the redundancy in the function of many cytokines, which suggested that blocking of one would leave the others to drive disease. It was therefore necessary to study cytokine regulation in disease in order to determine which, if any, of the cytokines involved could be targeted with success.

A typical example for cytokine redundancy was found in rheumatoid arthritis (RA). The first cytokine identified in the synovium of RA patients was interleukin (IL)-1, which was also shown to augment joint destruction in experimental models.[211,212] It was therefore widely believed that IL-1 might be the major driver of RA. However, soon after tumor necrosis factor α (TNFα) was discovered,[213] with largely overlapping properties, also present in rheumatic joints[214] and causing damage there.[215] It was therefore important to find out whether these two cytokines act independently or they function in an interrelated fashion. This question led to a series of studies investigating cytokine regulation in

RA, most of which were performed by Marc Feldmann and his colleagues in London.

The first surprising finding was that blocking of TNFα down-regulated IL-1 activity almost completely,[216] whereas blocking of IL-1 had no effect on TNFα.[217] TNFα was also found to influence the expression of additional cytokines[217,218] suggesting that it might be the privotal cytokine orchestrating the inflammatory cascade in RA, and as such a promising therapeutic target. Confirmation of the utility of anti-TNFα therapy was obtained in animal models,[219,220] and a chimeric monoclonal anti-TNFα antibody (infliximab or 'Remicade') proceeded to clinical trials[221] and was finally approved for the treatment of RA. Another therapeutic variant was a fusion protein of the TNF receptor and Ig-Fc (etanercept, or 'Enbrel'), which also succeeded in the clinic and was approved.[222]

> 'Marc Feldmann's scientific career, as that of many others in his time, went through three successive phases characterized by quantity, quality, and utility', adds Dr. G. 'What distinguished Mark from most of his colleagues was that he completed all three phases with success. As a young scientist he belonged to the most prolific authors in the field, he then made significant contributions to major histocompatibility complex restriction and anergy, and finally his RA studies resulted in a novel therapeutic. Who could wish for anything more?'

In contrast to the anti-TNFα therapy, targeting of IL-1 had only moderate success. The drug candidate resulting from this approach was a natural soluble antagonist able to bind to the IL-1 receptor without transmitting any signal.[223] The clinical evaluation of this antagonist in RA[224] showed some efficacy that was, however, clearly inferior to that of anti-TNFα.

Curiously, the presently available immunotherapies for multiple sclerosis (MS) have resulted from a trial-and-error type rather than scientific approach, yet they are not less successful than the ones with solid scientific rationale.

One of the most frequently used biotherapeutics in MS nowadays is the fibroblast interferon, IFNβ. Recombinant human IFNβ had been around in the clinic for a long time, and was extensively tested in a number of oncological indications, but it was not approved for any human disease. Nevertheless, its good tolerability tempted clinicians to further experiment with it, until it was found effective in relapsing-remitting MS.[225] Although IFNβ is not a cure for MS, it causes significant improvements in exacerbation rates and burden of disease. The mode of action has remained unknown. Because of its clinical (and economical) success, IFNβ is meanwhile available as three different preparations ('Avonex', 'Betaseron', and 'Rebif') made by three different companies.

The second successful immunotherapeutic for MS, Copolymer-1 (Cop-1) or 'Copaxone', had probably the most bizarre developmental history. As discussed before (Section 6.2.1), amino acid copolymers were produced by Michael Sela in the late 1950s for the purpose of testing out the lower limits of protein immunogenicity. They consisted of 2–4 amino acids at fixed ratios but in random sequence. Cop-1 is made up of four amino acids, alanine, glutamate, lysine and tyrosine. Because copolymers were extremely popular tools in immunology, it just appeared to be a matter of time before someone would test them in models of autoimmunity. This idea occurred to Michael Sela long before anyone else, and he was able to demonstrate that Cop-1 was effective in experimental auto-immune encephalitis.[226] Since this compound was virtually non-toxic nothing hindered its move to the clinic, and it was then found effective in relapsing-remitting MS.[227,228] The mode of action of Cop-1 has remained unclear. According to Jack Strominger the most likely mechanism may be inhibition of antigen presentation by class II major histocompatibility molecules,[229,230] but a number of additional, largely unclarified mechanisms, e.g., stimulation of myelin basic protein production, induction of suppressor T cells and anti-inflammatory cytokines, are also implicated.

10.4.6 The Take-Home Lesson

As illustrated in the previous sections, immunotherapeutic approaches to auto-immune diseases (AIDs) worked out with variable success. Immunologists were most disappointed by the failure of approaches targeting T-cell antigen recognition, for which detailed molecular information and strong proof of principle were available. On the other hand, some approaches that virtually lacked any rationale have resulted in functional drugs. Obviously there was a significant discrepancy between the expectations raised on scientific grounds, and what eventually materialized as pharmacological reality. To analyze the reasons for this discrepancy, one needs to look at the problem from both sides: from the standpoint of immunology and of pharmacology. A task like this suits Dr. G. perfectly, as he has ample experience in both areas.

'That the failure of the "trimolecular complex" (peptide+major histocompatibility molecule+T-cell receptor) as a pharmacological target was a sore point is understandable, because this was what immunologists knew most about, and so they were confident that it would work. I am not sure that it has failed for any specific reason, but there are some factors that might have contributed to the lack of success.'

'One potential problem was that the "trimolecular complex" was the earliest target candidate approached in the 1980s already, and at that time the industry had hardly any experience with protein-based drugs. Before the 1990s, drug development was an exercise for organic chemistry and the products were almost exclusively small molecules. But the experience collected in many decades was of no use, when it came to how to handle, manufacture and test protein drugs, what kind of toxicity profiles to expect, etc. Another issue was that the high-quality scientific information immunologists had, namely protein sequences, crystal structures, binding specificities, etc., did not necessarily permit to predict what could happen if one fumbled with these molecular interactions in vivo.

Furthermore, pharmacological experience tells that dead-sure targets may often cause the clearest side-effects. Fuzzy mechanisms are often easier to control by appropriate dosing. Admittedly, this latter argument stands half-way between science and superstition. The most likely answer comes from statistics that circulated in the industry in the 1990s, according to which 94% of pharmacological projects would never result in a drug. Thus, the probability of a hit is much like in roulette, and consequently, the failure of the trimolecular complex as a target might just have been incidental. The high failure rate in the industry is partially explained by the fact that each lead compound must pass through an obligatory testing schedule that consists of innumerable steps, any one of which can trigger a 'NO GO' decision. The other problem is that even at the age of genomics, it is still difficult to predict what processes a compound will affect at the level of the whole organism. Thus pharmacology remains a high-risk enterprise even in the twenty-first century.'

'An interesting conclusion born out of the efforts in immunotherapy concerns the importance of selectivity. At the beginning, every immunologist would have sworn on theoretical grounds that selective cellular expression of the target molecule was a pre-requisite for interfering with unwanted immune responses, while leaving the useful ones unaffected. However, this concept was not quite supported by reality. For example, the molecules successfully targeted for immunotherapy (Section 10.4.4) are broadly expressed: B7 is expressed on all B cells and antigen-presenting cells, CD2 is present on all T cells, and VLA-4 on most leukocytes in addition to activated/memory T cells. Yet, the protein therapeutics developed for these targets function with little immunological side-effects. Not to mention cytokines that are notoriously known for their multiple biological effects, and yet the therapies with interferon β and anti-tumor necrosis factor α are well tolerated. These examples suggest that pharmacological parameters, such as the route of administration and dosing schedules may be more important in avoiding side-effects than selective cellular expression of the target molecule.'

'To end with a positive note, I must point out that the success rate of immunotherapeutics, despite many failures, is still significantly higher than the industrial average. The possible reasons for this may again be manifold. One advantage is that protein leads are already the final drugs without the need for further optimization. Another important factor is that there is usually a clear mode of action of these biologicals, before the onset of pharmacological development. And finally the industry has meanwhile gained substantial interest as well as experience in this novel area.'

10.5 WHAT IS NEEDED FOR BETTER UNDERSTANDING OF AUTOIMMUNITY?

The attentive reader of this chapter will probably be left with the impression that the field of autoimmunity cannot be sufficiently understood, because far too many critical questions have remained open. Indeed this impression is justified, as autoimmunity is the least explored of all the topics covered in this book. This fact poses a specific problem: what can we offer as a final conclusion? Clearly, an all-embracing concept would be unrealistic to expect at this stage of the science. All we can try here is to raise some points of controversy, the clarification of which could further our understanding of the field.

'This is a sound approach, because the precise definition of what we don't understand is always the first step toward understanding', confirms Dr. G. 'However, in the case of autoimmunity this could become a horrendous task. Therefore I would suggest to discuss here only a few selected problems.'

'Let us start with a simple one that seems on the surface to be merely a question of terminology. This concerns the use of "autoimmune diseases" (AIDs) as a comprehensive term. It has hopefully become clear from this chapter that AIDs represent a rather loose assemblage of very different illnesses, and thus the term AIDs is not much more meaningful than "cancer". AIDs have only one thing in common: they are all manifested in immunopathology. However, immunopathology can also arise without autoimmunity, and thus the first task would be to firmly establish for each and every AID that it is triggered by an immune response to a self component. This has been reasonably well established for some AIDs but not for others. The work of separating autoimmune and non-autoimmune immunopathology may become like cleaning the stables of Augeas. But some guidelines can be used. For example, a disease caused by a mutation resulting in the overproduction of a destructive cytokine is likely to be non-autoimmune immunopathology. The real problem is posed by diseases where both autoimmune and non-autoimmune immunopathology occur. Here only a thorough analysis of each disease helps. All this may sound like splitting hairs, but the knowledge gained by such studies would not only promote our understanding, but also influence the therapeutic strategies to be employed.'

'The immunological community has recognized the inadequacy of AIDs as a general term, and uses "autoimmunity" instead. This use has also been adopted in the present chapter. Autoimmunity is defined as immunopathology initiated by a specific immune response to autologous components. Although this term may be satisfactory for everyday use, it has one shortcoming: it defines self from the immunologists' point of view. As discussed in the chapter, some AIDs are initiated by autoantigens that the immune system has never encountered before. From the system's perspective such antigens are foreign. Therefore, in a strict sense we can only talk about autoimmunity, if the components to which it is directed are considered by the immune system as self, in other words antigens or epitopes under self tolerance. Thus breaking of self tolerance should be an obligatory step preceding autoimmunity. Unfortunately, this definition of autoimmunity, although well understood, is not favored by the community.'

'This brings us to our next topic: the source of autoreactive cells. Thus far, two different sources have been identified, namely, cells that escaped self tolerance and cells rescued from tolerance. The former appear as "normal" members of the peripheral lymphocyte pool, and respond to self components as if they were foreign antigens. Such cells may be quite frequent in the B-cell repertoire, because the latter is not as stringently purged from autoreactivity at the site of its generation (in the bone marrow) as the T-cell pool in the thymus. However, because B-cell activation is strictly dependent on T helper (Th) cells, anti-self B cells normally enter a pathway of inactivation for lack of help. The situation is more dangerous, if the peripheral T-cell repertoire harbors non-tolerant Th cells, although they may be less frequent than non-tolerant B cells. As long as these Th cells are resting, they recirculate from blood to lymph, and have thus little chance to meet tissue-restricted antigens. However, once they become activated, usually by a mimicking epitope of a pathogen, they can migrate into tissues expressing the respective autoantigen, and become self-sustaining due to the continued presence of autoantigen. The pathology resulting from the response of such "ignorant" Th cells is usually considered AID, although the autoantigen they recognize is operationally non-self for the immune system. This mechanism seems to be involved, for example, in multiple sclerosis and insulin-dependent diabetes mellitus.'

'Autoimmunity, in a more strict sense, results from the reactivation of cells rescued from tolerance. The source of such cells is somewhat obscure. Under the two-signal model (Section 9.2.4), these are cells that have received signal-1 (antigen recognition), and are waiting for either signal-2 (activation), or inactivation. Although this "anticipatory" period is proposed to be short (at most 12 h), such cells should be present at a steady state (called the "autoimmune boundary"), and thus represent a source of potential autoreactivity. Another source may be provided by the dubious phenomenon of anergy (Section 9.3.3). Anergic cells arise by antigen stimulation in the absence of signal-2, but in contrast to cells in the "autoimmune boundary" they are long-lived. Lymphocytes can be anergized at any stage of their development, from early on in the thymus or bone marrow until after repeated activation with antigen. Because anergic cells are usually anti-self, and their unresponsive state is reversible, they may in fact be a major source of cells causing autoimmunity. It is another question why anergy is permitted at all, as it does not seem to bring any advantage and is in addition dangerous. There is no answer to this question yet, but anergy is an established fact and so we have to deal with it.'

'How can self tolerance be broken? This is easy to envisage in the case of B cells on the basis of classical experiments (see Section 9.1). All one needs is a cross-reacting antigen that shares some epitopes with the self molecule but differs at other epitopes. A tolerized B cells binds this antigen via the self-mimicking epitope, internalizes it and presents foreign (unshared) epitopes thereof to Th cells. The latter in turn help the B cell "wake up" from its unresponsive state and differentiate into an antibody-forming cell. Foreign antigens sharing epitopes with self are rather frequent, and thus autoantibodies accompanying infections are often demonstrable. However, this is normally a transient phenomenon, because after clearing of the infectious agent no more helper epitopes remain, and autoantibody production ceases. To make the autoimmune response self-sustaining, it is mandatory that the tolerant state of Th cells seeing the same autoantigen also be broken. How this exactly happens is unclear, one can only assume that it also requires the cross-reacting antigen, and an interaction between anti-foreign and anti-self Th cells. Breaking of Th cell tolerance may occur less frequently, judged by the observation that pathogen-induced autoantibody production develops only in certain cases into true AID.'

'Breaking of self tolerance should be a prerequisite for all diseases, in which the targeted autoantigen is ubiquitous and thus likely to be under self tolerance. Examples are ankylosing spondylitis and Reiter's syndrome where the autoantigen is a self major histocompatibility (MHC) class I molecule known to be under both

B- and T-cell tolerance. In these cases the cross-reactive antigen is provided by *Klebsiella* or *Yersinia* infection, which induces both B- and Th-cell response to self MHC. But in some instances, the same infection causes only autoantibody-mediated reactive arthritis that remits after infection, suggesting that only B-cell tolerance was broken.'

'What crystallizes out of this discussion is that the most likely protagonist of the autoimmune process is the activated (effector) Th cell. This statement receives indirect support from the observation that autoantibodies are formed in all AIDs, and a sustained autoantibody production is only possible in the presence of appropriate Th cells. The precursor of the effector Th cell can be either non-tolerant ("ignorant") or rescued from the tolerance pathway. The effector Th cell is, as a rule, specific for an autologous component. The only conceivable exception would be, if the Th cells were induced by a foreign antigen hiding in the body, e.g., derived from a pathogen causing latent chronic infection. But at the present state of molecular diagnostics the probability of an unnoticed infection is low. All additional aspects of autoimmunity, such as autoantibodies and different effector mechanisms, should be contingent on a self-sustaining pool of autoreactive Th cells that must be sufficiently large to keep the process going. The central role of Th cells in autoimmunity is indeed not too surprising, as Th cells are also the major regulators in responses to foreign antigens.'

'The initiation of autoimmunity often requires a cross-reacting antigen. Autologous proteins normally cannot do this, because they are either inaccessible for resting Th cells or are accessible but under self tolerance. The cross-reactive antigen is thus needed either for the priming of non-tolerant Th cells to an inaccessible self antigen, or for the breaking of Th cell tolerance to an accessible self antigen. However, the requirement for cross-reacting antigen is not absolute. At least two scenarios can be envisaged where autologous antigens may turn on the autoimmune process. First, a pathological change or genetic defect could render inaccessible self proteins accessible, and second, a defect of the tolerance mechanism could result in lack of tolerance to accessible self molecules. The cross-reacting antigen is usually "environmental", in most cases provided by an infectious agent. But in principle, a modified self protein could also serve the purpose.'

'The influence of genetic factors on autoimmunity also deserves a short discussion. Although the role of the MHC is reasonably well understood, the identity of additional genetic factors and the way they act in AIDs are largely unclear. Therefore I'll give here, for illustrative purposes, an *ad hoc* and surely incomplete list of genetic changes that could conceivably affect autoimmunity. There is a group of genes whose mutations can result in: impairment of tolerance mechanisms, change of antigen receptors from anti-foreign to anti-self, and change of the structure, quantity or accessibility of autoantigens. These mutations are assumed to promote autoimmunity selectively. Mutations in another group of genes can cause: changes in lymphocyte signalling, impairment of negative regulation, defects in apoptotic mechanisms, changes in cell adhesion and homing receptors, de-regulation of cytokine production, and possibly many other defects. This group of mutations would result in the impairment of general lymphocyte physiology, including lymphoproliferative disorders and immunopathology with possible autoimmune components. There is now evidence for mutations in both of these groups. AIDs are often accompanied by other disorders suggesting that mutations in the second group are frequently observable, probably because this group of genes is larger than the first one.'

'Finally we may address the question of why the immune clearance of certain self components appears as a physiological "housekeeping" function, whereas immunity to other self structures causes pathology. The only obvious difference between housekeeping and autoimmunity is that the former is directed to "autologous waste" that arises at a physiological rate. Elimination happens by complexing the waste with antibodies and subsequent phagocytosis of the complexes, i.e., by a process that usually does not entail pathology. In contrast, autoimmunity attacks viable self components and causes tissue destruction, which in turn may signal a different effector mechanism. Thus the difference between the two processes may have to do with the regulation of effector class, the latter being one of the last secrets in immunology.'

'Research efforts to dissect AIDs belong to the most important tasks of contemporary immunology. The utilitarian aspect of this work is strongly emphasized nowadays. Obviously, doctors are all eager to cure AIDs, and the frequent incidence of AIDs makes this indication area highly desirable for the pharmacological industry. But the scientific benefit is all too often overlooked, namely, that new insights into autoimmunity will inevitably lead to more profound understanding of the immune system as a whole.'

REFERENCES

1. Donath J, Landsteiner K. *Muench. Med. Wochenschr.* 1904;**51**:1590.
2. Silverstein AM. *A History of Immunology*. San Diego: Acad. Press; 1989.
3. Mackay IR, Burnet FM. *Autoimmune Diseases*. Springfield, Ill: Thomas; 1963.
4. Rose NR, Mackay IR. *The Autoimmune Diseases*. New York: Acad. Press; 1985.
5. Nepom GT, Erlich H. *Ann. Rev. Immunol.* 1991;**9**:493.
6. Cornelis F. In: Goronczy JJ, Weyand CM, editors. *Rheumatoid Arthritis. Curr. Dir. Autoimmun.* ;**3**Basel (: Karger; 2001. p. 1.
7. Nepom BS. *Clin. Immunol. Immunopathol.* 1993;**67**:850.
8. Breverton DA, Hart FD, Caffrey M, Nicholls A, James DCO, Sturrock RD. *Lancet* 1973;**i**:904.
9. Schlosstein L, Terasaki PI, Bluestone R, Pearson CM. *N. Engl. J. Med.* 1973;**288**:704.
10. Tiwari J, Terasaki PI. *HLA and Disease Associations*. New York: Springer-Verlag; 1985.
11. Bodmer JG, Marsh SGE, Albert ED, Bodmer WF, Dupont B, Erlich HA, et al. *Hum. Immunol.* 1994;**41**:1.
12. McMichael SJ, Sasazuki SJ, McDevitt HO, Payne RO. *Arthritis Rheum.* 1977;**20**:1037.
13. Stastny P. *N. Engl. J. Med.* 1978;**298**:869.
14. Nepom B, Nepom GT, Schaller J, Mickelson E, Antonelli P, Hansen J. *J. Clin. Invest.* 1984;**74**:287.
15. Zoschke D, Segall M. *Hum. Immunol.* 1986;**15**:118.
16. Arnett FC, Edworthy SM, Block DA, McShane DJ, Fries FJ, Cooper NS, et al. *Arthritis Rheum.* 1988;**31**:315.
17. Ohta N, Nishimura YK, Tanimoto K, Horiuchi Y, Abe C, Shiokawa Y, et al. *Hum. Immunol.* 1982;**5**:123.
18. Schiff B, Mizrachi Y, Orgad S, Yaron M, Gazit I. *Ann. Rheum. Dis.* 1982;**41**:403.
19. Wilkens RF, Nepom GT, Marks CR, Nettles JW, Nepom BS. *Arthritis Rheum.* 1991;**34**:43.
20. Gregersen PK, Silver J, Winchester RJ. *Arthritis Rheum.* 1987;**30**:1205.

21. Hiraiwa A, Yamanaka K, Kwok W, Mickelson EM, Masewicz S, Hansen JA, et al. *Proc. Natl. Acad. Sci. USA* 1990;**87**:8051.

22. Eisenbarth GS. *N. Engl. J. Med.* 1986;**314**:1360.

23. Thomson G, Robinson WP, Kuhner MK, Joe S, MacDonald MJ, Gotschall JL, et al. *Am. J. Hum. Genet.* 1988;**43**:799.

24. Rich SS. *LR Weitkamp J Barbosa, Am. J. Hum. Genet.* 1984;**36**:1015.

25. Nepom BS, Palmer J, Kim SJ, Hansen JA, Holbeck SL, Nepom GT. *J. Exp. Med.* 1986;**164**:345.

26. Baisch JM, Weeks T, Giles R, Hoover M, Stasny P, Capra JD. *N. Engl. J Med.* 1990;**322**:1836.

27. Todd JA, Bell JI, McDevitt HO. *Nature* 1987;**329**:599.

28. Scharf SJ, Horn GT, Erlich HA. *Science* 1986;**233**:1076.

29. Acha-Orbea H, McDevitt HO. *Proc. Natl. Acad. Sci. USA* 1987;**84**:2435.

30. Horn GT, Bugawan TL, Long CM, Erlich HA. *Proc. Natl. Acad. Sci. USA* 1988;**85**:6012.

31. Morel PA, Dorman JS, Todd JA, McDevitt HO, Trucco M. *Proc. Natl. Acad. Sci. USA* 1988;**85**:8111.

32. Awata T, Kuzuya T, Matsuda A, Iwamoto Y, Kanazawa Y, Okuyama M, et al. *Diabetes* 1990;**39**:266.

33. Rønningen KS, Iwe T, Halstensen TS, Spurkland A, Thorsby E. *Hum. Immunol.* 1989;**26**:215.

34. Amagai M, Klaus-Kovtun V, Stanley JR. *Cell* 1991;**67**:869.

35. Scharf SJ, Friedmann A, Steinmann L, Brautbar C, Erlich HA. *Proc. Natl. Acad. Sci. USA* 1989;**86**:6215.

36. Hammer J, Takacs B, Sinigaglia F. *J. Exp. Med.* 1992;**176**:1007.

37. Hammer J, Valsasini P, Tolba K, Bolin D, Higelin J, Takacs B, et al. *Cell* 1993;**74**:197.

38. Hammer J, Gallazzi F, Bono E, Karr RW, Guenot J, Valsasini P, et al. *J. Exp. Med.* 1995;**181**:1847.

39. Hammer J, Bono E, Gallazzi F, Belunis C, Nagy ZA, Sinigaglia F. *J. Exp. Med.* 1994;**180**:2353.

40. Stern LJ, Brown JH, Jardetzky TS, Gorga JC, Urban RG, Strominger JL, et al. *Nature* 1994;**368**:215.

41. Dessen A, Lawrence CM, Cupo S, Zaller DM, Wiley DC. *Immunity* 1997;**7**:473.

42. Fugger L, Rothbard JB, Sonderstrup-McDevitt G. *Eur. J. Immunol.* 1996;**26**:928.

43. Wucherpfennig KW, Yu B, Bhol K, Monos DS, Argyris E, Karr RW, et al. *Proc. Natl. Acad. Sci. USA* 1995;**92**:11935.

44. Gross DM, Forsthuber T, Tary-Lehmann M, Etling C, Ito K, Nagy ZA, et al. *Science* 1998;**281**:703.

45. Ota K, Matsui M, Milford EL, Mackin GA, Weiner HL, Hafler DA. *Nature* 1990;**346**:183.

46. Smith KJ, Pyrdol J, Gauthier L, Wiley DC, Wucherpfennig KW. *J. Exp. Med.* 1998;**188**:1511.

47. Wucherpfennig KW, Strominger JL. *J. Exp. Med.* 1995;**181**:1597.

48. Chicz RA, Urban RG, Gorga JC, Vignali DAA, Lane WS, Strominger JL. *J. Exp. Med.* 1993;**178**:27.

49. Chou CL, Sadegh-Nasseri S. *j. Exp. Med.* 2000;**192**:1697.

50. Nelson CA, Petzold SJ, Unanue ER. *Nature* 1994;**371**:250.

51. Nepom BS, Nepom GT, Coleman M, Kwok WW. *Proc. Natl. Acad. Sci. USA* 1996;**93**:7202.

52. Brown JH, Jardetzky TS, Gorga JC, Stern LJ, Urban RG, Strominger JL, et al. *Nature* 1993;**364**:33.

53. Lee KH, Wucherpfennig KW, Wiley DC. *Nature Immunol.* 2001;**2**:501.

54. Corper AL, Stratmann T, Apostolopoulos V, Scott CA, Garcia KC, Kang AS, et al. *Science* 2000;**288**:505.

55. Quinn A, Sercarz EE. *J. Autoimmun.* 1996;**9**:365.

56. Abraham RS, Wen L, Marietta EV, David CS. *J. Immunol.* 2001;**166**:1370.

57. Chao CC, Sytwu HK, Chen EL, Toma J, McDevitt HO. *Proc. Natl. Acad. Sci. USA* 1999;**96**:9299.

58. Kim C-Y, Quarstein H, Bergseng E, Khosla C, Sollid LM. *Proc. Natl. Acad. Sci. USA* 2004;**101**:4175.

59. Ridgway WM, Fasso M, Lanctot A, Garvey C, Fathman CG. *J. Exp. Med.* 1996;**183**:1657.

60. Thomas-Vaslin V, Damotte D, Coltey M, Le Douarin NM, Coutinho A, Salaün J. *Proc. Natl. Acad. Sci. USA* 1997;**94**:4598.

61. Reich EP, Sherwin RS, Kanagawa O, Janeway Jr CA. *Nature* 1989;**341**:326.

62. Böhme J, Schuhbaur B, Kanagawa O, Benoist C, Mathis D. *Science* 1990;**249**:293.

63. Lühder Fl., Katz J, Benoist C, Mathis D. *J: Exp. Med.* 1998;**187**:379.

64. Goronczy JJ, Bartz-Bazzanella P, Hu W, Jendro MC, Walser-Kuntz DR, Weyand CM. *J. Clin. Invest.* 1994;**94**:2068.

65. Yang H, Rittner H, Weyand CM, Goronczy JJ. *J. Investig. Med.* 1999;**47**:236.

66. Wagner UG, Koetz K, Weyand CM, Goronczy JJ. *Proc. Natl. Acad. Sci. USA* 1998;**95**:14447.

67. Schmidt D, Goronczy JJ, Weyand CM. *J. Clin. Invest.* 1996;**97**:2027.

68. Weyand CM, Goronczy JJ. *Curr. Opin. Rheumatol.* 1999;**11**:210.

69. Brewerton DA, Caffrey M, Nicholls A. *Lancet* 1973;**2**:996.

70. Chen JH, Kono DH, Yong Z, Park MS, Oldstone MMBA, Yu DTY. *J. Immunol.* 1987;**139**:3003.

71. Albani S, Tuckwell JE, Esparza L, Carson DA, Roudier J. *J. Clin. Invest.* 1992;**89**:327.

72. Kouskoff V, Korganow AS, Duchatelle V, Degott C, Benoist C, Mathis D. *Cell* 1996;**87**:811.

73. Müller U, Jongeneel CV, Nedospasov SA, Fischer Lindahl K, Steinmetz M. *Nature* 1987;**325**:265.

74. Spies T, Morton CC, Nedospasov SA, Fiers W, Pious D, Strominger JL. *Proc. Natl. Acad. Sci. USA* 1986;**83**:8699.

75. Jacob CO, McDevitt HO. *Nature* 1988;**331**:356.

76. Jacob CO, Fronek Z, Lewis GD, Koo M, Hansen JA, McDevitt HO. *Proc. Natl. Acad. Sci. USA* 1990;**87**:1233.

77. Wicker LS, Appel MC, Dotta F, Pressey A, Miller BJ, DeLarato NH, et al. *J. Exp. Med.* 1992;**176**:67.

78. Ghosh S, Palmer SM, Rodriques NR, Cordell HJ, Hearne CM, Cornall RJ, et al. *Nat. Genet.* 1993;**4**:404.

79. Kono DH, Burlingame RW, Owens DG, Kuramochi A, Banderas RS, Balomenos D, et al. *Proc. Natl. Acad. Sci. USA* 1994;**91**:10168.

80. Scott B, Liblau R, Degermann S, Marconi LA, Ogata L, Caton AJ, et al. *Immunity* 1994;**1**:73.

81. Cornall RJ, Prins JB, Todd JA, Pressey A, DeLarato NH, Wicker LS, et al. *Nature* 1991;**353**:262.

82. Prins JB, Todd JA, Rodrigues NR, Ghosh S, Hogarth PM, Wicker LS, et al. *Science* 1993;**260**:695.

83. Nistico L, Buzzetti R, Pritchard LE, Van der Auwera B, Giovanni C, Bosi E, et al. *Hum. Mol. Genet.* 1996;**5**:1075.

84. Julier C, Hyer RN, Davies J, Merlin F, Soularue P, Briant L, et al. *Nature* 1991;**354**:155.

85. Bennett ST, Lucassen AM, Gough SC, Powell EE, Undlien DE, Pritchard LE, et al. *Nat. Genet.* 1995;**9**:284.

86. Davies JL, Kawaguchi Y, Bennett ST, Copeman JB, Cordell HJ, Pritchard LE, et al. *Nature* 1994;**371**:130.

87. Hashimoto L, Habita C, Beressi JP, Delepine M, Besse C, Cambon-Thomsen A, et al. *Nature* 1994;**371**:161.

88. Todd JA, Aitman TJ, Cornall RJ, Ghosh S, Hall JR, Hearne CM, et al. *Nature* 1991;**351**:542.

89. Gonzalez A, Katz JD, Mattei MG, Kikutani H, Benoist C, Mathis D. *Immunity* 1997;**7**:873.

90. Todd JA. *Proc. Natl. Acad. Sci. USA* 1995;**92**:8560.

91. Rosatelli MC, Meloni A, Meloni A, Devoto M, Cao A, Scott HS, et al. *K Nagamine J Kudoh, N Shimizu, SE Antonarakis, Hum. Genet.* 1998;**103**:428.

92. Björses P, Halonen M, Palvimo JJ, Kolmer M, Aaltonen J, Ellonen P, et al. *Am. J. Hum. Genet.* 2000;**66**:378.

93. Anderson MS, Venanzi ES, Klein L, Chen Z, Berzins SP, Turley SJ, et al. *Science* 2002;**298**:1395.

94. Derbinski J, Gäbler J, Brors B, Tierling S, Jonnakuty S, Hergenhahn M, et al. *J. Exp. Med.* 2005;**202**:33.

95. Kyewski B, Derbinski J. *Nat. Rev. / Immunol.* 2004;**4**:688.

96. DeVoss J, Hou Y, Johannes K, Lu W, Liou GI, Rinn J, et al. *J. Exp. Med.* 2006;**203**:2727.

97. Gotter J, Brors B, Hergenhahn M, Kyewski B. *j. Exp. Med.* 2004;**199**:155.

98. Klein L, Klugmann M, Nave KA, Tuohy VK, Kyewski B. *Nat. Med.* 2000;**6**:56.

99. Anderson AC, Nicholson LB, Legge KL, Turchin V, Zaghouani H, Kuchroo VK. *J. Exp. Med.* 2000;**191**:761.

100. Katz JD, Wang B, Haskins K, Benoist C, Mathis D. *Cell* 1993;**74**:1089.

101. Scott B, Liblau R, Degermann S, Marconi LA, Ogata L, Caton AJ, et al. *Immunity* 1994;**1**:73.

102. Weigle WO. *J. Immunol.* 1964;**92**:791.

103. Humphrey JH. *Immunol.* 1964;**7**:449.

104. Schwimmbeck PL, Yu DTY, Oldstone MBA. *J. Exp. Med.* 1987;**166**:173.

105. Rosloniec EF, Brand DD, Myers LK, Esaki Y, Whittington KB, Zaller DM, et al. *J. Immunol.* 1998;**160**:2573.

106. Andersson M, Holmdahl R. *Eur. J. Immunol.* 1990;**20**:1061.

107. Malmström V, Michaelsson E, Burkhardt H, Mattsson R, Vuorio E, Holmdahl R. *Proc. Natl. Acad. Sci. USA* 1996;**93**:4480.

108. Malmström V, Kiellen P, Holmdahl R. *J. Autoimmun.* 1998;**11**:213.

109. Larsson P, Kleinau S, Holmdahl R, Klareskog L. *Arthritis Rheum.* 1990;**33**:693.

110. Lehmann PV, Forsthuber T, Miller A, Sercarz EE. *Nature* 1992;**358**:155.

111. Kaufmann DL, Clare-Salzler M, Tian J, Forsthuber T, Ting GSP, Robinson P, et al. *Nature* 1993;**366**:69.

112. Krusius FF. *Arch. Augenheilkd.* 1910;**67**:6.

113. Hickey WF, Hsu BL, Kimura H. *J. Neurosci. Res.* 1991;**28**:254.

114. Burns J, Rosenzweig A, Zweiman B, Lisak RP. *Cell. Immunol.* 1983;**81**:435.

115. Hickey WF, Hsu BL, Kimura H. *J. Neurosci. Res.* 1991;**28**:254.

116. Crawford L, Leppard K, Lane D, Harlow E. *j. Virol.* 1982;**42**:612.

117. Tardieu M, Powers ML, Hafler DA, Hauser SL, Weiner HL. *Eur. J. Immunol.* 1984;**14**:561 β-cell.

118. Clarke MF, Gelmann EP, Reitz Jr MS. *Nature* 1983;**305**:60.

119. Sheshberadaran H, Norrby E. *J. Virol.* 1984;**52**:995.

120. Dales S, Fujinami RS, MBA Oldstone. *J. Immunol.* 1983;**134**:1546.

121. Fujinami RS, Oldstone MBA, Wroblewska Z, Frankel ME, Koprowski H. *Proc. Natl. Acad. Sci. USA* 1983;**80**:2346.

122. Haspel MV, Onodera T, Prabhakar BS, Horita M, Suzuki H, Notkins AL. *Science* 1983;**220**:403.

123. Kagnoff MF, Austin RK, Hubert JJ, Bernardin JE, Kasarda DD. *J. Exp. Med.* 1984;**160**:1544.

124. Fujinami RS, Oldstone MBA. *Science* 1985;**230**:1043.

125. Oldstone MBA. *Cell* 1987;**50**:819.

126. Wucherpfennig KW, Strominger JL. *Cell* 1995;**80**:695.

127. Zhao ZS, Granucci F, Yeh L, Schaffer PA, Cantor H. *Science* 1998;**279**:1344.

128. Bachmaier K, Neu N, de la Maza LM, Pal S, Hessel A, Penninger JM. *Science* 1999;**283**:133.

129. Atkinson MA, Bowman MA, Campbell L, Darrow BL, Kaufman DL, Maclaren NK. *J. Clin. Invest.* 1994;**94**:2125.

130. Ohashi PS, Oehen S, Buerki K, Pircher H, Ohashi CT, Odermatt B, et al. *Cell* 1991;**65**:305.

131. Oldstone MB, Nerenberg M, Southern P, Price J, Lewicki H. *Cell* 1991;**65**:319.

132. Miller SD, Vanderlugt CL, Begolka WS, Pao W, Yauch RL, Neville KL, et al. *Nat. Med.* 1997;**3**:1133.

133. Kukreja A, Maclaren NK. *Cell. Mol. Life Sci.* 2000;**4**:534.

134. Horwitz MS, Bradley LM, Harbertson J, Krahl T, Lee J, Sarvetnick N. *Nat. Med.* 1998;**4**:781.

135. Brocke S, Gaur A, Piercy C, Gautam A, Gijbels K, Fathman CG, et al. *Nature* 1993;**365**:642.

136. Gray DH, Gavanescu I, Benoist C, Mathis D. *Proc. Natl. Acad. Sci. USA* 2007;**104**:18193.

137. Karjalainen J, Martin JM, Knip M, Ilonen J, Robinson BH, Savilahti E, et al. *New Engl. J. Med.* 1992;**327**:302.

138. Cohn M. *Mol. Immunol.* 2005;**42**:651.

139. Newsom-Davis J, Harcourt G, Sommer N, Beeson D, Willcox N, Rothbard JB. *J. Autoimmunity* 1989;**2**(Suppl.):101.

140. Satyamurti S, Drachman DB, Slone F. *Science* 1975;**187**:955.

141. Fambourgh DM. *DB Drachman S Satyamurti, Science* 1973;**182**:293.

142. Toyka KV, Drachman DB, Pestonk A, Kao I. *Science* 1975;**190**:397.

143. Zamvil S, Nelson P, Trotter J, Mitchell D, Knobler R, Fritz R, et al. *Nature* 1985;**317**:355.

144. Koh DR, Fung-Leung WP, Ho A, Gray D, Acha-Orbea H, Mak TW. *Science* 1992;**256**:1210.

145. Miller BL, Appel MC, O'Neil JJ, Wicker LS. *J. Immunol.* 1988;**140**:52.

146. Wang Y, Pontesilli O, Gill RG, La Rosa FG, Lafferty KJ. *Proc. Natl. Acad. Sci. USA* 1991;**88**:527.

147. Bucala R, Ritchlin C, Winchester R, Cerami A. *J. Exp. Med.* 1991;**173**:569.

148. Liblau RS, Singer SM, McDevitt HO. *Immunol. Today* 1995;**16**:34.

149. Baron JL, Madri JA, Ruddle NH, Hashim G, Janeway Jr CA. *J. Exp. Med.* 1993;**177**:57.

150. Merrill JE, Kono DH, Clayton J, Ando DG, Hinton DR, Hofman FM. *Proc. Natl. Acad. Sci. USA* 1992;**89**:574.

151. Kennedy MK, Torrance DS, Picha KS, Mohler KM. *J. Immunol.* 1992;**149**:2496.

152. Ruddle NH, Bergman CM, McGrath KM, Lingenheld EG, Grunnet ML, Padula SJ, et al. *J. Exp. Med.* 1990;**172**:1193.

153. van der Veen RC, Stohlman SA. *J. Neuroimmunol.* 1993;**48**:213.

154. Lafaille JJ, van de Keere F, Hsu AL, Baron JL, Haas W, Raine CS, et al. *J. Exp. Med.* 1997;**186**:307.

155. Karpus WJ, Gould KE, Swanborg RH. *Eur. J. Immunol.* 1992;**22**:1757.

156. Chen Y, Kuchroo VK, Inobe J, Hafler DA, Weiner HL. *Science* 1994;**265**:1237.

157. van de Keere F, Tonegawa S. *J. Exp. Med.* 1998;**188**:1875.

158. Campbell IL, Kay TW, Oxbrow L, Harrison LC. *J. Clin. Invest.* 1991;**87**:739.

159. Shehadeh NN, LaRosa F, Lafferty KJ. *J. Autoimmunity* 1993;**6**:291.

160. Katz JD, Benoist C, Mathis D. *Science* 1995;**268**:1185.

161. Wraith DC, McDevitt HO, Steinman L, Acha-Orbea H. *Cell* 1989;**57**:709.

162. Feldmann M, Maini RN. *Annu. Rev. Immunol.* 2001;**19**:163.

163. Steinman L, Rosenbaum JT, Sriram S, McDevitt HO. *Proc. Natl. Acad. Sci. USA* 1981;**78**:7111.

164. Waldor MK, Sriram S, McDevitt HO, Steinman L. *Proc. Natl. Acad. Sci. USA* 1983;**80**:2713.

165. McDevitt HO, Perry R, Steinman LA. *Autoimmunity and autoimmune disease*. Chichester: Wiley; 1987, 184.

166. Boitard C, Bendelac A, Richard MF, Carnaud C, Bach JF. *Proc. Natl. Acad. Sci. USA* 1988;**85**:9719.

167. Billing R, Chatterjee S. *Transplant. Proc.* 1983;**15**:649.

168. Jonker M, Nooij FJM, den Butter G, van Lambalgen R, Fuccello AJ. *Transpl.* 1988;**45**:677.

169. Adorini L, Muller S, Cardniaux F, Lehmann PV, Falcioni F, Nagy ZA. *Nature* 1988;**334**:623.

170. Wraith DC, Smilek DE, Mitchell DJ, Steinman L, McDevitt HO. *Cell* 1989;**59**:247.

171. Sakai K, Zamvil SS, Mitchell DJ, Hodgkinson S, Rothbard JB, Steinman L. *Proc. Natl. Acad. Sci. USA* 1989;**86**:9470.

172. Hurtenbach U, Lier E, Adorini L, Nagy ZA. *J. Exp. Med.* 1993;**177**:1499.

173. Myers LK, Rosloniec EF, Seyer JM, Stuart JM, Kang AH. *J. Immunol.* 1993;**150**:4652.

174. Ishioka G, Adorini L, Guery JC, Gaeta FCA, LaFond R, Alexander J, et al. *J. Immunol.* 1994;**152**:4310.

175. Falcioni F, Ito K, Vidovic D, Belunis C, Campbell R, Berthel SJ, et al. *Nat. Biotech.* 1999;**17**:562.

176. Rosloniec EF, Brandstetter T, Leyer S, Schwaiger FW, Nagy ZA. *J. Autoimmun.* 2006;**27**:182.

177. Oki A, Sercarz E. *J. Exp. Med.* 1985;**161**:897.

178. Nihira SI, Falcioni F, Juretic A, Nagy ZA. *Eur. J. Immunol.* 1996;**26**:1736.

179. Clayton JP, Gammon GM, Ando DG, Kono DH, Hood L, Sercarz EE. *J. Exp. Med.* 1989;**169**:1681.

180. Gaur A, Wiers B, Liu A, Rothbard J, Fathman CG. *Science* 1992;**258**:1491.

181. Marusic S, Tonegawa S. *J. Exp. Med.* 1997;**186**:507.

182. Sharma SD, Nag B, Su XM, Green D, Spack E, Clark BR, et al. *Proc. Natl. Acad. Sci. USA* 1991;**88**:11465.

183. Miller A, Lider O, Weiner HL. *J. Exp. Med.* 1991;**174**:791.

184. Metzler B, Wraith DC. *Internatl. Immunol.* 1993;**5**:1159.

185. Blanas E, Carbone FR, Allison J, Miller JFAP, Heath WR. *Science* 1996;**274**:1707.

186. Smilek DE, Wraith DC, Hodgkinson S, Dwivedy S, Steinman L, McDevitt HO. *Proc. Natl. Acad. Sci. USA* 1991;**88**:9633.

187. Brocke S, Gijbels K, Allegretta M, Ferber I, Piercy C, Blankenstein T, et al. *Nature* 1996;**379**:343.

188. Gaur A, Boehme SA, Chalmers D, Crowe PD, Pahuja A, Ling N, et al. *J. Neuroimmunol.* 1997;**74**:149.

189. Posnett DN, Singha R, Kabak C, Russo J. *J. Exp. Med.* 1994;**179**:609.

190. Sempe P, Bedossa P, Richard MF, Villa MC, Bach JF, Boitard C. *Eur. J. Immunol.* 1991;**21**:1163.

191. Goldschmidt TJ, Holmdahl R. *Eur. J. Immunol.* 1991;**21**:1327.

192. Yoshino S, Cleland LG, Mayrhofer G, Brown RR, Schwab JH. *J. Immunol.* 1991;**146**:4187.

193. Acha-Orbea H, Mitchell DJ, Timmermann L, Wraith DC, Tausch GS, Waldor MK, et al. *Cell* 1988;**54**:263.

194. Oksenberg JR, Stuart S, Begovich AB, Bell RB, Erlich HA, Steinman L, et al. *Nature* 1990;**345**:344.

195. Kotzin BL, Katuturi S, Chou YK, Lafferty J, Forrester JM, Better M, et al. *Proc. Natl. Acad. Sci. USA* 1991;**88**:9161.

196. Falcioni F, Dembic Z, Muller S, Lehmann PV, Nagy ZA. *J. Exp. Med.* 1990;**171**:1665.

197. Howell MD, Winters ST, Olee T, Powell HC, Carlo DJ, Borstoff SW. *Science* 1989;**246**:668.

198. Offner H, Hashim GA, Vandenbark AA. *Science* 1991;**251**:430.

199. Sriram S, Ranges GE. *Concepts Immunopathol.* 1987;**4**:275.

200. Tak PP, van der Lubbe PA, Cauli A, Daha MR, Smeets TJM, Kluin PM, et al. *Arthritis Rheum.* 1995;**38**:1457.

201. Choy EH, Adjaye J, Forrest L, Kingsley GH, Panay GS. *Eur. J. Immunol.* 1993;**23**:2676.
202. Cobbold SP, Martin G, Qin S, Waldman H. *Nature* 1986;**323**:164.
203. Fessel WJ, Anderson B, Follansbee SE, Winters MA, Lewis ST, Weinheimer SP, et al. *Antiviral Res.* 2011;**92**:484.
204. Lenschow DJ, Zeng Y, Thislcthwaite JR, Montag A, Brady W, Gibson MG, et al. *Science* 1992;**257**:789.
205. Linsley PS, Wallace PM, Johnson J, Gibson MG, Greene JL, Ledbetter JA, et al. *Science* 1992;**257**:792.
206. Miller GT, Hochman PS, Meier W, Tizard R, Bixler SA, Rosa MD, et al. *J. Exp. Med.* 1993;**178**:211.
207. Hynes RO. *Cell* 2002,**110**:673.
208. Miller DH, Khan OA, Sheremata WA, Blumhardt LD, Rice GP, Libonati MA, ct al. *N. Engl. J. Med.* 2003;**348**:15.
209. Polman CH, O'Connor PW, Havrdova E, Hutchinson M, Kappos L, Miller DH, et al. *N. Engl. J. Med.* 2006;**354**:899.
210. Stüve O, Marra CM, Jerome KR, Cook L, Cravens PD, Cepok S, et al. *BHemmer, NL Monson, MK Racke, Ann. Neurol.* 2006;**59**:743.
211. Fontana A, Hengartner H, Fehr K, Grob PJ, Cohen G. *Rheumatol. Int.* 1982;**2**:49.
212. Gowen M, Wood DD, Ihrie EJ, McGuire MKB, Russel RG. *Nature* 1983;**306**:378.
213. Pennica D, Nedwin GE, Hayflick JS, Seeburg PH, Derynck R, Palladino MA, et al. *Nature* 1984;**312**:724.
214. Buchan G, Barrett K, Turner M, Chantry D, Maini RN, Feldmann M. *Clin. Exp. Immunol.* 1988;**73**:449.
215. Saklatvala J. *Nature* 1986;**322**:547.
216. Brennan FM, Chantry D, Jackson AM, Maini R, Feldmann M. *Lancet* 1989;**ii**:244.
217. Butler DM, Maini RN, Feldmann M, Brennan FM. *Eur. Cytokine Netw.* 1995;**6**:225.
218. Haworth C, Brennan FM, Chantry D, Turner M, Maini RN, Feldmann M. *Eur. J. Immunol.* 1991;**21**:2575.
219. Thorbecke GJ, Shah R, Leu CH, Kuruvilla AP, Hardison AM, Palladino MA. *Proc. Natl. Acad. Sci. USA* 1992;**89**:7375.
220. Willams RO, Feldmann M, Maini RN. *Proc. Natl. Acad. Sci. USA* 1992;**89**:9784.
221. Maini RN, Breeveld FC, Kalden JR, Smolen JS, Davis D, Macfarlane JD, et al. *Arthritis Rheum.* 1998;**41**:1552.
222. Moreland LW, Baumgartner SW, Schiff MH, Tindall EA, Fleischmann RM, Weaver AL, et al. *N. Engl. J. Med.* 1997;**337**:141.
223. Arend WP, Welgus HG, Thompson RC, Eisenberg SP. *J. Clin. Invest.* 1990;**85**:1694.
224. Bresnihan B, Alvaro-Gracia JM, Cobby M, Doherty M, Domjan Z, Emery P, et al. *Arthritis Rheum.* 1998;**41**:2196.
225. IFNB Multiple Sclerosis Study Group. *Neurology* 1993;**43**:655.
226. Teitelbaum D, Meshmorer A, Hirshfeld T, Arnon R, Sela M. *Eur. J. Immunol* 1971;**1**:242.
227. Bornstein MB, Miller A, Slagle S, Weitzman M, Crystal H, Drexler E, et al. *N. Engl. J. Med.* 1987;**317**:408.
228. Johson KP, Brooks BR, Cohen JA, Ford CC, Goldstein J, Lisak RP, et al. *Neurology* 1995;**45**:1268.
229. Fridkis-Hateli M, Strominger JL. *J. Immunol.* 1998;**160**:4386.
230. Fridkis-Hateli M, Rosloniec EF, Fugger L, Strominger JL. *Proc. Natl. Acad. Sci. USA* 1998;**95**:12528.

$$\overbrace{\text{Concluding Remarks}}$$

The last third of the twentieth century was the period when the 100-year-old pursuit for the meaning and molecular basis of immunological specificity was finally crowned with success, and it was therefore a time of crucial importance in the history of immunology The highlights of the first decade were the clarification of immunoglobulin structure, the interaction of antibody with antigen, and the mechanisms for generation of antibody diversity, and in the following 20 years, the T-cell antigen receptor and the nature of its ligand were discovered. Beyond doubt, these three decades represented the unsurpassable peak of research into the adaptive (i.e., somatically generated) immune system. By the mid-1990s, practically everything had become known about antigen recognition, and although there is disagreement on some details, it is no longer expected that new facts could fundamentally change our view, in other words, the study of adaptive immune system can be regarded as (more or less) complete.

The knowledge gained about antigen recognition then gave impetus to other research areas. For example, the information on immunoglobulin gene structure triggered a technological course of development that culminated in the production of synthetic human antibodies without immunization. Furthermore, the characterization of T-cell recognition enabled from the 1980s on a renaissance of tolerance and autoimmunity studies that had to do largely with the clarification of the role T cells play in these two processes. But mechanistic studies into tolerance and autoimmunity are still relatively recent, and thus much remains to be done before our understanding of these fields reaches the level of knowledge on antigen recognition.

Self tolerance and autoimmunity are the immediate consequences of somatically generated antigen recognition repertoires: as the latter are random, they inevitably comprise specificities against self structures. This necessitated the evolution of another somatic process – acquisition of self tolerance – that removes anti-self from the repertoire, and the limitations of this process are marked by autoimmunity. One could thus say that the historical development of research followed the internal logic of the immune system.

Before the 1970s, the effector response was the stepchild of immunology research. All we knew at that time was that B cells produce antibodies, and T cells 'help' B cells in doing so or participate in delayed-type hypersensitivity reactions. Studies of the effector response have taken a more analytical course from the 1970s on, thanks to the discovery that different T-cell functions, namely help and cytotoxicity, are mediated by distinct T-cell subpopulations. These kinds of studies have continued all through the rest of the century, and resulted in an increasing number of T-cell subsets performing defined protective functions. The only subset that has remained problematic is regulatory (sup-pressor) T cells, whose place in the immune system is still unclear.

A new level of complexity has been added to effector functions with the discovery that T cells secrete many biologically active proteins, or induce other cell types to do so. These proteins, collectively termed cytokines, perform a wide spectrum of activities often in a redundant manner, i.e., different cytokines may appear to have the same effect, while a single cytokine may have diverse effects on different target cells. It is therefore extremely difficult to disentangle the ways the cytokine network functions, and how its function is regulated. Another interesting aspect that has arisen in this period is that effector responses are shared between the adaptive (somatically generated) and innate (germ-line-encoded) immune system. But the ways these two systems may interact are largely unknown.

The open questions concerning the effector response remain challenging tasks for the new millennium.

The leitmotif all through the book was understanding, but I made no attempt to clarify what the latter was meant to be. To define understanding is not easy, yet I must take now the last opportunity to at least outline its meaning in science. In the sense used in this book, understanding is the result of a mental evaluation of observed phenomena. To illustrate with a commonplace example, it is like finding out who the murderer was on the basis of material evidence in a criminal investigation. This element of 'searching for the truth' makes scientific pursuit a fascinating occupation. Of course, facts in science just like in everyday life are mute, and thus often misleading or interpreted falsely. A good example for this is presented by major histocompatibility complex (MHC) molecules that were discovered as blood group antigens in 1936, later they were considered transplantation antigens, until the first hint to their true immunological function came 38 years later.

As a rule, understanding starts with forming a hypothesis, and each new fact is then to be scrutinized whether it fits into the hypothesis or not. Hypotheses therefore may go through several cycles of amendment, or they may be rejected and new ones formed before reaching a sufficient level of understanding. This mental exercise is further complicated by the usual practice of proposing at least two competing hypotheses for each set of observations. It is therefore not surprising that the phase of mental evaluation between a key observation and its understanding can be quite long.

History provided numerous examples to illustrate this. Consider again the MHC that was discovered in 1936, but answers to the most important what?, how?, and why? questions concerning its function came as late as the mid-1990s. Another example is T cells that were discovered and shown to be antigen-specific in 1961, but sufficient understanding of how they recognize antigen was not achieved before the late 1990s. The case of self tolerance is similar: it was discovered around 1950, and as of the 2013, a few critical elements for its understanding are still missing. Thus in the investigated period of time, several decades were necessary to achieve sufficient understanding of a key discovery. The evaluation process will possibly be accelerated in the future by technical development, which permits a faster output of critical data. On the other hand, the biological problems to be analyzed will be vastly more complex, because to find out how the now-known elements of life work in concert in a cell or a whole organism will not be possible by simple linear logic. Computers will certainly be useful in this analysis, but we still have to instruct the machine how to think before it can tell us what to think. Thus biological understanding will foreseeably take its time also in the future.

As repeatedly emphasized in the book, the most important touchstone in testing the validity of a biological hypothesis is evolution. This is because every biological mechanism that we observe owes its existence to an evolutionary need. Thus, it is a good sign if we can rationalize the evolutionary driver for a mechanism. In the opposite case, chances are high that we have overlooked or misinterpreted something.

It is important to realize that understanding is not absolute, it is like everything else in science, a quantitative category. Its useful extent is determined by the system investigated. Probably the best sign of sufficient understanding is when a phenomenon 'falls into place' naturally and precisely, like a perfectly carved stone into the wall of an Inca building, the latter being in this case immunology. Before this happens, the construction of the building cannot be continued, and this is why understanding is indispensable.

Finally, I must point out that understanding, being a mental category, always has subjective elements, as it depends on education, way of thinking, cultural background, and other personal features and preferences. Thus the writer of a scientific text will inevitably transmit his personal understanding to the reader. This is a natural consequence of the author's obligation to form his own understanding of the topic. For understanding is a fundamental requirement also for the clear and authentic formulation of a text.

Index

Note: Page numbers followed by "f" denote figures; "t" tables.

Printed and bound by CPI Group (UK) Ltd, Croydon, CR0 4YY

03/10/2024

01040422-0010